Essential Medical Imaging

CD cataloged as 'Medical Imaging' C20460039

CD-ROM operating instructions

Instructions

1. Insert CD
2. *Macintosh*: Double click the CD "MI" icon on the desktop
   Windows PC: Double click the CD "MI" icon in "My Computer"
3. *Macintosh*: Double click on "Medical Imaging"
   Windows PC: Double click on "Medical Imaging.exe"

Medical Imaging requires QuickTime* to operate.
If you do not have QuickTime available on your PC then use either the Mac or PC installers included on this CD (or download QuickTime from the web at http://www.apple.com/quicktime/download/).

Installing QuickTime

1. Select and open the folder with the QuickTime installer for your operating system.
2. *Macintosh*: Double click the "Quicktime.pkg" icon
   Windows PC: Double click the "Quicktimeinstaller.exe" icon
3. Follow the instructions within the QuickTime installer

*QuickTime and the QuickTime logo are trademarks used under license. The QuickTime logo is registered in the U.S. and other countries.

Minimum requirements

256 MB RAM, Screen Resolution 800×600, CD-ROM drive.

Windows

450 MHz Intel Pentium II processor (or equivalent)
Win 2000: Internet Explorer 5.01x, QuickTime 6
Win XP: Internet Explorer 6x, QuickTime 6

Macintosh

500 MHz PowerPc G3, OS 10.3.9 or above, Safari 2.0, QuickTime 6

Essential Medical Imaging

Edited by
Robert N. Gibson
Associate Editor
Anne Mitchell

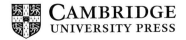
CAMBRIDGE
UNIVERSITY PRESS

CAMBRIDGE UNIVERSITY PRESS
Cambridge, New York, Melbourne, Madrid, Cape Town, Singapore,
São Paulo, Delhi

Cambridge University Press
The Edinburgh Building, Cambridge CB2 8RU, UK

Published in the United States of America by Cambridge University
Press, New York

www.cambridge.org
Information on this title: www.cambridge.org/9780521709118

First published 2009

Printed in the United Kingdom at the University Press, Cambridge

A catalog record for this publication is available from the British Library

Library of Congress Cataloging-in-Publication Data

Essential medical imaging / edited by Robert Gibson.
    p. ; cm.
  Includes index.
  ISBN 978-0-521-70911-8 (pbk.)
1. Diagnostic imaging–Textbooks.   I. Gibson, Robert, 1952–
[DNLM: 1. Diagnostic Imaging.   2. Anatomy. WN 180 E78 2009]
  RC78.7.D53E867 2009
  616.07′54–dc22
                                                              2008038895

ISBN 978-0-521-70911-8 paperback

Contents

Contents

Contributors

Editor
Professor Robert N. Gibson
Department of Radiology
Royal Melbourne Hospital
University of Melbourne
Parkville, Australia

Associate Editor
Dr. L. Anne Mitchell
Department of Radiology
Austin Hospital
University of Melbourne
Heidelberg, Australia

Dr. Nik Barnes
Department of Radiology
Royal Liverpool Children's Hospital
Liverpool, UK

Dr. Jacqueline Brown
Department of Radiology
University of Melbourne
Parkville, Australia

Dr. Mark Brooks
Department of Radiology
Austin Hospital
Heidelberg, Australia

Dr. Tony Cullen
Department of Radiology
Austin Hospital
Heidelberg, Australia

Professor Patricia Desmond
Department of Radiology
Royal Melbourne Hospital
University of Melbourne
Parkville, Australia

Dr. A. Michelle Fink
Department of Radiology
Royal Children's Hospital
University of Melbourne
Parkville, Australia

Associate Professor Dr. Stefan Heinze
Department of Radiology
Royal Melbourne Hospital
University of Melbourne
Parkville, Australia

Professor Oliver Hennessy
Department of Radiology
St. Vincent's Hospital
University of Melbourne
Fitzroy, Australia

Dr. Renata Kukuruzovic
Department of General Medicine
Royal Children's Hospital
University of Melbourne
Parkville, Australia

Dr. Louise Kornman
Department of Obstetrics and Gynaecology
Royal Women's Hospital
University of Melbourne
Parkville, Australia

Dr. Elizabeth McCarthy
Department of Obstetrics and Gynaecology
Mercy Hospital for Women
University of Melbourne
Heidelberg, Australia

Associate Professor Peter Mitchell
Department of Radiology
Royal Melbourne Hospital
University of Melbourne
Parkville, Australia

Dr. Graeme O'Keefe
Nuclear Medicine and Centre for PET
Austin Hospital
University of Melbourne
Heidelberg, Australia

Dr. Natalie Okun
Department of Radiology
University of Melbourne
Parkville, Australia

Dr. Patrick Page
Department of Radiology
University of Melbourne
Parkville, Australia

Professor Michael Permezel
Department of Obstetrics and Gynaecology
Mercy Hospital for Women
University of Melbourne
Heidelberg, Australia

Dr. Aurora Poon
Nuclear Medicine and Centre for PET
Austin Hospital
Heidelberg, Australia

Associate Professor Christopher Rowe
Nuclear Medicine and Centre for PET
Austin Hospital
University of Melbourne
Heidelberg, Australia

Dr. Damien Stella
Department of Radiology
Royal Melbourne Hospital
University of Melbourne
Parkville, Australia

Dr. Colin Styles
Department of Radiology
Peter MacCallum Cancer Centre
University of Melbourne
East Melbourne, Australia

Dr. Paul Tauro
Department of Radiology
University of Melbourne
Parkville, Australia

Professor Brian Tress
Department of Radiology
Royal Melbourne Hospital
University of Melbourne
Parkville, Australia

Dr. Rohan White
Department of Radiology
University of Melbourne
Parkville, Australia

Dr. Kerry Whyte
Department of Radiology
Austin Hospital
Heidelberg, Australia

Dr. Susan Walker
Department of Obstetrics and Gynaecology
Mercy Hospital for Women
University of Melbourne
Heidelberg, Australia

Preface

Medical imaging has come to occupy a pivotal role in the delivery of patient care. Apart from the major area of medical diagnosis, imaging is integrated into basic and clinical research and in the teaching of anatomy.

This text evolved from the development of an integrated medical imaging curriculum for undergraduate medical students at The University of Melbourne. The contents also meet the needs of a much broader group of readers, including trainee physicians and surgeons, general practitioners, junior radiology trainees, and nursing and allied health professionals. As the curriculum is delivered via a web-browser interface, a CD-ROM is included, which includes an expanded version of the text and images, as well as a search engine.

The aim of this text is to provide a comprehensive but manageable coverage of medical imaging in clinical medicine, and assumes no prior knowledge of imaging modalities. All areas of general and specialist adult medicine and surgery are included, as well as obstetrics and gynecology, and pediatrics.

The emphasis is on placing medical imaging in clinical context and enabling the reader to learn how best to use imaging. The topics describe the role of imaging in common clinical presentations, and the important imaging features of common or important diseases. In addition, substantial sections outline the principles of image generation and interpretation, risks, benefits, and costs. We have included a comprehensive overview of nuclear medicine techniques and some of its common clinical applications, an area sometimes not covered in similar texts.

A section with annotated normal radiological images is included to act as a reference with which to compare the abnormal and to aid in the learning of anatomy. This section can be viewed on the CD-ROM in self-test mode.

Readers can use this text from any starting point, depending on the clinical situation. A useful place to start for many will be with the sections outlining how images are produced, how normal images appear, and how to develop a systematic way of looking at images.

The accompanying CD-ROM is an expanded version of the text. It is a comprehensive resource that provides a number of ways to browse its content and locate relevant information. Users should spend a few minutes reading the introduction for orientation and can then select topics of current interest, use the search engine to generate links to particular subjects, and use the library of normal images as a reference as well as using it in self-test mode.

Robert N. Gibson
and
L. Anne Mitchell
(Associate Editor)

Acknowledgments

This text has been reliant on the contributions from numerous expert people in medical imaging, listed in the contributors' list. Pivotal support for development of the curriculum, and hence the content of this text and accompanying CD-ROM, was provided by Brian Tress, Richard Larkins, Susan Elliott, and Peter Harris in the Faculty of Medicine, Dentistry, and Health Sciences of The University of Melbourne.

I am very grateful for the support of my Associate Editor, Anne Mitchell and the assistance of Merilyn Denning, Angela Alexiou, and Annabella Zupan.

Many people in the Faculty brought the CD-ROM to fruition and they are listed in its credits. Special thanks are due to Melinda Jones, Natalie Okun, Tom Petrovic, Kevin Sweeney, Greg Nelson, Stephanie Bysouth, Terry Judd, Andrew Bonollo, and Wai Chan.

Thank you to the patient staff of Cambridge University Press.

Finally, I am forever grateful to my family and to Bill Hare, who have supported me and inspired me.

Robert N. Gibson

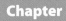
Radiation and radiology – the basics

Contents

Ionizing radiation

Ionization may be simply defined as any process by which an atom or molecule gains an electric charge. Any radiation which is capable of causing this effect is known as ionizing radiation. Non-ionizing radiations include such things as light and microwaves. Ionizing radiations emitted from radioactive atoms or produced by devices such as X-ray tubes include:

- Alpha particles
- Beta particles
- Gamma rays
- X-rays

Alpha particles

Alpha particles are identical with helium nuclei, having two protons and two neutrons. Alpha particles are usually emitted by heavy radioactive atoms such as uranium and radium. Being large and relatively slow, they quickly dissipate their energy by colliding with the atoms of the material through which they travel causing ionization to take place. Alpha particles thus have very little power of penetration and are stopped completely by a thin sheet of paper, the outer layer of human skin, or a few centimeters of air. Alpha emitters are most damaging when incorporated into the body, and are not normally used unless securely sealed.

Beta particles

Beta particles are high-speed electrons emitted from the nuclei of radioactive atoms. Having low mass, and emitted with a speed close to that of light, beta particles have greater penetrating ability than alpha particles of the same energy, but still will be stopped by a few millimeters of aluminum, a centimeter or so of human tissue or a few meters of air, dependent on their energy. Beta emitters are most hazardous when ingested, but can cause skin and eye damage. Beta emitters are frequently used therapeutically.

Gamma rays

Gamma rays are a form of electromagnetic radiation (as is visible light). They may be extremely penetrating and can pass through several hundreds of meters of air or many centimeters of dense materials such as iron or lead. Gamma emitters are hazardous internally and externally, although less damaging than the particle sources alpha and beta particles.

X-rays

X-rays are physically identical to gamma rays although of lower energy. They differ in their means of production, which is usually by means of electrons striking a dense material such as occurs in diagnostic or therapeutic X-ray tubes.

Radiation hazards and protection

X-rays (ionizing radiation) can produce harmful effects, which can be divided into two types:

- Those that inhibit cell growth and lead to cell death and
- Those that modify cell DNA (chromosomes) increasing the probability of cancer and the incidence of fetal damage and genetic defects.

These hazardous effects occur as a result of direct damage to cells caused by ionization. Ionization results in the production of free radicals – atoms which have a single unpaired electron in the outer electron orbit. Free radical interactions are the primary mechanism of radiation damage to organic molecules such as DNA.

There are no data available to determine whether there may be a threshold below which no effects occur, therefore there is no proven totally "safe" dose.

Effects of radiation

Stochastic effects

Stochastic effects are effects that occur on a random basis with the effect being independent of the size of dose. The effect typically has no threshold and is based on probabilities, with the chances of seeing the effect increasing with dose. Cancer, leukemia, and genetic mutations are stochastic effects.

Non-stochastic effects

Non-stochastic effects are related directly to the dose received. They typically have a threshold below which the effect will not occur and the effect is more severe with a higher dose. Skin burns and other skin changes, cataracts and decreased fertility are examples of non-stochastic effects.

The nature and degree of cell damage vary according to: the radiation dose, the dose rate, irradiated volume, and type of radiation.

The aim of radiotherapy is to cause cell death and inhibition of cell growth. It causes these effects by breaking one or both of the DNA strands within the cell, which will die when attempting to divide. DNA rupture results from damage caused by free radicals produced from the water that makes up 80% of the cell, or directly from the radiation. Radiotherapy operates at much higher energies (up to 10 000 000 volts) than diagnostic radiology (e.g. 100 000 volts).

Diagnostic radiology is not so much concerned about cell death and inhibition of growth as with the possibility of creating a free radical, and producing cancer or other chromosomal disease.

Man-made radiation contributes approximately 15% to the total population dose, of which 97% is from diagnostic radiology. The other 85% comes from natural background sources.

Background radiation

Everyone receives a dose of radiation from naturally occurring radiation sources in the environment and from cosmic rays. This amounts to approximately 2 mSv/year. The sources include cosmic radiation from the sky, inhaled air, and diet.

Radiation doses from common diagnostic investigations

Doses from diagnostic X-ray procedures vary widely according to the type of examination, patient thickness and the choice of technique. The average or typical radiation doses for a variety of examinations are shown in Table 1.1.

Table 1.1. Typical radiation doses for a range of examinations and the approximate time taken to receive the same dose from natural background radiation

Radiological examination	Effective dose (mSv)	Equivalent time at natural background levels (2 mSv/year)
Abdomen AP	0.41	10 weeks
Chest PA	0.013	3 days
Thoracic spine		
-AP	0.20	5 weeks
-Lateral	0.10	2.5 weeks
Coronary angiogram	3.1	1.5 years
Barium meal	2.6	1.3 years
CT (chest)	10.7	5.4 years
CT (abdomen)	17.5	9 years
CT (Liver)	13.4	6.7 years
^{99m}Tc lung scan	2.7	1.3 years

Radiation dose units

Gray (Gy)

The Gray is a unit used to measure a quantity called absorbed dose. This relates to the amount of energy actually absorbed in some material, and is used for any type of radiation and any material. One Gray is equal to one joule of energy deposited in one kg of a material. The unit Gray can be used for any radiation, but it does not describe the biological effects of the different radiations. Absorbed dose is often expressed in terms of hundredths of a Gray, or centi-Grays.

Sievert (Sv)

The Sievert is a unit used to derive a quantity called equivalent dose. This relates the absorbed dose in human tissue to the effective biological damage of the radiation. Not all radiation has the same biological effect, even for the same amount of absorbed dose. Equivalent dose is often expressed in terms of millionths of a Sievert, or micro-Sievert. To determine equivalent dose (Sv), you multiply absorbed dose (Gy) by a quality factor (Q) that is unique to the incident radiation. Equivalent dose takes into account the type of radiation, rate at which it is received and other factors. Effective dose takes into account the biological effects of the radiation on the tissue. It is the sum of the equivalent doses in all tissues and organs of the body weighted for tissue effects of radiation.

Protection in radiological practice

The risks of cancer due to radiological imaging are extremely low and population studies have not confirmed any increase in genetic defects in exposed populations. Nonetheless, it is important to keep radiation doses as low as reasonably possible so as to minimize risks.

Certain tissues are more sensitive to damage from X-rays, especially thyroid, breast, the lens of the eye, and rapidly dividing cells (gonads, bone marrow, lymph glands, and the developing fetus). Particular care is taken to protect these regions. The protective measures are primarily the responsibility of the radiology department; however, there are ways in which referring clinicians can contribute.

- Order only the minimum number of tests that use ionizing radiation
- Request the use of mobile equipment as little as possible
- Ask about possible pregnancy
  Explanation of radiation risks to patients should include:
- Risks versus potential benefits
- Comparison with natural background radiation

Protection of patients

Aims and principles of radiation protection are:

- To prevent harmful effects by keeping all justifiable exposure as low as reasonably achievable (ALARA principle).
- To prevent non-stochastic effects and to limit the chance of stochastic effects to an acceptable level.
- No practice is accepted unless its introduction results in a benefit that outweighs its detriment. Specifically:
- Each film should be justified
- Focus beam accurately to area of interest and shield relevant sensitive areas
- Minimize use of mobile equipment
- Use ultrasound or MRI where appropriate and possible
- Ensure good equipment is used and is regularly tested
- Ensure only trained personnel operate equipment.
- Take care with women of reproductive age

Protection of staff

- Only necessary staff should be present in a radiology procedure room. If viewing monitors are in use outside the screening room, staff may observe the procedure at a safe distance. If not, staff need to wear the appropriate protective clothing including lead aprons and thyroid shields.
- At no time should staff be directly irradiated by the primary X-ray beam. Where necessary, lead gloves should be worn if hands are at risk of irradiation (e.g. in reducing a fracture under fluoroscopic guidance in theater).
- All X-ray rooms should be fully lead lined.
- If a mobile image intensifier or X-ray machine is in use, all staff and students should stand well behind the portable unit so as not to be in the direct radiation or scatter field. The further away from the X-ray source, the less risk of exposure (several meters is adequate). The inverse square rule states that dose is inversely proportional to the distance (squared) away from the source.
- Rotate places of work, so that the same staff are not constantly working in areas that lead them to have higher levels of radiation exposure (e.g. angiography).
- Personnel radiation dose monitoring.

Radiation and the pregnant patient
Avoiding radiation exposure in pregnancy

A number of particular precautions should be taken when irradiation of women of reproductive age is contemplated. The aim is to minimize or avoid any exposure of the unborn fetus given that fetal tissues are thought to be more radiosensitive than those of mature adults.

Radiation exposure of the lower abdomen and pelvis of women of reproductive capacity should be kept to a minimum. During pregnancy, radiation exposure to these regions should only occur if the procedure cannot be postponed because of the urgent nature of the investigation.

It is prudent to consider as pregnant any woman of reproductive capacity whose menstrual period is overdue or clearly missed at the time of presenting for radiological examinations. The primary responsibility for identification of patients at risk rests with the referring doctor, but prior to any procedure involving ionizing radiation, all women of reproductive age should be asked about the possibility of being pregnant. If pregnancy is confirmed, consideration must be given to the possibility of delaying the procedure at

3

least until such time as the fetal sensitivity is reduced (post-24 weeks).

When radiography of areas remote from the fetus is needed, such as head, chest, or extremities, these can be undertaken with negligible exposure to the fetus at any time during pregnancy provided proper X-ray beam collimation is used. The use of protective drapes may be helpful also.

The following guidelines and precautions are useful in minimizing irradiation of the embryo or fetus, even though inadvertent exposure in utero from a diagnostic radiological examination is unlikely to result in an absorbed dose in excess of 20 mGy which is well below the probable threshold for the induction of malformations or mental retardation.

Points to remember
- Indicate on request form whether patient is pregnant or potentially pregnant.
- Avoid ionizing radiation procedures not essential for optimal medical care. This is good practice in any event. Substitute a non-radiological procedure (ultrasound, MRI, laboratory test) if possible.
- If a patient is pregnant or a procedure must be performed before pregnancy can be ruled out, consider the relative importance of the examination and risks to the mother and child.
- If pregnancy is confirmed and the procedure must be performed, the minimum amount of exposure that provides diagnostic information is used.

Procedure when patient is found to be pregnant after an X-ray

Occasionally, a patient will not be aware of a pregnancy at the time of an X-ray examination, and may become very concerned when the pregnancy becomes known.

In such cases, estimation of the radiation dose to the fetus should be obtained. A radiation safety officer should be consulted for advice in these circumstances. The patient can then be better advised as to the risks involved in the procedure. In many cases there is very little risk as the irradiation will have occurred in the first 3 weeks following conception. In a few cases, however, the fetus will be older and the dose involved may be considerable. It is, however, extremely rare for the dose to be large enough to warrant advising the patient to consider termination.

Fetal irradiation – current knowledge

There is some evidence to suggest that the fetus is more susceptible to the harmful effects of ionizing radiation than is the mature human being (Table 1.2). Certainly, any effect of irradiation in utero will be dependent on stage of development. In the first few days following fertilization the most likely effect is death with little or no chance of malformation. Subsequently, during the period of early organogenesis, malformation, and growth retardation may be expected.

The International Community for Radiological Protection (ICRP) have suggested that these effects are deterministic with an estimated threshold in humans of at least 100 mSv. From 8 weeks to 25 weeks following fertilization, the most likely effect will be an increased incidence of mental retardation although growth retardation at relatively high doses (>200 mSv) may occur.

However, human abnormalities, explicitly identified as due to radiation, are impossible to isolate given that the spontaneous incidence of all such effects is about 6%. In comparison, it is estimated that an effective dose of 10 mSv delivered over the whole

Table 1.2. Types of effects following irradiation in utero compared where appropriate with the normal incidence (modified from International Commission on Radiation Protection)

Time after conception	Effect	Normal incidence
First 3 weeks	None in live-born. Failure to implant may result in an undetectable death. Almost certainly a threshold of approximately 100 mSv	30% to 50% of impregnations may result in spontaneous abortion
3rd to 8th week	Potential for malformations of organs with a probable threshold of 100 mSv	4–6%
8th to 15th week	Potential for severe mental retardation – no observed effect below 100 mSv	0.5–1%
16th to 25th week	Reduced potential for severe mental retardation	
4th week until term	Possibility of growth retardation	
4th week until term	Cancer in childhood or adult life. Risk is likely to be two to three times higher than for the general population	0.1% for childhood cancer and 0.04% for childhood leukemia*

*The percentages reflect death rates, not incident rates, which are about 70% higher.

pregnancy would add a probability of an adverse health effect in the live born of less than 0.2%.

There is some evidence of increased levels of childhood leukemia and cancer following in utero irradiation at any stage of development after the third week. There is some evidence to suggest that the major part of the risk is associated with irradiation during the latter part of the first trimester.

Since the doses from diagnostic radiological procedures (typically a few mSv) and from occupational exposures (typically a few mSv per year) are small, it should be clear that the risks to the unborn child from diagnostic and occupational levels of radiation exposure are very small. Nevertheless, the deliberate irradiation of pregnant and potentially pregnant female patients naturally requires some caution. The general rule is to ask the patient if she is, or could be, pregnant.

Guidelines for administration of radionuclides to pregnant patients

Nuclear medicine studies in a pregnant woman, because they have the potential to irradiate the whole body, are best avoided entirely but they are not absolutely contraindicated. When a patient is pregnant, indications for the study should be discussed with the nuclear medicine specialist and the fact that the patient is pregnant should be clearly marked on the request form. A smaller than normal dose of radioisotope may be administered.

It is worth noting that the fetal irradiation does not arise just from uptake of radionuclide by the mother. Depending on the degree of organogenesis that has occurred, radionuclides may be concentrated in specific fetal organs resulting in substantial radiation burden to the fetus. A most obvious case of this is thyroid scanning with ^{131}I or ^{99m}Tc-pertechnetate but even bone agents will be taken up in the fetal skeleton if organogenesis is complete. As a rule, a pregnant woman should not be treated with a radioactive substance unless the therapy is required to treat a life-threatening condition. In that event the fetal dose should be estimated and consideration given to terminating the pregnancy.

The radiology department

The many types of radiology departments range in size from small private centers, which may specialize in imaging specific organs (e.g. mammography breast screening clinics) to large departments in major hospitals. These may have multiple subsections and subspecialists who engage in a wide spectrum of clinical imaging, interventional procedures, and research projects. Radiology departments are also called Medical Imaging departments or similar names. There are several features which most departments have in common:

- Imaging rooms and the equipment for each imaging modality
- Darkroom or processor where films are developed or processed (unless entirely digital)
- Filing room where films are recorded, stored, and retrieved; or more commonly now, servers and archives for digital images
- Reporting rooms where films or digital images are interpreted by radiologists
- Patient care facilities where patients in need of close attention can be monitored

In large hospital centers the radiology department is not usually confined to a single area within the hospital, but involves other departments of the hospital. These include:

- The emergency department – where X-rays, US, and often CT are performed
- The wards and ICU (intensive care unit) – where portable X-rays and US are performed on patients too sick to be moved
- The operating rooms where portable fluoroscopy units are used in surgical procedures

Radiology staff

The professional staff within a department include the following groups.

Radiologists and trainee radiologists

Radiologists are the specialists trained to interpret images and to perform radiological procedures. As the hospital size and range of services increase, radiologists tend to become experts in one or more subspecialty areas. The responsibility for interpreting examinations rests with the radiologist.

Radiology tends to attract doctors who like the challenge involved in reaching a diagnosis. It is an attractive area for those seeking to be involved in many disciplines in medicine.

Radiology is no longer a "hands-off" specialty of medicine, dedicated to the interpretation of films. It has entered the treatment realm with interventional procedures offering an alternative or supplementary treatment option to surgery, in many instances reducing complications and length of hospital stay. The rapid enlargement of the radiologist's field has seen the specialty change tremendously in the last few decades. Procedures involving direct patient contact make up a large part of a radiologists work. The training program for radiology is about 5 years in most Western countries usually after at least 2 clinical resident years.

Radiographers (medical imaging technologists)

These are the staff who perform the acquisition of the images or assist the radiologist in image acquisition for the procedural studies. They are trained in radiation, MRI and ultrasound physics and image processing, as well as in anatomy and pathology. They work with radiologists to ensure quality control.

Many departments also have trainee radiographers who rotate through the various specialty areas.

Radiation physicist

Physicists are concerned with patient and staff radiation safety issues and related quality control within the department, and more broadly within a hospital.

Radiology nursing staff

These are specially trained nurses working within the department. They are responsible for monitoring patients in need of close attention and for assisting with diagnostic and interventional procedures. They also ensure that emergency carts, appropriate medications, and patient monitoring devices are available for patient care.

A department in a hospital performing 100 000 radiological examinations per year would typically have approximately 15 radiologists, 15 trainee radiologists, 50 radiographers, 10 trainee radiographers, 15 nursing staff, 5 assistants for patient transport, 20 administration and clerical staff, 5 audiotypists (unless voice recognition software is used), 2 or 3 IT staff to support information systems and PACS (see below), and a physicist.

Picture archive and communication systems (PACS)

Traditionally imaging departments have produced the record of the examination on film as a hard copy X-ray. As a result of the introduction of digital imaging, images can now be acquired, archived and transferred electronically. This has allowed more efficient and reliable access to images from multiple locations. Images can be manipulated in many ways on dedicated workstations, which is how radiologists report them, and also can be viewed remotely on routine computer monitors and even hand-held devices usually using, for example, web browser technology. Radiology departments now tend to make use of this in systems known as Picture Archive and Communication Systems (PACS).

Requesting radiology tests

When requesting radiology studies there are a range of issues to consider.

Communication with the radiologist

- Relevant clinical information needs to be made available to the radiologist before imaging tests are performed so that the examination can best answer the specific clinical problem.
- The selection of imaging test, the way in which it is performed and its interpretation can all be critically affected by clinical information provided.
- When requesting complex imaging, it can be very useful to speak directly with a radiologist to discuss imaging planning.

Guidelines to help determine the usefulness of an imaging test or procedure

Imaging examinations should not be requested without considering the impact of the result on patient management.

The referring clinician should make clear the clinical question that needs to be answered.

To help prevent unnecessary or inappropriate requests some basic questions should be considered:
- Is the test suitable for the patient?
  - In particular, does the examination image the area of interest and will it yield the needed diagnostic information?
- Is the patient suitable for the test?
  - Is the patient able to co-operate to lie still or breath-hold for a CT or MRI scan?
  - Does the patient have a pacemaker, for example, that would make them unsuitable for MRI?
  - Is the patient pregnant?
  - Is the patient allergic to radiographic intravascular contrast agents?
  - Can the patient tolerate the examination?
  - Does the patient have renal impairment, which may preclude the use of intravascular contrast agents?

- Is the patient a diabetic taking metformin, which may preclude the use of intravascular contrast agents?
- Can the same information be obtained by other methods that are cheaper, more available or safer?
- Has the patient previously had the examination?

  If an examination does need to be repeated then the previous images are invaluable to the radiologist to assess any change.
- Will the examination interfere with other planned examinations?

  For example, a barium study of the gastrointestinal tract can degrade a CT image so that interpretation is impossible.
- Is the patient properly prepared for the examination?

  This not only includes physical preparation (e.g. fasting prior to an abdominal US) but also mental preparation, that is, what to expect with the examination or procedure.

Consent

Consent should be obtained for any radiological procedure which carries a material risk.

The legal responsibility for informed consent of a patient lies with the person performing the procedure, namely the radiologist. However, the referring clinician may also be legally accountable if the indication for the procedure is questionable or the procedure is particularly hazardous for that patient.

Furthermore, the process of the referring clinician obtaining consent helps ensure good communication with the patient so that they are informed well ahead of the procedure being performed and know what to expect. So the provision of informed consent is the domain of both the clinician and the radiologist. Radiology departments and practices need to attempt to provide information in suitable format about common examinations and procedures both to referring clinicians and to patients.

Follow-up arrangements

It is most important for the referring doctor to actively check the results of any tests ordered to avoid a missed diagnosis.

Risk versus benefit

The potential benefit of the examination must always outweigh the risk in order to justify a test.

This depends in part on the pre-test probability of the provisional diagnosis and how important it is to confirm this diagnosis. For example, where the provisional diagnosis is lung cancer, one would want to be almost 100% certain of the diagnosis before embarking on hazardous treatment. However, where the provisional diagnosis is sinusitis, one might start antibiotic treatment when one is only 75% certain of the diagnosis and not request paranasal sinus X-rays to confirm the hypothesis. Ordering tests should not be about reaching a diagnosis at any cost, but rather be aimed at gaining information which has a reasonable likelihood of affecting patient care.

2 Imaging modalities and contrast agents

Contents

Plain films

Plain films are what are generally meant when referring patients for "X-rays." Plain radiography requires less sophisticated equipment compared to other methods of imaging. The physics of X-ray production is beyond the scope of this text. A basic description of plain film production is outlined below.

Equipment

Plain film production requires an X-ray tube, filters, grids, a film in a light-tight film holder, or a digital recording medium, and controls for determining radiographic exposures (Fig. 2.1).

High energy X-rays are produced in an X-ray tube and travel toward the patient. A filter is placed between the patient and the tube to remove unwanted low energy X-rays that do not contribute to the final image but would add to the radiation dose the patient receives.

Then the X-rays pass through the patient, exiting as a pattern of X-ray intensities (subject image) dependent on the type of tissue traversed. The X-rays then pass through a grid, which filters out scattered radiation, producing a clearer image.

The pattern of X-ray intensities (which represents the image of the body part) is then recorded by a number of means

- Traditional film cassette where they stimulate chemicals in the film screen to fluoresce. It is this fluorescence that exposes the film rather than the X-rays themselves. This results in traditional hard copy films.
- Digital recording – this may then be converted to film or retained purely as a digital "soft copy" to be viewed on a monitor.

Differentiation of tissues

The absorption of the X-ray beam is directly proportional to the physical thickness and density of the tissue it traverses, and more importantly, to the atomic number of the elements in the beam. Thus the following densities, in increasing order of absorption can be identified on plain films:

- Air
- Fat
- Soft tissues (including body fluids)
- Calcifications
- Teeth
- Metal (e.g. surgical plates and screws)

Costs and utility

Plain film imaging is cheaper than more sophisticated radiological modalities, but nonetheless accounts for a huge proportion of diagnostic imaging expenditure, simply by virtue of the enormous number of examinations performed.

Doctors should not request a radiographic examination unless it will have an effect on patient management. It is important to avoid an unnecessary radiation dose to the patient, and minimise unnecessary costs. Clinicians bear the responsibility for knowing when plain films are indicated, as most are performed without radiologist input prior to the performance of the test.

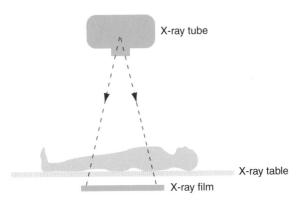

Fig. 2.1. Plain X-ray schematic.

Plain film projections

A number of projections or views are commonly used.

If the beam passes through the patient's ventral (anterior) surface first, and then through the dorsal (posterior) surface to reach the film, it is called an anteroposterior (AP) projection.

Conversely, if the beam passes from dorsal to ventral through the body, then a posteroanterior (PA) view is obtained.

Lateral and oblique films are named according to which part of the body is closest to the film. For instance, a left lateral projection indicates that the left side of the body is closest to the film. When the right anterior part of the body is placed adjacent to the film it is called a right anterior oblique (RAO) view.

A lateral decubitus film (chest or abdomen) is obtained with the patient lying on their side and the film is placed vertically, with the X-ray beam being horizontal. Left side down is referred to as left lateral decubitus.

Tomography

Tomography allows imaging of a selected section or "layer" of a patient. Only structures within the focal plane are clearly visualized, and those outside it are blurred. This sometimes assists in clarifying uncertainties on plain films.

It is performed by moving the X-ray tube and the film cassette about an adjustable fulcrum during exposure. The fulcrum point defines the focal plane where structures are kept "in focus."

Tomography is commonly used for renal evaluation as part of an intravenous pyelogram.

Computed tomography has almost totally replaced conventional tomography.

Fluoroscopy

Fluoroscopy uses low intensity X-ray beams to continuously visualize the area of interest in "real time."

The fluoroscopy system consists of an X-ray tube and on the opposite side of the patient a means of X-ray detection to generate an image; increasingly this is done by digital flat panel detectors. The image is viewed "live" on a computer or television monitor. Recordings of each study can be made using a range of storage media. The system and/or the patient can be moved to examine any body part of interest.

Indications

Fluoroscopy is routinely used to monitor contrast studies and angiograms. It is also used in innumerable other procedures requiring continuous visualization including endoscopy, bronchoscopy, orthopedic surgery, myelography, diaphragmatic motion studies, arthrography, and urethrography.

Radiation risks

The radiation dose from modern fluoroscopic equipment is relatively low, but the amount of fluoroscopy time is monitored for each patient, as the dose is related to total fluoroscopy time so has the potential to be unacceptably high.

Portable fluoroscopy

Portable C-arm units are often used in operating rooms, e.g. to assess orthopedic alignment or for intraoperative cholangiography. Imaging on these units is usually of adequate quality, but in general, standard fluoroscopic units in radiology departments offer superior image quality and optimal radiation protection.

Computed tomography (CT)

Image production

The basis of CT image generation is that a narrow beam of X-rays is transmitted through the patient and received by radiation detectors that transmit the data in digital form into a computer. The X-ray tube rotates around the body as it generates the X-ray beam and the amount of X-ray transmission through the body is recorded at numerous points by the detector ring that lies on the outside of the ring that is the path of motion of the X-ray tube. The measurement of transmitted X-ray energy at many points in the rotation is then translated by the computer into a "map" of X-ray absorption of the tissue slice. The patient lies on a special table that can be moved in steps for each X-ray tube rotation or can be moved continuously as the X-ray tube also rotates continuously, so-called spiral or helical CT.

Terms
- Increased attenuation or hyperdensity = whiter (more X-rays are absorbed)
- Decreased attenuation or hypodensity = darker (fewer X-rays are absorbed)

CT image display
- The computer mathematically reconstructs a digitized image of the "slice" of the body part being studied.
- The slices are made up of small volumes ("voxels"), which are precisely placed in space and have an attenuation value ascribed to them in Hounsfield Units (HU) based on how much X-ray energy each voxel absorbs.
- Tissue attenuation or density is therefore measured in Hounsfield Units (HU), named after the inventor of CT. A scale of arbitrary numbers is used to display this information, from −1000 HU (air) to +1000 HU (cortical bone) with zero HU, the center, representing the attenuation value of water.
- These density values are displayed as shades of gray (gray-scale) with dense structures (e.g. bone) shown as white, and least dense shown as black (air). The voxels are displayed in two dimensions as an array of pixels with their gray-scale depending on the HU of the voxel as well as on "windowing" (see below). These pixel values are directly related to the attenuation coefficients of the tissue at corresponding locations within the slice.
- Approximate density measurements are shown in Table 2.1.

Image display: windowing
By changing the settings of the gray-scale display (the window "width" and window "level"), one can change the appearance of the image, in order to demonstrate specific anatomy or pathology. There are a number of standardized windows including those optimized for looking at bones, brain, lungs, and soft tissues (Figs. 2.2, 2.3).

Table 2.1. Approximate CT density measurements in Hounsfield Units (HU)

Air	−1000 HU
Fat	−100 HU
Water	0 HU
Body fluids	< 25 HU
Soft tissues	25–90 HU
Calcification	> 100 HU
Bone	1000 HU

CT scanners now have the ability to generate multiple slices with each rotation and combined with spiral scanning now have the ability to rapidly collect data from a volume of tissue which, with software functions, allows displays in a variety of planes (multiplanar reformatting), and three-dimensional displays (Fig. 2.4), used, for example, in CT angiography, CT cholangiography, and CT colonography.

Intravascular contrast
Intravenous (IV) water-soluble iodinated contrast media is often administered as the scanning is started to allow:
- Identification of vascular structures
- Detection of avascular tissue
- Delineation of the extent of abnormal tissue/tumor.

Studies where contrast has been administered are usually labeled as such, with the annotation "C" or "C+" on the image.

The scans can be timed to coincide with maximum arterial or venous opacification as well as more delayed scans, for example, to assess the urinary tract.

Gastrointestinal contrast
For abdominal and pelvic studies, gastrointestinal contrast is usually given to delineate normal bowel from possible masses, as well as to help identify bowel pathology.

Oral contrast is usually given up to an hour before the examination.

Rectal contrast (via a rectal tube) is sometimes administered in pelvic examinations, to better delineate rectum from surrounding structures.

Computed tomography angiography (CTA)
Computed tomography angiography (CTA) may be used to show vascular anatomy. CT slices are made after the rapid i.v. injection of a large bolus of contrast.

Dynamic scans can be performed for assessment of, for example, aortic dissection, arterial stenoses and

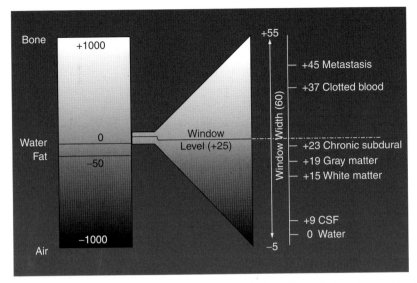

Fig. 2.2. Hounsfield Units (HU) of various tissues in the body and how window width and level can be selected to optimally use the gray-scale display to best show the differences.

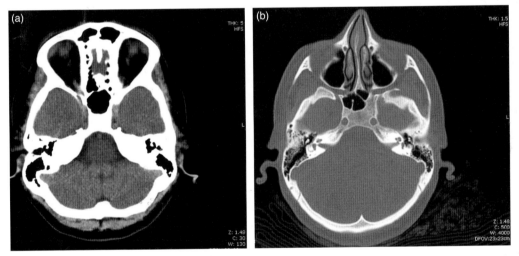

Fig. 2.3. CT of brain using (a) brain windows for display, and (b) bone windows. Note the difference in appearance of the posterior fossa when the window settings have been changed. The brain is optimally demonstrated in the brain window, but bone detail can be better appreciated in the bone window (with loss of brain detail).

aneurysms, arterial injuries or active bleeding, and pulmonary embolism.

CTA is replacing conventional angiography in many clinical situations.

Advantages of CT
- Readily available
- The contrast resolution is approximately 500 times better than conventional radiography, allowing distinction of tissues with subtle density differences, e.g. cerebral gray and white matter.
- Relatively non-invasive, quick, and painless.
- Images not degraded by bowel gas or obesity
- Imaging in transverse and other planes

Limitations of CT
- Relatively high radiation dose – this is very important to consider, particularly for young patients (see Chapter 1).
- Artifacts can totally degrade images. These are often caused by patient motion and metal objects.

11

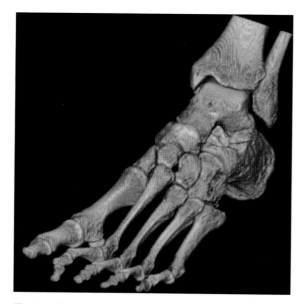

Fig. 2.4. Foot CT with 3D reconstruction.

- Adverse intravascular contrast effects. Non-contrast scans can be performed, but are not optimal for many indications.
- Higher costs compared with, for example, ultrasound.

Ultrasound (US)

Basic principles

Ultrasound creates images of the body by receiving echoes from tissue interfaces, using a narrow beam of high frequency sound. The US frequency range is usually in the range 3–15 MHz (audible sound range is 10–20 kHz).

Sound is transmitted into the body by a small transducer containing a piezoelectric crystal. When a voltage is applied to this crystal, its shape changes and this generates a sound wave.

The transducer has a second function, namely, to detect returning echoes. After each US pulse is generated, there is a "listening" period in which returning US signals are detected.

As US passes through the body, echoes reflect back from every tissue interface. An interface is a boundary between two tissues of differing acoustic impedance (the relative resistance of the tissue to sound transmission). The amount of US reflected depends on the difference in impedance at an interface.

For example, at an air/soft tissue interface, most of the beam is reflected back to the transducer, hence the need for good contact between the transducer and the patient's skin, through use of a gel coupling material.

US is highly effective for imaging most soft tissues, but bowel gas, aerated lung and bone are all barriers to US because their acoustic impedances differ markedly from soft tissue.

To date, no biological effects have been confirmed at diagnostic levels. This is also true for the growing fetus.

Advantages
- No radiation
- Real time (examines things as they happen, e.g. vascular flow, tendon movements)
- Portable
- Non-invasive
- Relatively low cost

Disadvantages
- Operator dependent
- Limited field of view
- Patient preparation
- Blind spots – some areas are poorly seen because of overlying bowel gas or bone, e.g. central to lower abdomen
- Body habitus (fat attenuates the US beam, hence thin patients are better candidates for US than obese individuals)

Terms
- "Hyperechoic" or "more echogenic" = whiter (produces more echoes; more US waves are reflected back)
- "Hypoechoic" or "less echogenic" = darker (produces fewer echoes; fewer US waves are reflected back)
- "Anechoic" = pure black and usually implies "clear" fluid (produces no echoes)
- "Real time imaging" = the image information is updated 20–40 times per second so it is perceived as instantaneous, rather than as a series of consecutive static images. Most US is real time imaging.

Image display

Each US examination involves methodical scanning of specific structures or areas of interest in at least two planes perpendicular to each other. Sections generally include sagittal (longitudinal), transverse and coronal planes.

When looking at US images, sagittal images are conventionally displayed as if the patient's head is on the left of the screen and the patient's feet on the right (Figs. 2.5, 2.6). When viewing transverse images, it is conventional for the image to be oriented as if one is looking at the patient as though you were standing at the patient's feet so that the left side of the patient is displayed on the right side of the image (as for CT).

Calculi

The difference in acoustic impedance between calculi (calcified or not) and other tissues is great, so the US beam is reflected, yielding the echogenic (white)

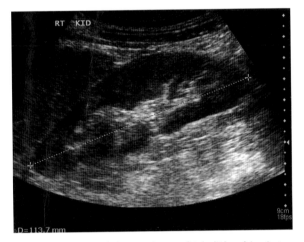

Fig. 2.5. Longitudinal ultrasound scan of right kidney lying just inferior to the liver. Note callipers used to measure renal length. The kidney hilum is echogenic relative to the renal parenchyma due to pelvicalyceal system walls, fat and connective tissue within the renal pelvis.

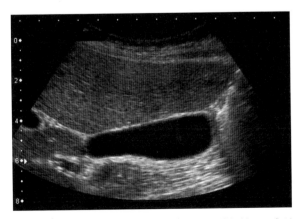

Fig. 2.6. Longitudinal scan of gallbladder. The gallbladder is a fluid filled and anechoic (black) sac with a thin echogenic (white) wall.

appearance of calculi. Very little sound energy passes through calculi, so there is an acoustic shadow (black).

Cyst versus solid

Simple uncomplicated cysts are filled with clear fluid; these therefore are anechoic (black) on US. Fluid absorbs less sound so echoes from tissues beyond a cyst (or other fluid filled structure) are brighter. This is referred to as posterior enhancement.

If a cyst-like lesion (i.e. with posterior enhancement) contains echoes one should consider:

- Hemorrhage
- Pus
- Neoplasm, especially lymphoma
  Features of cysts:
- Thin, smooth wall with no irregularity
- Anechoic contents
- Increased through transmission (posterior enhancement/whiter posterior to the cyst)

Doppler ultrasound

Doppler ultrasound relies on the Doppler effect which describes the change in perceived frequency of sound emitted by a moving source. Most people notice the Doppler effect (perhaps unknowingly) when an ambulance siren speeds past. As the siren travels towards the listener, the frequency of the sound seems higher, and when it has passed the listener, the frequency seems lower.

Moving blood cells act as a moving source of sound as they generate echoes. Blood that is flowing towards the US probe produces echoes with higher frequency, and that flowing away produces echoes with lower frequency. This frequency change or shift (the Doppler shift) can be calculated, allowing quantitation of blood flow velocity. This can be displayed as a spectrum of velocity plotted against time (spectral Doppler) (Fig. 2.7).

Color Doppler extends these principles to color code blood flow direction and speed, and displays this in a relatively large section of tissue. Colors are displayed on the conventional gray-scale image so that direction of flow can be assessed in real time (Fig. 2.8).

Color Doppler is used extensively in echocardiography, in the abdomen and in peripheral vessels. It allows the operator to assess whether flow is present, in which direction it is moving, and to calculate the flow rate. It is an important tool when looking for arterial or venous stenosis or occlusion. It is often

13

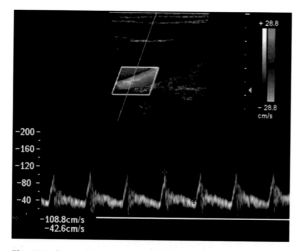

Fig. 2.7. Spectral Doppler shows velocity trace obtained from the internal carotid artery.

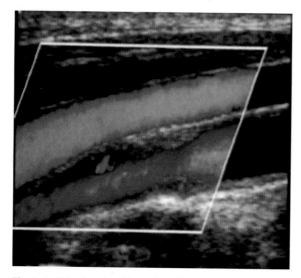

Fig. 2.8. Color Doppler of internal jugular vein with direction of flow displayed as blue, and internal carotid artery with opposite direction of flow displayed as red. Note atheromatous plaque in the proximal internal carotid artery (arrow).

combined with spectral Doppler (commonly referred to as duplex ultrasound).

Magnetic resonance imaging (MRI)

MRI uses a strong magnetic field and radiofrequency (RF) pulses to generate sectional images of the body in almost any plane.

The patient lies in the center of a very strong magnet. Atoms that have nuclei with an odd number of protons act like tiny magnets and align themselves along the direction of the magnetic field. The atom most commonly imaged is hydrogen because it has only one proton and is abundant in the human body in water. An RF pulse is applied at the resonant frequency of the hydrogen nuclei. It excites the nuclei and changes their alignment. When the pulse is stopped, the nuclei return to initial alignment (relaxation). In doing so, they emit a radiofrequency signal. The anatomical origin and the strength of these signals determine the image. The image is made up of pixels of varying shades of gray corresponding to signal strength.

Several factors determine the brightness or darkness of each pixel:

- The density of hydrogen protons or water molecules within the tissue
- The nature of nearby molecules
- Motion of the hydrogen protons (e.g. in flowing blood)
- The presence of MR contrast agents

The T1 and T2 relaxation times relate to the times for the nuclei to return to their original alignment in the longitudinal axis (T1) and in the transverse axis (T2) of the magnetic field.

A variety of radiofrequency pulse sequences are available which vary in their T1- and T2-weighting thus emphasizing different contrast properties of the tissue. In general, T1-weighted scans demonstrate anatomy best whilst pathology is best viewed on T2-weighted scans (most pathology shows up as high signal or white). Stationary or near stationary fluid (e.g. CSF, urine) shows as low signal (dark) on T1-weighted scans and as high signal (white) on T2-weighted scan (Figs. 2.9(a),(b)).

MRI has superior soft tissue contrast resolution compared to other imaging modalities. However, bone does not produce significant signal and appears black. CT is the investigation of choice for fine bony detail (although soft tissue tumors arising from bone are best evaluated with MRI).

Contrast media

To highlight pathological tissue, paramagnetic intravenous contrast agents are often used (see above).

Gadolinium causes increased signal on T1-weighted images, hence pathological areas show up white on these scans (Fig. 2.9(c)).

EPI – echoplanar imaging

EPI is an ultra-fast MRI technique that results in reduced motion artifact. It has also made possible new functional applications, including diffusion and perfusion-weighted scans and spectroscopy (MRS).

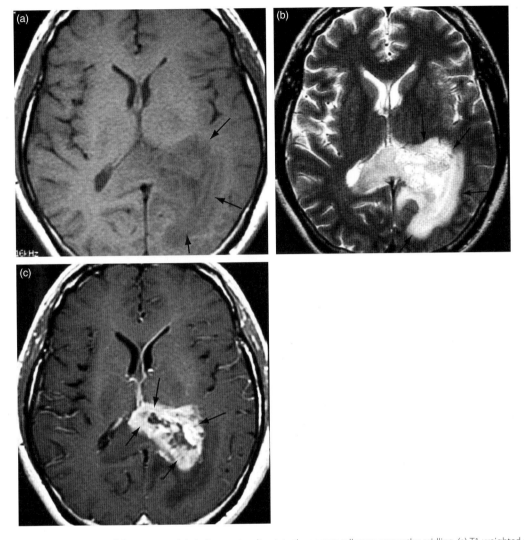

Fig. 2.9. MR showing left parieto-occipital glioma extending into the corpus callosum across the midline. (a) T1-weighted axial section. Note that the CSF is low signal (dark). There is a poorly circumscribed area of low signal surrounding the region of the posterior horn of the left lateral ventricle (arrows). This represents tumor plus surrounding vasogenic edema. (b) T2-weighted scan on which CSF shows up as high signal (white). The high signal area represents tumor plus surrounding vasogenic edema (arrows). (c) Gadolinium contrast-enhanced T1-weighted scan shows the tumor (arrows) enhances (high signal), whilst the surrounding edema does not.

Diffusion scans (diffusion weighted imaging – DWI)

Newer scanners can image the diffusion of protons within tissues, thus making MRI the only imaging modality currently capable of demonstrating cerebral infarcts less than 6 hours old.

Perfusion scans

Cerebral perfusion can be measured following injection of gadolinium. It can be used to determine areas of reduced perfusion, for example in infarcts.

Magnetic resonance spectroscopy (MRS)

MRS has long been used by physicists to analyze organic compounds and is now used in some diagnostic medical imaging to detect in vivo biochemical markers of disease processes.

MRCP

Magnetic resonance cholangiopancreatography allows imaging of the biliary system and pancreatic ducts, without requiring contrast medium.

MRA

Magnetic resonance angiograms are images of flow within blood vessels, displayed without the background soft tissues. This method is non-invasive, with excellent spatial resolution. Intravenous MR contrast is often used to improve definition.

Important contraindications for MRI

- Cardiac pacemakers, ferromagnetic intracranial aneurysm clips, cochlear implants. Some implantable devices are MRI compatible but this needs to be checked in each case.
- Intravenous or intra-arterial stainless steel stents inserted in the preceding 6 weeks
- Shrapnel/metallic foreign bodies, e.g. in orbit
- Marked obesity – patient girth and weight limits vary significantly between scanners

Relative contraindications

- Claustrophobia – Most magnets require the patient to be placed in a confined space. This is not always tolerated, even with the use of sedation. Up to 10% of patients require sedation and appropriate monitoring.

MRI advantages

- High sensitivity to a wide range of pathology
- No ionizing radiation
- No iodinated contrast media used. IV contrast (gadolinium) has a lower risk of death (1 in 1 000 000) compared with iodinated contrast used with CT (1 in 250 000). Gadolinium does nevertheless carry a risk in patients with marked renal impairment (see below).
- Soft tissue contrast resolution superior to CT
- Can display images in any plane
- Can produce an angiogram/venogram/cholangiogram without using injected contrast

MRI disadvantages

- Cost
- Less widespread availability compared with CT
- Claustrophobia
- Patients must remain still for a prolonged period. Sedation and occasionally general anesthetic (particularly in children) is needed for this reason.
- CT is better for trauma, it is quicker and easier to monitor the patient, and is better at displaying fractures, chest and abdominal injuries. MRI, however, is better than CT for display of soft tissue and spinal cord injuries.

Biological effects of MRI

- There are no known deleterious biological effects caused by standard clinical MRI.
- Hazards exist from the effect of the magnetic field on metallic implants and devices.

- High auditory noise levels within the scanner are lessened by earplugs or headphones.
- There are no known adverse effects of MRI in pregnancy.

Angiography and interventional radiology

Angiography with fluoroscopic imaging uses contrast material injected to demonstrate vascular structures: intra-arterial injection for angiography, intravenous for venography. Digital subtraction angiography (DSA) is now standard with digital image acquisition and display on monitors, and the digital acquisition allows digital subtraction of tissues which do not contain the injected contrast (e.g. bone) (Fig. 2.10).

Types of angiography and typical applications

- Aortogram – aneurysms, dissection
- Cerebral (carotid and/or vertebral arteries) – subarachnoid or cerebral hemorrhage, cerebral ischemic events
- Renal – stenosis, hemorrhage
- Mesenteric – hemorrhage, ischemia
- Peripheral (limb vessels) – stenosis, occlusion, aneurysm
- Coronary – stenosis, occlusion
- Selective angiography – this term is used when one specific vessel or its branches are catheterized.

Vascular access and technique

- Arterial sites – common femoral artery (commonest access site), brachial
- Venous sites – femoral, jugular, subclavian, brachial

Vascular interventional radiology

The term refers to many radiological procedures including angioplasty, stent insertion, thrombolysis, embolization, and infusion of therapeutic agents.
  Potential benefits include:
- Reduced risk and cost compared to surgery
- Stabilization prior to definitive surgery (decrease bleeding)
- Reduced length of hospital stay
- Preservation of organ function
  Some definitions:
- Angioplasty, percutaneous transluminal angioplasty (PTA) – balloon dilatation of a vascular stenosis

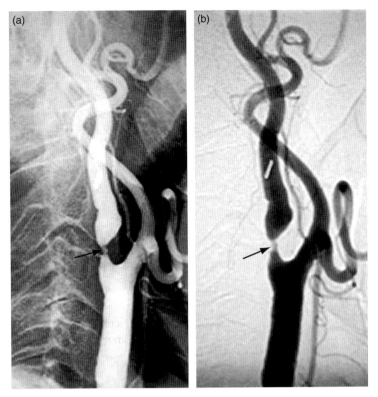

(a) (b)

Fig. 2.10. Lateral view of carotid digital subtraction angiogram with background mask (a) unsubtracted and (b) subtracted. Note severe internal carotid artery stenosis (arrow).

- Vascular stent – implanted metallic device for maintaining vascular lumen after angioplasty
- Thrombolysis – dissolution of clot, usually using pharmacological lytic agents but may be mechanical
- Thrombectomy/embolectomy – removal of clot
- Atherectomy – removal of atheroma
- Embolization – occlusion of vessel(s) using coils, particles, alcohol, glue

Balloon angioplasty and vascular stents
Stenoses within arteries and veins can sometimes be managed with balloon angioplasty alone but often a stent is required to maintain vessel patency (Fig. 2.11).

Embolization
- Introduction of foreign material into a vessel to induce thrombosis and cause occlusion
- Used to treat aneurysms, active hemorrhage, arteriovenous malformations (AVMs)

Venous access
These are usually performed with ultrasound and fluoroscopic guidance and include:
- Peripherally inserted central catheter (PICC)
- Tunneled central lines and port insertions

Angiography – complications
- Related to puncture site:
  - Hematoma
  - False aneurysm
  - Thrombosis
- Related to use of catheter, balloon or guide wires:
  - Dissection of vessel wall, stenosis, and occlusion
  - Thromboembolism to a distant site
  - Cholesterol emboli
  - Vessel perforation or rupture
- Contrast reactions
- Radiation
  - Radiation skin burn (necrosis) if patient radiation level not adequately monitored

Non-vascular interventional radiology – procedures
- Biopsy – CT, US guided
- External drainage – abscess, renal (nephrostomy), biliary, stomach (gastrostomy)
- Internal drainage – ureteric and biliary stents

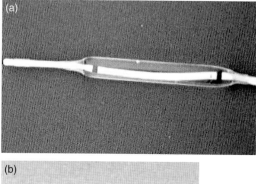

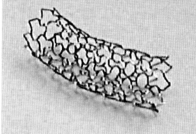

Fig. 2.11. (a) Angiographic balloon catheter with balloon inflated. (b) Vascular stent; these come in various sizes and shapes and are similar to stents used elsewhere, for example, for treatment of malignant bile duct obstruction.

- Tumor ablation
- Drainage of pleural effusions and ascites
  Some definitions:
- Fine needle aspiration (FNA) – cellular material or fluid is aspirated, e.g. for cytopathology
- Core biopsy – solid core of tissue suitable for histological examination
- PTC – percutaneous transhepatic cholangiogram (usually as part of a biliary drainage tube or stent placement)
- Antegrade pyelogram – needle injection of contrast into pelvicalyceal system
- Nephrostomy – insertion of drainage catheter into pelvicalyceal system

Mammography
Basic principles
Mammography must be performed with equipment that is specifically dedicated to breast imaging. Conventional X-ray equipment produces inferior breast images and should never be used for mammography. A dedicated mammography unit uses a special X-ray tube which operates at a low energy (kV) range to produce high-contrast images with excellent soft tissue detail.

Images are captured either using high-resolution film and screens, resulting in extremely high spatial resolution images, or by using digital capture (digital mammography).

The breast must be compressed between two plates in order to achieve the best possible quality images. The firmer the compression, the better the image. The examination is often uncomfortable but should not be painful. Try to avoid mammography just before the onset of menses to decrease the level of discomfort.

Standard views include the superoinferior (or craniocaudal) view and the mediolateral oblique. Coned magnified views of a suspicious region may also be performed.

Accuracy and limitations
Mammography is sensitive in breast cancer detection (95% sensitive combined with clinical examination findings, 80%–85% sensitive without physical examination).

A normal mammogram, however, does not exclude carcinoma. About 10% of breast cancers are not visible with mammography, even knowing that a cancer is present, and sometimes even in the presence of a palpable mass.

Ionizing radiation carries a low risk of inducing cancer. This is outweighed in the older female population by the benefits of breast cancer detection and treatment.

Advantages and disadvantages of imaging modalities (Table 2.2)

Contrast media
Iodinated contrast media
Iodinated contrast agents are routinely used as intravascular agents for angiography, CT, intravenous pyelography, as well as for direct injection into such things as biliary and urinary tracts, sinus tracts, and fistulas.

Non-ionic, low osmolar compounds are now routinely used, with a low rate of contrast-related adverse reactions. Older "ionic" agents, i.e. sodium or meglumine salts of iodinated acids have a higher rate of adverse reactions.

Table 2.2. Advantages and disadvantages of imaging modalities

	Plain films	Fluoroscopy	Ultrasound	CT	Angiography	MRI	Nuclear medicine
Advantages	Cheap, readily available	Relatively inexpensive	No ionizing radiation	Readily available	High resolution vascular imaging	No ionizing radiation	Readily available
	Especially good for chest and skeletal system	Readily available	Relatively inexpensive	Minimally invasive	Allows vascular intervention	High soft tissue contrast resolution	Minimally invasive
		Can be portable	Portable	Cross-sectional imaging		Multiplanar imaging	Functional/molecular imaging
	Low radiation dose	"Real-time" imaging	Non-invasive	Multiplanar reformatting and 3D reconstruction		Functional imaging	
	Non-invasive	Assists in interventions	Assists in interventions	Assists in interventions			
		Useful in operating theater					
Disadvantages	Two-dimensional imaging only	Potentially high radiation dose	Bone and gas obscure anatomy	Intermediate to high radiation dose	Intermediate to high radiation dose	Less readily available	Intermediate to high radiation dose
	Poor soft tissue contrast	Usually lower resolution	High operator dependence	Expensive	Expensive	Expensive	Expensive
		No cross-sectional imaging			High level of technical expertise required	Limited use in unstable patients	Poor anatomical detail
					Invasive	Claustrophobia often a problem	
						Contraindicated with pacemakers and some surgical devices	

Excretion

Excretion of intravascular agents is normally almost entirely via the kidneys. These compounds undergo glomerular filtration and concentration by tubular resorption of water. There is an insignificant amount of tubular secretion.

Reactions and side effects

Most patients tolerate these injected agents without adverse effects. Some patients, however, suffer idiosyncratic reactions ranging from slight nausea or sensation of heat, to anaphylactic shock and death. The mechanism of reactions, such as urticaria, angioneurotic edema, bronchospasm, vasomotor collapse, and respiratory arrest is poorly understood.

The incidence of severe reactions with non-ionic contrast media is of the order of 1 in 1000 and the incidence of death probably of the order of 1 in 250 000.

Risk factors

There is usually no way of predicting who will react adversely to an IV contrast injection. Certain groups of patients have increased risk, e.g. those with a history of past reaction, asthma, allergies, renal or cardiac impairment, diabetes, and myeloma. Resuscitation from a severe reaction may be more difficult in elderly patients.

If there is a history of reaction to contrast agents, then the need for the test must be balanced against the risk of a life-threatening reaction. It may be possible to obtain the diagnostic information in other ways (e.g. non-contrast CT scan, ultrasound, MRI).

Special precautions must be taken in patients with impaired renal function, myeloma, or diabetes. The risk of renal impairment is increased with high cumulative doses from studies performed in close succession.

Nephrotoxicity

An important aspect of the use of iodinated contrast agents is their potential effect on renal function, which may worsen after their use.

The major risk factors for nephrotoxicity, in addition to pre-existing renal dysfunction, are diabetes mellitus and dehydration. Pre-investigation administration of N-acetylcysteine and increased hydration appear to provide some protection in these patients. It is important to be aware of the risk of high cumulative doses if studies are performed in close succession.

Baseline serum creatinine values should be obtained in patients who are recognized at risk of pre-existing renal impairment. Calculated creatinine clearance is a better way of identifying renal dysfunction and this can be determined using serum creatinine, patient gender, age and weight.

Metformin-associated lactic acidosis (MALA)

A specific further risk in diabetics taking metformin is "metformin-associated lactic acidosis" (MALA). MALA is an uncommon but important hazard when metformin is used in the presence of renal impairment. The potential for nephrotoxicity resulting from intravascular iodinated contrast agents makes this a potential side effect of these contrast agents.

In patients taking metformin, it is important to determine renal function (calculated creatinine clearance is generally used) and to avoid the use of intravascular iodinated contrast agents (especially if there is significant renal dysfunction) or to withhold metformin for a period of time around the study.

Local guidelines should be followed as to how to approach this problem in diabetics taking metformin and the risks need to be balanced against the potential benefit of using intravascular iodinated contrast agents in a given clinical setting.

Patients without pre-existing renal dysfunction appear at very low risk of developing MALA.

Contrast agent administration

Intra-arterial and intravenous contrast

These are water-soluble non-ionic agents for evaluation of the venous and arterial systems. They are injected either directly into the veins (e.g. for intravenous pyelography, venography, or CT) or intra-arterially (e.g. for evaluation of carotid, renal, coronary, abdominal, and limb arteries).

Intrathecal contrast

Water-soluble intra-thecal agents are used to evaluate the cervical, thoracic, and lumbar subarachnoid space (myelography). They are occasionally associated with both minor and major reactions ranging from nausea, headache (which is occasionally severe), and hypertension, to more severe reactions, particularly seizures.

Oral and rectal contrast

Barium sulphate preparations are used for the detailed evaluation of the gastrointestinal tract. These are not water soluble and are rarely associated with any contrast reactions.

If there is any risk of leakage from the gastrointestinal tract (e.g. suspected perforated bowel), barium is contraindicated, because of the risk of inducing severe fibrosing peritonitis. In this situation, water-soluble contrast should be used.

Water-soluble agents are also used to evaluate the gastrointestinal tract but provide less detail. They can be ingested orally or administered rectally. Bowel opacification for CT studies utilizes water-soluble contrast agents.

Water-soluble contrast agents are rarely associated with any contrast reactions when given by these routes.

If there is any risk of tracheal aspiration or of a tracheo-esophageal fistula, standard water-soluble contrast agents are contraindicated because they can cause pulmonary edema.

Biliary and renal contrast

Non-ionic contrast agents are used in such procedures as ERCP (endoscopic retrograde cholangiopancreatography), PTC (percutaneous transhepatic cholangiography), and nephrostograms where contrast is injected into the biliary, pancreatic, and renal tracts. These routes of administration are rarely associated with adverse reactions.

Contrast agents for other imaging modalities

Magnetic resonance imaging contrast (paramagnetic contrast)

These are usually chelates of the rare earth element gadolinium (a paramagnetic substance).

When an external magnetic field is present, the magnetic moments of different atoms align with the field inducing local magnetic fields. Substances with unpaired electrons, e.g. gadolinium, produce strong local magnetic fields, and affect the magnetic relaxation properties of nearby tissues. With IV gadolinium enhancement, the magnetization properties of tissue water are altered, making it appear brighter or more intense on T1-weighted images.

It is not the actual gadolinium that alters image intensity, but the altered relaxation characteristics of adjacent protons, thus gadolinium only indirectly affects image intensity.

Gadolinium has a much lower incidence of adverse reactions than iodine-based contrast. Moreover, most reactions are minor, e.g. nausea, vomiting, urticaria, and local injection site reactions. Mortality from injection is around 1 in 1 000 000.

Nephrogenic systemic fibrosis

This is a rare but severe progressive and sometimes fatal side effect of some gadolinium-based agents when used in patients with pre-existing severe renal impairment. Gadolinium agents must therefore be avoided in this group of patients.

Ultrasound contrast

Ultrasound contrast agents are now sometimes used in cardiac and other areas of ultrasound (e.g. liver and kidney imaging). These agents are stabilized microbubbles, which are injected intravenously and resonate or collapse when hit by an ultrasound pulse and thereby enhance the echo signal.

Treatment of contrast reactions

Major reactions

The essential treatment elements include:

- Stop contrast administration
- Oxygen
- IV access and fluids
- Adrenaline
- Monitor with ECG, BP, oximetry

Minor reactions

- Observe closely
- Consider IV access
- Oral or parenteral antihistamines

Patients must be informed about the specific contrast agent and nature of the reaction for future medical care. The medical records should document the adverse reaction, with a suitable alert for future care.

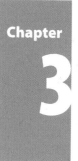

Chapter

3 Normal images

Contents

Head
Head CT

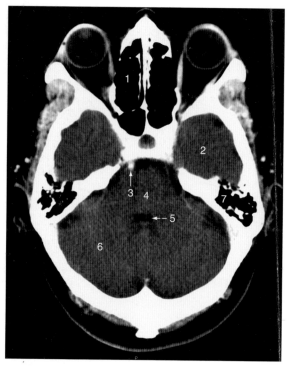

Fig. 3.1. Axial CT head (contrast enhanced)
1. Ethmoidal air cells
2. Left temporal lobe
3. Basilar artery
4. Pons
5. Fourth ventricle
6. Right cerebellar hemisphere
7. Mastoid air cells

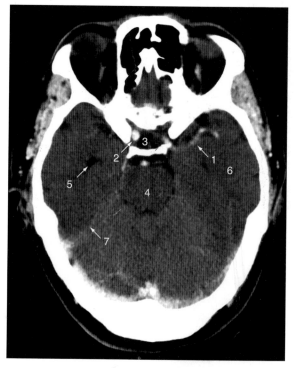

Fig. 3.2. Axial CT head (contrast enhanced)
1. Left middle cerebral artery
2. Terminal right internal carotid artery
3. Pituitary fossa
4. Midbrain
5. Temporal horn of right lateral ventricle
6. Left temporal lobe in middle cranial fossa
7. Tentorium cerebelli

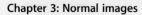

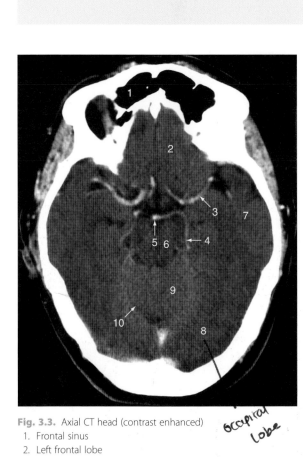

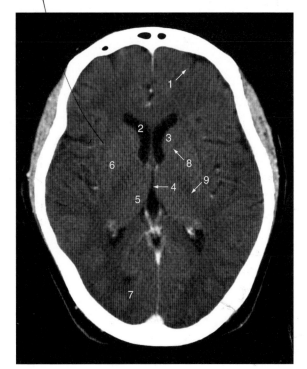

Fig. 3.3. Axial CT head (contrast enhanced) *Occipital Lobe*
1. Frontal sinus
2. Left frontal lobe
3. Left middle cerebral artery
4. Left posterior cerebral artery
5. Terminal portion basilar artery
6. Midbrain
7. Left temporal lobe
8. Left occipital lobe
9. Cerebellum
10. Tentorium cerebelli

Fig. 3.4. Axial CT head (contrast enhanced)
1. Gray matter in left frontal lobe
2. Frontal horn of lateral ventricle
3. Head of caudate nucleus
4. Third ventricle
5. Thalamus
6. Lentiform nucleus
7. Occipital lobe
8. Anterior limb of left internal capsule
9. Posterior limb of left internal capsule

lentiform nucleus

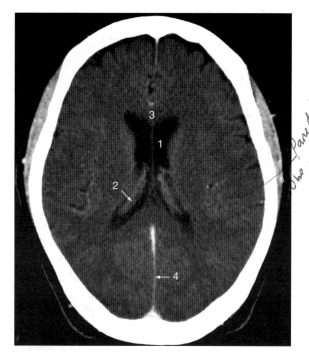

Fig. 3.5. Axial CT head (contrast enhanced)
1. Body left lateral ventricle
2. Choroid plexus in right lateral ventricle
3. Genu of the corpus callosum
4. Falx cerebri – posterior aspect

Head MR

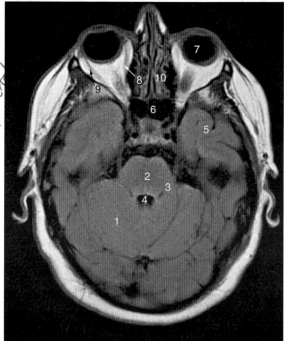

Fig. 3.7. T1 axial MR brain
1. Right cerebellar hemisphere
2. Pons
3. Left cerebellar peduncle
4. Fourth ventricle
5. Left temporal lobe in middle cranial fossa
6. Sphenoid sinus
7. Left globe
8. Right medial rectus
9. Right lateral rectus
10. Left ethmoid sinus

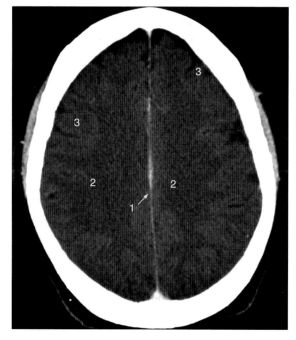

Fig. 3.6. Axial CT head (contrast enhanced)
1. Falx cerebri
2. White matter
3. Gray matter

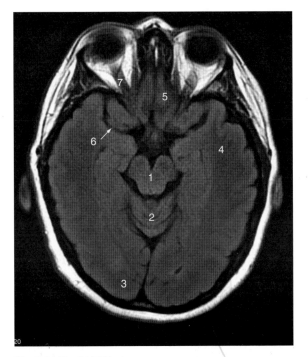

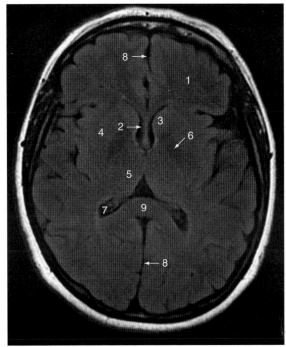

Fig. 3.8. T1 axial MR brain
1. Midbrain
2. Superior cerebellar vermis
3. Right occipital lobe
4. Left temporal lobe
5. Left frontal lobe
6. Right Sylvian tissue
7. Right optic nerve

Fig. 3.9. T1 axial MR brain
1. Left frontal lobe
2. Frontal horn right lateral ventricle
3. Head of caudate nucleus
4. Lentiform nucleus
5. Thalamus
6. Posterior limb internal capsule
7. Trigone right lateral ventricle
8. Interhemispheric fissure
9. Corpus callosum (splenium)

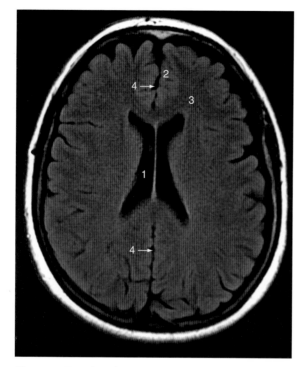

Fig. 3.10. T1 axial MR brain
1. Body of right lateral ventricle
2. Frontal lobe gray matter
3. Frontal lobe white matter
4. Interhemispheric fissure

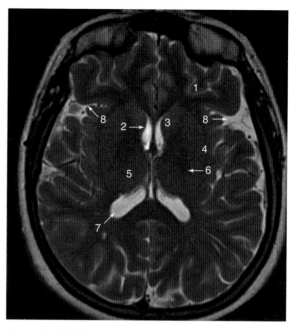

Fig. 3.12. T2 MR brain
1. Left frontal lobe
2. Frontal horn right lateral ventricle
3. Head of caudate nucleus
4. Lentiform nucleus
5. Thalamus
6. Posterior limb internal capsule
7. Trigone right lateral ventricle
8. Sylvian fissure

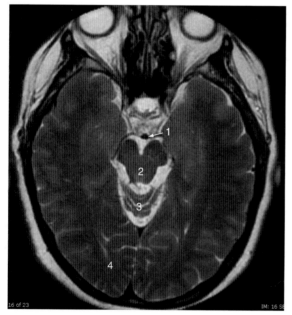
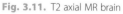

Fig. 3.11. T2 axial MR brain
1. Basilar artery
2. Midbrain
3. Superior cerebellar vermis
4. Occipital lobe

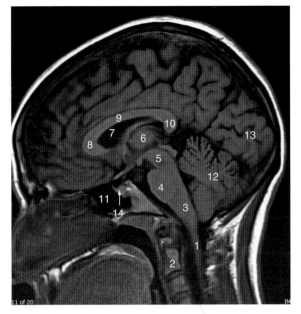

Fig. 3.13. Midline sagittal T1 MR brain
1. Spinal cord
2. Second cervical vertebra
3. Medulla
4. Pons
5. Midbrain
6. Massa intermedia (thalami)
7. Lateral ventricle
8. Genu of the corpus callosum
9. Body of the corpus callosum
10. Splenium of the corpus callosum
11. Sphenoid sinus
12. Cerebellum
13. Occipital lobe
14. Pituitary gland

Head angiography

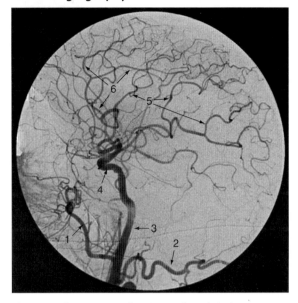

Fig. 3.14. Common carotid angiogram (lateral view)
1. Maxillary artery
2. Occipital artery
3. Internal carotid artery
4. Cavernous portion of internal carotid artery
5. Middle cerebral artery branches
6. Anterior cerebral artery branches

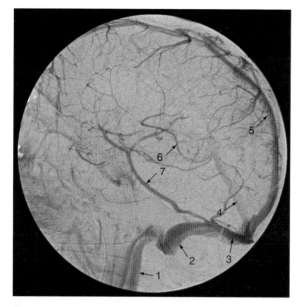

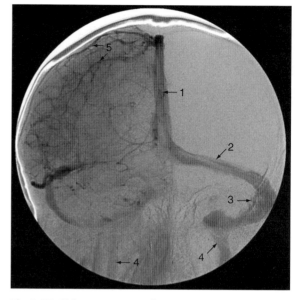

Fig. 3.15. Carotid angiogram – lateral view of venous phase
1. Internal jugular vein
2. Sigmoid sinus
3. Transverse sinus
4. Straight sinus
5. Superior sagittal sinus
6. Internal cerebral vein
7. Superficial cerebral vein

Fig. 3.17. Right common carotid angiogram – anteroposterior view of venous phase
1. Superior sagittal sinus
2. Transverse sinus
3. Sigmoid sinus
4. Internal jugular vein
5. Superficial cerebral veins

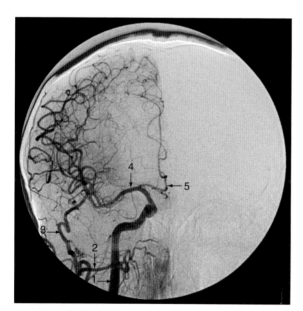

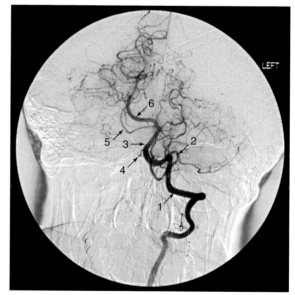

Fig. 3.16. Right common carotid angiogram (anteroposterior view)
1. Internal carotid artery
2. Maxillary artery
3. Occipital artery
4. Middle cerebral artery
5. Anterior cerebral artery

Fig. 3.18. Left vertebral angiogram – anteroposterior view
1. Left vertebral artery
2. Left posterior inferior cerebellar artery
3. Basilar artery
4. Right anterior inferior cerebellar artery
5. Right superior cerebellar artery
6. Right posterior cerebral artery

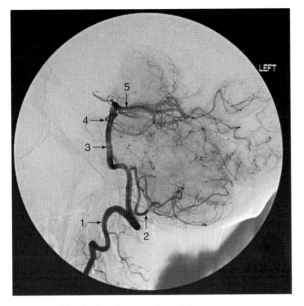

Fig. 3.19. Vertebral angiogram – lateral view
1. Vertebral artery
2. Posterior inferior cerebellar artery
3. Basilar artery
4. Superior cerebellar artery
5. Posterior cerebral artery

Spine

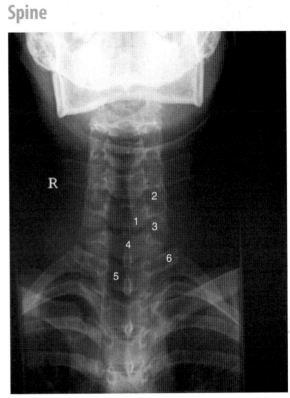

Fig. 3.20. Cervical spine – anteroposterior view
1. Body of sixth cervical vertebra
2. Superior articular process
3. Inferior articular process
4. Spinous process
5. Trachea
6. Transverse process of first thoracic vertebra

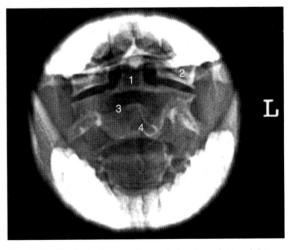

Fig. 3.21. Cervical spine – anteroposterior view of C1 and C2
1. Odontoid process of C2
2. Lateral mass of C1
3. Vertebral body of C2
4. Spinous process of C2

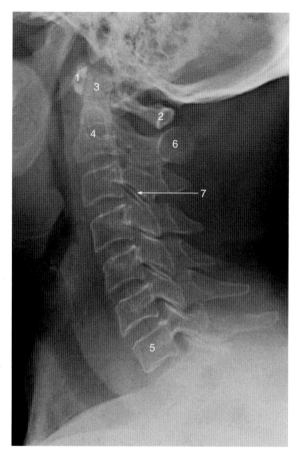

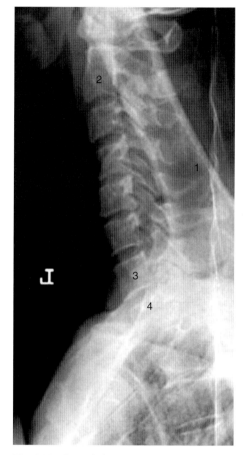

Fig. 3.22. Cervical spine – lateral
1. Anterior arch of first cervical vertebra
2. Posterior arch of first cervical vertebra
3. Odontoid process (dens) of second cervical vertebra
4. Body of second cervical vertebra
5. Body of seventh cervical vertebra
6. Spinous process of second cervical vertebra
7. Facet joint between C3 and C4

Fig. 3.23. Cervical spine – Lateral swimmer's view
1. Humerus
2. Body of second cervical vertebra
3. Body of seventh cervical vertebra
4. Body of first thoracic vertebra

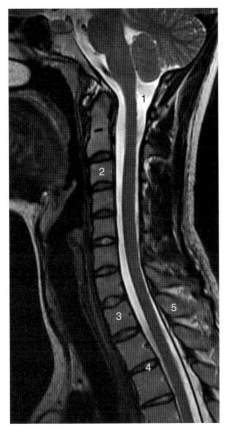

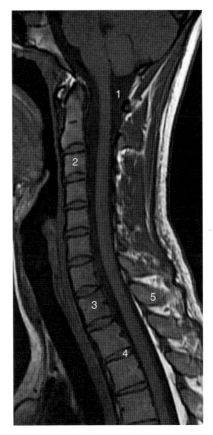

Fig. 3.24. Cervical spine T2 sagittal MR
1. CSF in subarachnoid space
2. Third cervical vertebra
3. First thoracic vertebra
4. Intervertebral disk
5. T1 spinous process

Fig. 3.25. Cervical spine T1 sagittal MR
1. CSF In subarachnoid space
2. Third cervical vertebra
3. First thoracic vertebra
4. Intervertebral disk
5. T1 spinous process

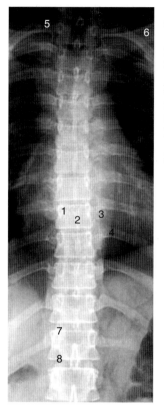

Fig. 3.26. Thoracic spine – anteroposterior view
1. Right T8 pedicle
2. T7 spinous process
3. Left T8 transverse process
4. Left ninth rib
5. Right first rib
6. Left clavicle
7. Superior endplate of T12 vertebral body
8. Inferior endplate of T12 vertebral body

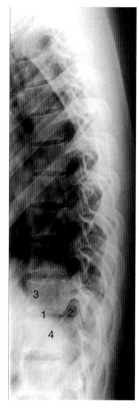

Fig. 3.27. Thoracic spine – lateral view
1. T10–11 intervertebral disk-space
2. T10–11 intervertebral foramen
3. T10 vertebral body
4. T11 vertebral body

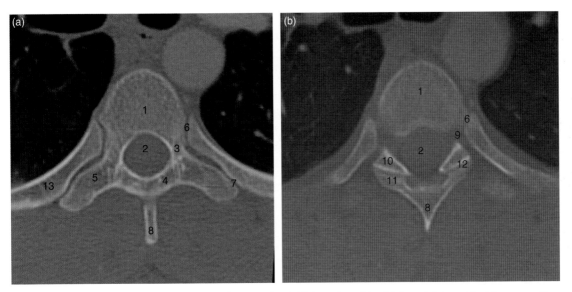

Fig. 3.28. CT thoracic spine – mid thoracic levels (bone windows): (a) through pedicles (b) through intervertebral foramen-section superior to (a)

1. Vertebral body
2. Dural sac
3. Left pedicle
4. Left lamina
5. Right transverse process
6. Costovertebral joint
7. Costotransverse joint
8. Spinous process of vertebra above
9. Intervertebral foramen
10. Superior articular process of vertebra
11. Inferior articular process of vertebra above
12. Articular facet joint
13. Rib

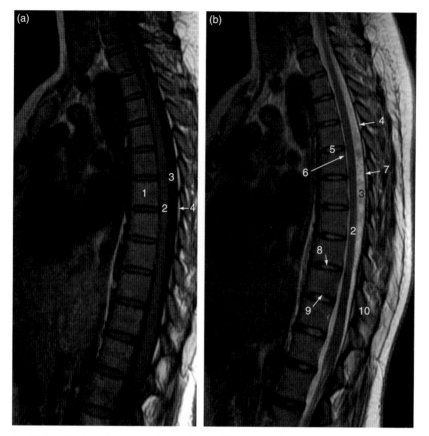

Fig. 3.29. MRI thoracic spine – midsagittal view. (a) T1-weighted image, (b) T2-weighted image

1. Vertebral body bone marrow
2. Spinal cord
3. Cerebrospinal fluid
4. Epidural fat
5. Intervertebral disk
6. Anterior dura and posterior longitudinal ligament
7. Posterior dura
8. Superior vertebral endplate
9. Inferior vertebral endplate
10. Spinous process

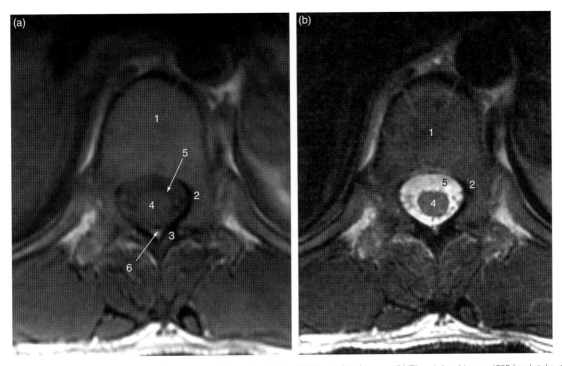

Fig. 3.30. MRI thoracic spine – axial images mid thoracic vertebra. (a) T1-weighted image, (b) T2-weighted image (CSF has bright signal)
1. Vertebral body
2. Pedicle
3. Lamina
4. Spinal cord
5. Cerebrospinal fluid
6. Epidural space (containing fat)

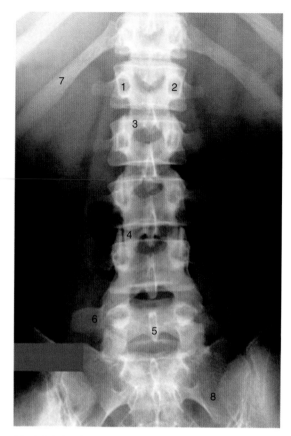

Fig. 3.31. Lumbar spine – AP view
1. Right pedicle L1
2. Left pedicle L1
3. Right inferior articular process
4. L3/4 right articular facet joint (apophyseal joint)
5. L5 spinous process
6. L5 right transverse process
7. Right 12th rib
8. Alar of sacrum

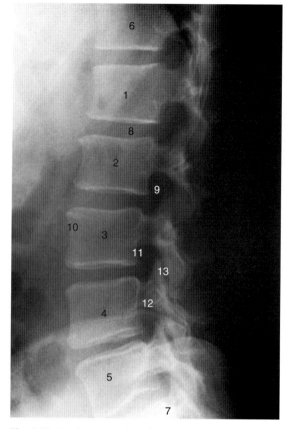

Fig. 3.32. Lumbar spine – lateral view
1. L1 vertebral body
2. L2 vertebral body
3. L3 vertebral body
4. L4 vertebral body
5. L5 vertebral body
6. T12 vertebral body
7. S1
8. L1/2 intervertebral disk space
9. L2/3 intervertebral foramen
10. Anterior margin of body L3
11. Posterior margin of body L3
12. L4 pedicle
13. L3–L4 articular facet joint (apophyseal joint)

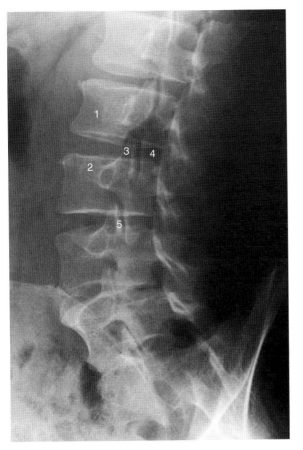

Fig. 3.33. Lumbar spine
Oblique view (right posterior oblique)
1.   L2 vertebral body
2.   Right L3 transverse process
3.   Right L3 superior articular process
4.   Right L2 inferior articular process
5.   L3–L4 right articular facet joint

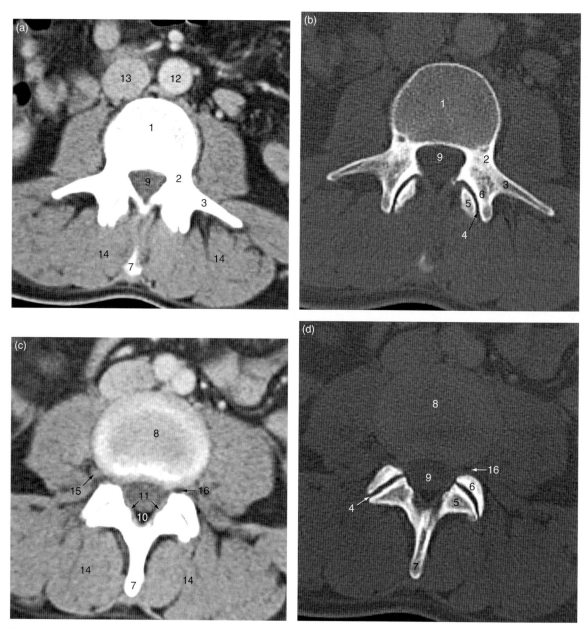

Fig. 3.34. CT lumbar spine – mid lumbar level. Soft tissue (a) and (c) and bone (b) and (d) windows at levels of pedicles (a) and (b) and intervertebral disks (c) and (d)

1. Vertebral body
2. Pedicle
3. Transverse process
4. Articular facet joint
5. Inferior articular process
6. Superior articular process
7. Spinous process
8. L3–4 intervertebral disk

9. Dural sac
10. Epidural fat
11. Ligamentum flava
12. Abdominal aorta
13. Inferior vena cava
14. Paraspinal musculature
15. Emerging spinal nerve
16. Intervertebral foramen

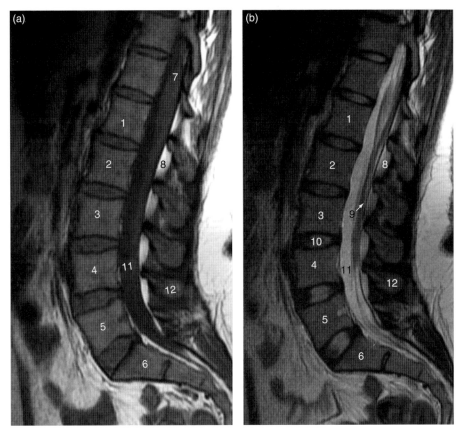

Fig. 3.35. MRI lumbar spine – midsagittal view. (a) T1-weighted image, (b) T2-weighted image

1. Vertebral body L1
2. Vertebral body L2
3. Vertebral body L3
4. Vertebral body L4
5. Vertebral body L5
6. Vertebral segment S1
7. Spinal cord
8. Epidural fat
9. Cauda equina in CSF
10. Intervertebral disk nucleus pulposus
11. Cerebrospinal fluid
12. L4 spinous process

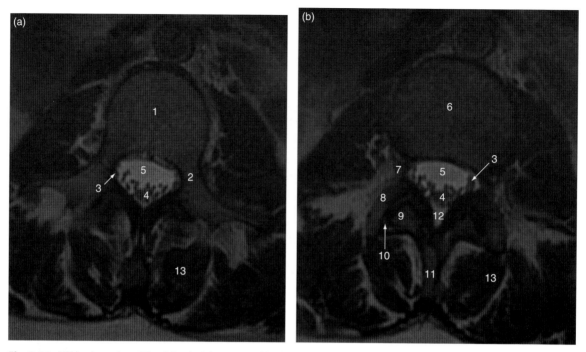

Fig. 3.36. MRI lumbar spine – T2-weighted axial images mid lumbar spine. (a) at level of pedicles, (b) at level of intervertebral disk

1. Vertebral body
2. Pedicle
3. Nerve roots in lateral aspect of dural sac
4. Cauda equina
5. Cerebrospinal fluid
6. Intervertebral disk
7. Intervertebral foramen
8. Superior articular process
9. Inferior articular process
10. Articular facet joint
11. Spinous process
12. Epidural fat
13. Intrinsic muscles of back

Chest

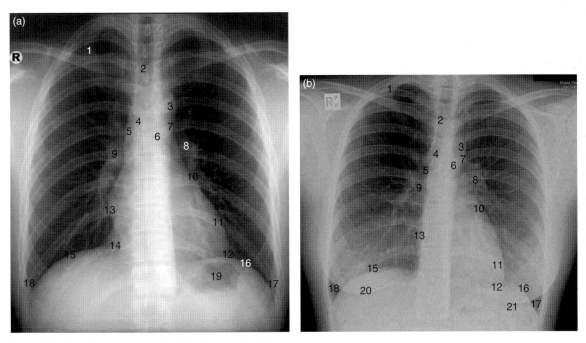

Fig. 3.37. Chest X-ray posteroanterior (PA) view (a) male, (b) female

1. Right 1st rib
2. Trachea
3. Aortic arch
4. Carina
5. Right main bronchus
6. Left main bronchus
7. Aortopulmonary window
8. Left pulmonary artery
9. Right pulmonary artery
10. Margin of left atrium
11. Margin of left ventricle
12. Apex of heart
13. Margin of right atrium
14. Margin of inferior vena cava
15. Dome of right hemidiaphragm
16. Dome of left hemidiaphragm
17. Left costophrenic angle
18. Right costophrenic angle
19. Air in the stomach
20. Right breast shadow
21. Left breast shadow

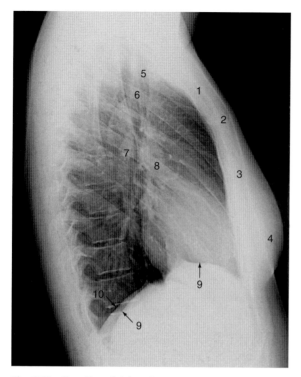

Fig. 3.38. Chest X-ray (left lateral view – taken with the patient's left side against the film)

1. Sternum (manubrium)
2. Sternal angle
3. Sternum (body)
4. Breast shadow
5. Trachea
6. Aortic arch
7. Left pulmonary artery
8. Right pulmonary artery
9. Right hemidiaphragm
10. Left hemidiaphragm

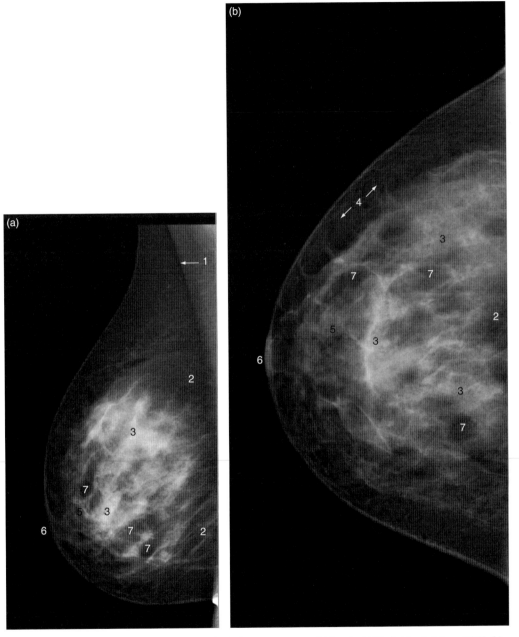

Fig. 3.39. Mammogram – two standard views of right breast in 35-year-old female. (a) Mediolateral oblique (MLO), (b) craniocaudal (CC)

1. Edge of pectoralis major muscle
2. Retromammary fat
3. Breast parenchyma
4. Suspensory ligaments
5. Subareolar ducts and parenchyma
6. Nipple
7. Fat (between breast parenchyma)

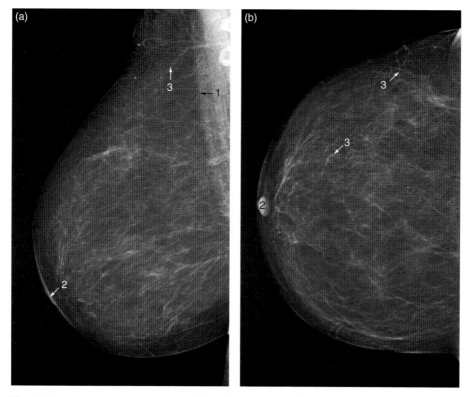

Fig. 3.40. Mammogram – post-menopausal. There is involution of glandular tissue and replacement with low density adipose tissue.
(a) Mediolateral oblique, (b) craniocaudal
1.   Edge of pectoralis major muscle
2.   Nipple
3.   Veins

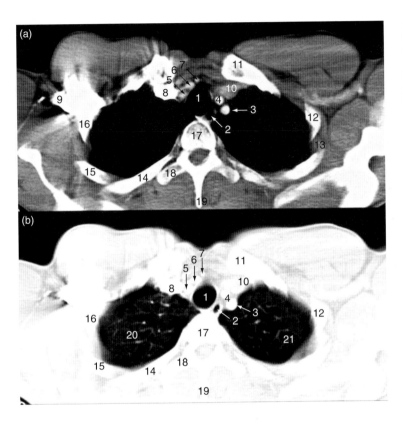

Fig. 3.41. Contrast-enhanced CT chest at level of thoracic inlet. Contrast is being injected in a right arm vein. (a) Mediastinal window – demonstrates the mediastinal structures rather than the lung parenchyma. (b) Lung window – demonstrates the lung parenchyma rather than the greater density mediastinal structures

1. Trachea
2. Esophagus
3. Left subclavian artery
4. Left common carotid artery
5. Right subclavian artery
6. Right common carotid artery
7. Inferior thyroid vein
8. Right brachiocephalic vein
9. Right axillary vein
10. Left brachiocephalic vein
11. Medial end of left clavicle
12. Left second rib
13. Intercostal muscles
14. Right fourth rib
15. Right third rib
16. Right second rib
17. Vertebral body T4
18. Vertebral right transverse process
19. Vertebral spinous process
20. Right lung upper lobe
21. Left lung upper lobe

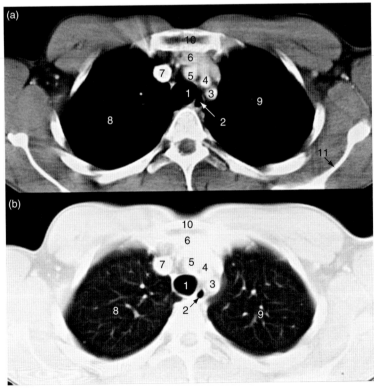

Fig. 3.42. Contrast-enhanced CT chest; T3 level (above aortic arch). (a) mediastinal window, (b) lung window

1. Trachea
2. Esophagus
3. Left subclavian artery
4. Left common carotid artery
5. Brachiocephalic trunk artery
6. Left brachiocephalic vein
7. Right brachiocephalic vein
8. Right lung upper lobe
9. Left lung upper lobe
10. Sternum (manubrium)
11. Left scapula

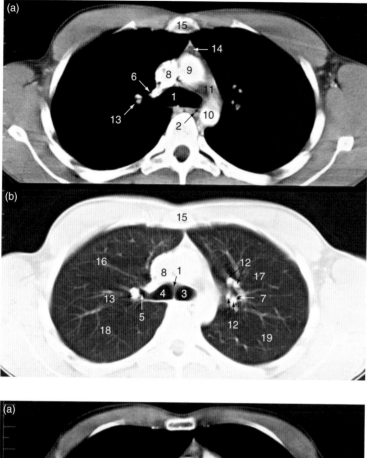

Fig. 3.43. Contrast-enhanced CT chest; level of T4–5 (tracheal bifurcation). (a) Mediastinal window, (b) lung window
1. Tracheal bifurcation, carinal ridge
2. Esophagus
3. Left main bronchus
4. Right main bronchus
5. Right upper lobe bronchus
6. Azygos vein
7. Left upper lobe bronchus
8. Superior vena cava
9. Ascending aorta
10. Descending (thoracic) aorta
11. Aortopulmonary window
12. Left upper lobe vessels
13. Right upper lobe vessels
14. Residual thymus (anterior mediastinal fat)
15. Sternum (body)
16. Right lung upper lobe
17. Left lung upper lobe
18. Position of right oblique (major) fissure
19. Position of left oblique (major) fissure

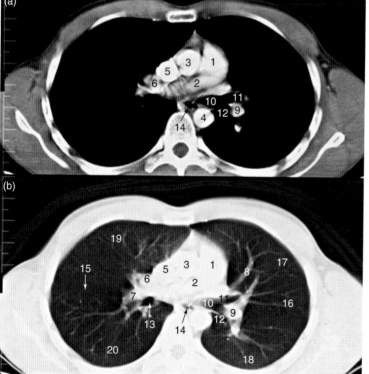

Fig. 3.44. Contrast-enhanced CT chest; level of T5. (a) Mediastinal window, (b) lung window
1. Pulmonary trunk
2. Right pulmonary artery
3. Ascending aorta
4. Descending aorta
5. Superior vena cava
6. Right upper lobe pulmonary vein
7. Right upper lobe pulmonary artery
8. Left upper lobe pulmonary vein
9. Left upper lobe pulmonary artery
10. Left main bronchus
11. Left upper lobe bronchus
12. Left lower lobe bronchus
13. Bronchus intermedius
14. Esophagus
15. Position of right oblique fissure
16. Position of left oblique fissure
17. Left lung upper lobe
18. Left lung lower lobe
19. Right lung upper lobe
20. Right lung lower lobe

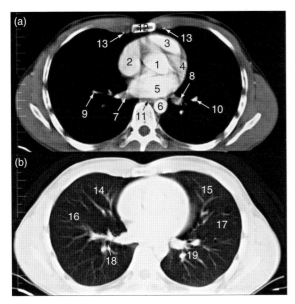

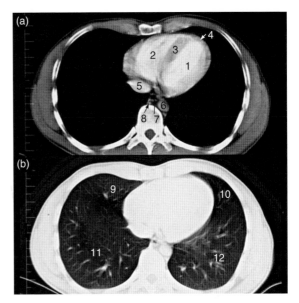

Fig. 3.45. Contrast-enhanced CT chest; level of T6 level (aortic origin). (a) mediastinal window, (b) lung window

1. Ascending aorta, origin
2. Right atrium
3. Right ventricle, infundibulum
4. Left atrium, auricle
5. Left atrium, body
6. Descending aorta
7. Right lower lobe pulmonary vein
8. Left lower lobe pulmonary vein
9. Right lower lobe pulmonary arteries
10. Left lower lobe pulmonary arteries
11. Esophagus
12. Sternum
13. Internal thoracic vessels
14. Right middle lobe
15. Lingula of left upper lobe
16. Position of right oblique fissure
17. Position of left oblique fissure
18. Right lower lobe bronchi
19. Left lower lobe bronchi

Fig. 3.46. Contrast-enhanced CT chest; level of T7. (a) mediastinal window, (b) lung window

1. Left ventricle
2. Right ventricle
3. Interventricular septum
4. Apex of heart
5. Inferior vena cava
6. Descending aorta
7. Esophagus
8. Azygos vein
9. Right middle lobe
10. Lingula of left upper lobe
11. Right lower lobe
12. Left lower lobe

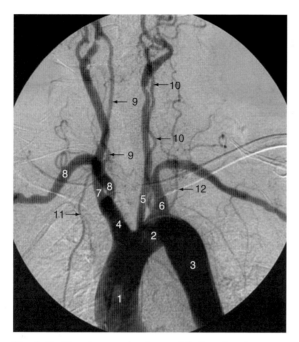

Fig. 3.47. Thoracic aortogram (some of the branches show atheromatous irregularity)

1. Ascending aorta
2. Aortic arch
3. Descending aorta
4. Brachiocephalic trunk
5. Left common carotid artery
6. Left sublavian artery
7. Right common carotid artery
8. Right subclavian artery
9. Right vertebral artery
10. Left vertebral artery
11. Right internal thoracic artery
12. Left internal thoracic artery

Abdomen

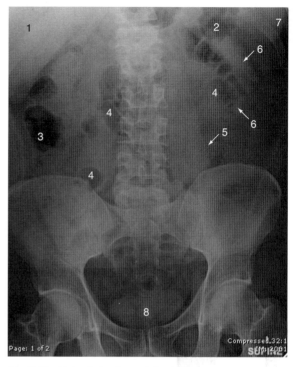

Fig. 3.48. Abdominal radiograph (supine)

1. Liver
2. Gas in stomach
3. Gas in ascending colon
4. Gas in small bowel
5. Left psoas
6. Left kidney
7. Spleen
8. Urinary bladder

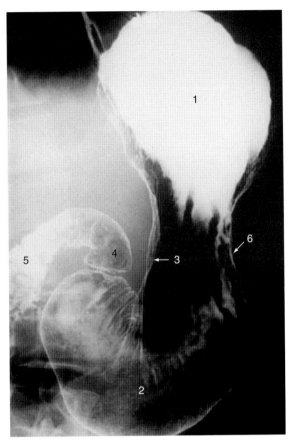

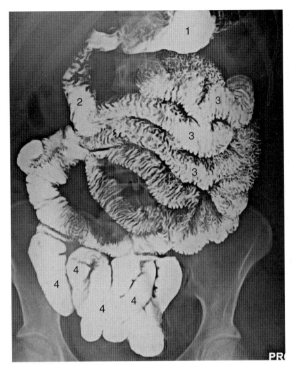

Fig. 3.50. Barium small bowel follow-through
1. Stomach
2. Duodenum
3. Jejunum
4. Ileum

Fig. 3.49. Barium meal (double contrast)
1. Barium in gastric fundus
2. Gastric antrum
3. Lesser curve of stomach
4. First part of duodenum
5. Second part of duodenum
6. Greater curve of stomach

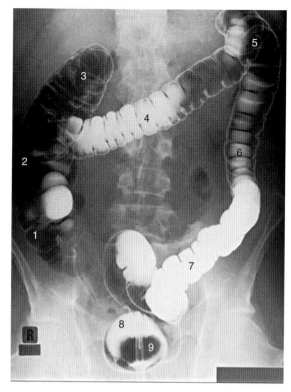

Fig. 3.51. Double-contrast barium enema
1. Cecum
2. Ascending colon
3. Hepatic flexure
4. Transverse colon
5. Splenic flexure
6. Descending colon
7. Sigmoid colon
8. Rectum
9. Rectal tube with retaining balloon

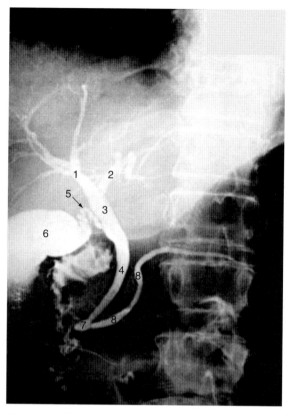

Fig. 3.52. Endoscopic retrograde cholangiopancreatogram (ERCP) (endoscope has been removed)
1. Right hepatic duct
2. Left hepatic duct
3. Common hepatic duct
4. Common bile duct
5. Cystic duct
6. Gallbladder
7. Ampulla of Vater
8. Pancreatic duct

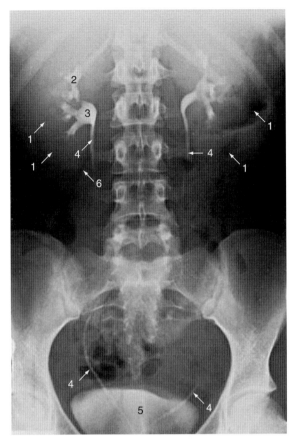

Fig. 3.53. Intravenous pyelogram (IVP)
1. Renal outline
2. Upper pole calyx
3. Renal pelvis
4. Ureter
5. Bladder
6. Right psoas outline

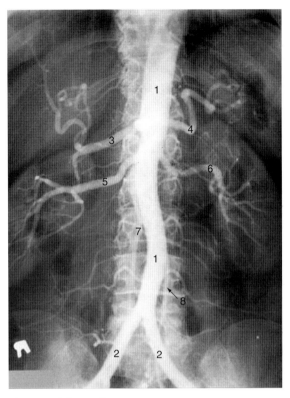

Fig. 3.54. Adbominal aortogram
1. Aorta
2. Common iliac artery
3. Common hepatic artery
4. Splenic artery
5. Right renal artery
6. Left renal artery
7. Superior mesenteric artery
8. Inferior mesenteric artery

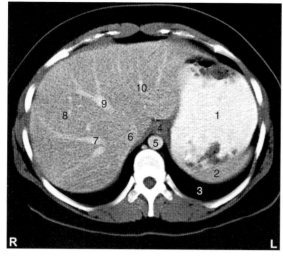

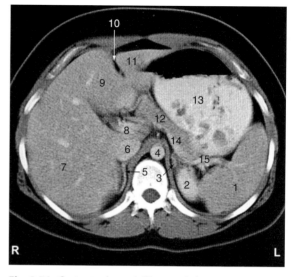

Fig. 3.55. Contrast-enhanced CT upper abdomen. Subsequent figures progress inferiorly through the abdomen and pelvis.
1. Oral contrast in stomach
2. Spleen
3. Left lung base
4. Lower end of esophagus passing through diaphragm
5. Aorta
6. Inferior vena cava (little contrast within it on this section)
7. Right hepatic vein
8. Right lobe of liver
9. Middle hepatic vein
10. Left hepatic vein

Fig. 3.56. Contrast-enhanced CT upper abdomen
1. Spleen
2. Upper pole of left kidney
3. Left adrenal gland
4. Aorta
5. Right adrenal gland
6. Inferior vena cava (IVC)
7. Right lobe of liver
8. Main portal vein
9. Quadrate lobe of liver
10. Umbilical fissure of liver
11. Left lateral segments of liver
12. Body of pancreas
13. Stomach
14. Splenic vein
15. Splenic artery

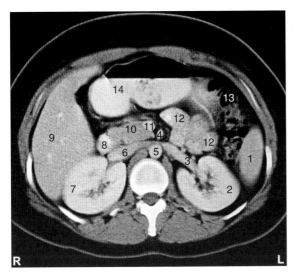

Fig. 3.57. Contrast-enhanced CT upper abdomen
1. Spleen
2. Left kidney
3. Left renal vein
4. Superior mesenteric artery
5. Aorta
6. Inferior vena cava
7. Right kidney
8. Duodenum (second part)
9. Right lobe of liver
10. Head of pancreas
11. Superior mesenteric vein
12. Proximal loops of jejunum
13. Splenic flexure of colon
14. Stomach

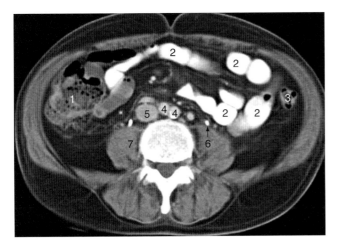

Fig. 3.58. Contrast-enhanced CT upper abdomen
1. Proximal ascending colon
2. Small bowel
3. Descending colon
4. Right and left common iliac arteries
5. Lower end of inferior vena cava
6. Left ureter
7. Right psoas

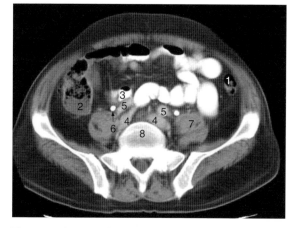

Fig. 3.59. Contrast-enhanced CT pelvis
1. Descending colon
2. Cecum
3. Ileum
4. Common iliac veins
5. Common iliac arteries
6. Right ureter
7. Left psoas
8. Fifth lumbar vertebrae

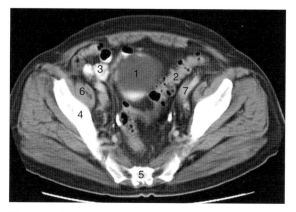

Fig. 3.61. Contrast-enhanced CT – male pelvis
1. Bladder (containing small amount of contrast)
2. Sigmoid colon
3. Small bowel (containing oral contrast)
4. Right iliac bone
5. Sacrum
6. Right psoas muscle
7. Left iliac vessels

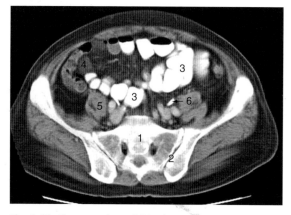

Fig. 3.60. Contrast-enhanced CT pelvis
1. Sacrum
2. Left sacroiliac joint
3. Small bowel (opacified)
4. Distal small bowel (non-opacified)
5. Right psoas
6. Left ureter

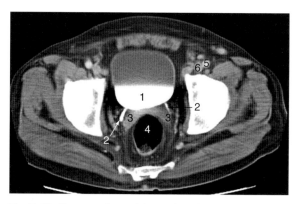

Fig. 3.62. Contrast-enhanced CT – male pelvis
1. Bladder (containing contrast)
2. Distal ureters
3. Seminal vesicles
4. Rectum
5. Left femoral artery
6. Left femoral vein

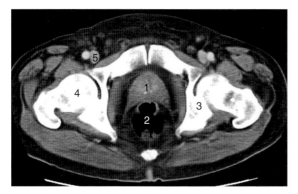

Fig. 3.63. Contrast-enhanced CT – male pelvis
1. Prostate
2. Rectum
3. Left acetabulum
4. Right femoral head
5. Right femoral vein (not opacified at the time of scan) – adjacent to opacified femoral artery

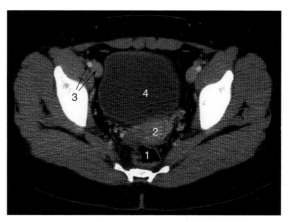

Fig. 3.65. Contrast-enhanced CT – female pelvis
1. Rectum
2. Uterus
3. Iliac vessels
4. Bladder

Upper limb

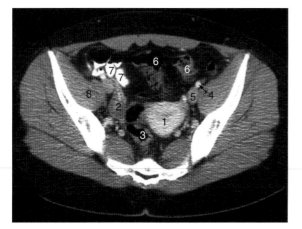

Fig. 3.64. Contrast-enhanced CT – female pelvis
1. Body of uterus
2. Right ovary
3. Rectum
4. Left common iliac artery
5. Left common iliac vein
6. Sigmoid colon
7. Small bowel (ileum)
8. Right iliopsoas muscle

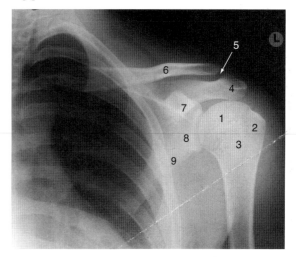

Fig. 3.66. Left shoulder – anteroposterior view
1. Head of humerus
2. Greater tuberosity of humerus
3. Surgical neck of humerus
4. Acromion process
5. Acromioclavicular joint
6. Clavicle
7. Coracoid process
8. Glenoid fossa of scapula
9. Scapula

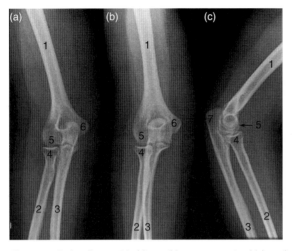

Fig. 3.67. Right elbow – (a) oblique, (b) anteroposterior, (c) lateral
1. Humerus
2. Radius
3. Ulnar
4. Head of radius
5. Capitellum
6. Medial epicondyle of humerus
7. Olecranon process of ulnar

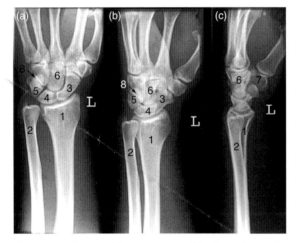

Fig. 3.68. Left wrist – (a) posteroanterior, (b) oblique, (c) lateral
1. Radius
2. Ulnar
3. Scaphoid
4. Lunate
5. Triquetrum
6. Capitate
7. Trapezium
8. Pisiform

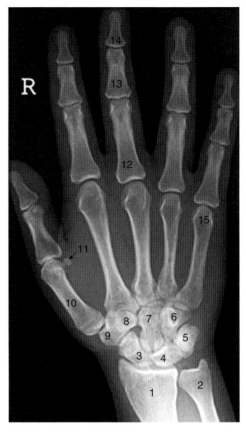

Fig. 3.69. Right hand – posteroanterior
1. Radius
2. Ulnar
3. Scaphoid
4. Lunate
5. Pisiform + triquetrum (superimposed)
6. Hamate
7. Capitate
8. Trapezoid
9. Trapezium
10. First metacarpal
11. Sesamoid bone
12. Proximal phalanx
13. Middle phalanx
14. Distal phalanx
15. Head of fifth metacarpal

Pelvis and lower limb

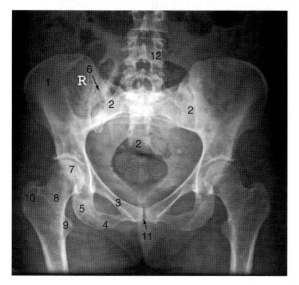

Fig. 3.70. Pelvis
1. Right Ilium
2. Sacrum
3. Superior pubic ramus
4. Inferior pubic ramus
5. Ischium
6. Right sacroiliac joint
7. Femoral head
8. Neck of femur
9. Lesser trochanter
10. Greater trochanter
11. Pubic symphysis
12. 4th lumbar vertebra

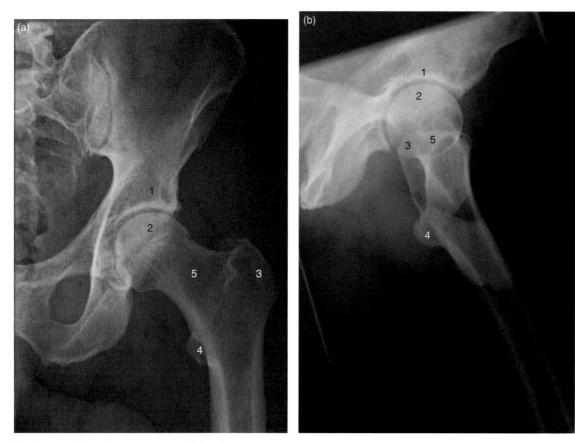

Fig. 3.71. Left hip – (a) anteroposterior, (b) lateral
1. Acetabulum
2. Femoral head
3. Greater trochanter
4. Lesser trochanter
5. Femoral neck

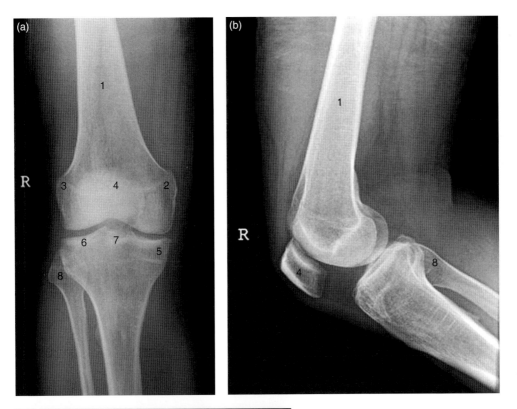

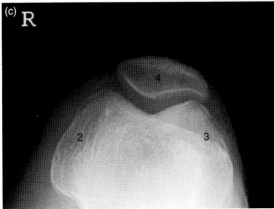

Fig. 3.72. Right knee – (a) anteroposterior, (b) lateral, (c) skyline view

1. Femoral shaft
2. Medial femoral condyle
3. Lateral femoral condyle
4. Patella
5. Medial tibial condyle
6. Lateral tibial condyle
7. Intercondylar eminence (and tubercles)
8. Head of fibula

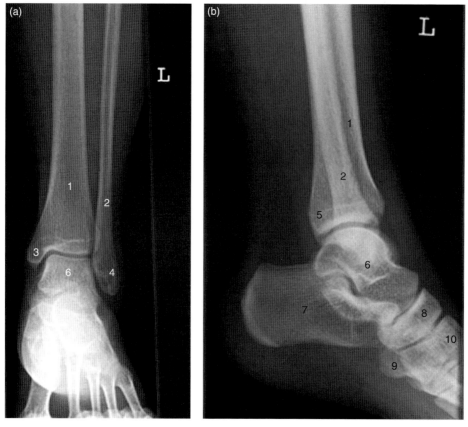

Fig. 3.73. Ankle – (a) anteroposterior, (b) lateral
 1. Tibia
 2. Fibula
 3. Medial malleolus
 4. Lateral malleolus
 5. Posterior malleolus
 6. Talus
 7. Calcaneus
 8. Navicular
 9. Cuboid
10. Medial cuneiform

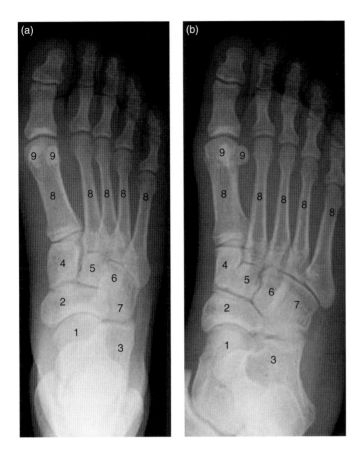

Fig. 3.74. Right foot – (a) posteroanterior, (b) oblique

1. Talus
2. Navicular
3. Calcaneus
4. Medial cuneiform
5. Intermediate cuneiform
6. Lateral cuneiform
7. Cuboid
8. 1st to 5th metatarsals
9. Sesamoid bones

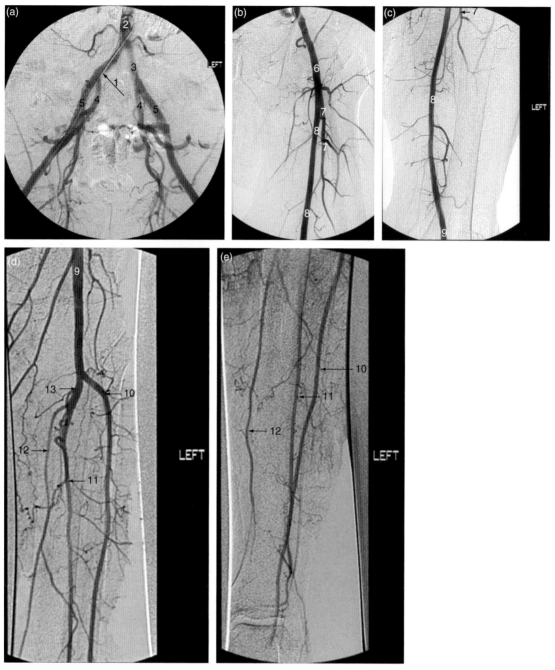

Fig. 3.75. (a)–(e) Aortogram and left femoral angiogram

1. Angiogram catheter (inserted via right femoral artery)
2. Aorta
3. Common iliac artery
4. Internal iliac artery
5. External iliac artery
6. Common femoral artery
7. Profunda femoris artery
8. Superficial femoral artery
9. Popliteal artery
10. Anterior tibial artery
11. Peroneal artery
12. Posterior tibial artery
13. Tibioperoneal trunk

Approach to systems imaging

Contents

Chest X-ray

The plain chest X-ray (CXR) is the most widely ordered radiological test and yet one of the most complex to interpret. Approach to interpretation of a CXR should be systematic and aim to inspect all areas. One approach, sometimes called the "outside-to-in" approach, is outlined below.

Terminology

Although there are general descriptive terms that can be used throughout radiology, each modality also has its own special set of terms. For plain radiography, these include the following:

- "Opacity" or "density" for any object that appears whiter than surrounding tissues
- "Lucency" for anything that appears darker

"Outside-to-in" approach

- This approach is for the PA or anteroposterior (AP) views (collectively referred to as "frontal" CXRs) using the lateral CXR as an adjunct when an abnormality needs better localization
- The periphery of the film or image is looked at first, before the more central areas

- The advantage of this approach is that areas that are often given little attention are examined first and not forgotten in the routine

Image label

- Always begin by checking the film or image label
- The label usually has the date of the examination, the patient's age and sex, as well as their name
- This will ensure that you look at the correct patient and the correct examination for that patient and avoid simple but potentially damaging mistakes

Effect of projection and degree of inspiration

- Establish whether the examination has been performed PA (posteroanterior) or AP (anteroposterior).
- A posteroanterior image is taken with the patient facing the X-ray image and the X-ray source behind him/her (the X-ray beam therefore travelling posterior-to-anterior through the patient). PA films are taken erect in the radiology department.
- An anteroposterior image is the reverse, with the patient facing the X-ray source and his/her back against the film/image detector. This is important because an AP image magnifies the cardiac outline and may give the incorrect impression of cardiomegaly (Fig. 4.1).
- AP image labels are usually labelled "AP" (to distinguish them from a PA image) and may be "erect" or "supine", or "portable" (same as "mobile").
- Supine films tend to make the heart look larger, the superior mediastinum wider, and the lung vasculature appears more prominent and lung volumes are often smaller (Fig. 4.2).
- Assess whether the film has been taken with good inspiration (the normal standard). A poor degree of inspiration is common in very ill patients. This makes the heart appear larger and

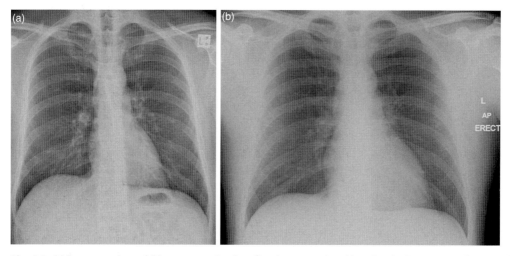

Fig. 4.1. (a) Posteroanterior and (b) anteroposterior chest films in same patient. Note that the heart appears larger on the anteroposterior (AP) projection.

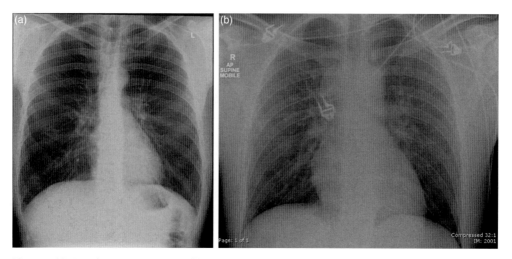

Fig. 4.2. (a) Normal posteroanterior view. (b) Anteroposterior supine view in the same patient. The heart appears larger, the superior mediastinum larger, and the pulmonary vessels appear congested. All of these effects are normal. Monitoring leads are in place.

the lungs appear congested (Fig. 4.3). Expiratory films are taken deliberately to look for pneumothoraces.

Bones and soft tissues
- Bony structures – include clavicles, shoulder joints, ribs, lower cervical spine, and thoracic spine.
- Soft tissue structures – breast shadows, diaphragm, subdiaphragmatic areas, axillae and soft tissues of the neck.

Lung volumes
- Common disease processes may alter lung volumes dramatically, especially in their late stages. Remember that ill patients may not be able to co-operate enough to take a good inspiration.

- Pulmonary fibrosis leads to low volume lungs because of diffuse scarring; emphysema leads to markedly hyperinflated lungs due to gas trapping and bullus formation (Fig. 4.4).
- Count the number of anterior ribs displayed. As a rough rule the anterior aspect of the seventh rib should intersect with the dome of the right hemidiaphragm.

Locating abnormal findings
- When describing the position of an abnormal finding on a single view, e.g. on a posteroanterior (PA) CXR, it is best to use the phrase "projected over"; for example, "a rounded opacity is projected over the right lower zone."

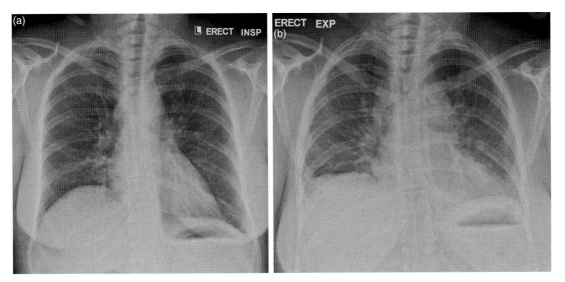

Fig. 4.3. Chest films taken in (a) inspiration and (b) expiration. Note that, in the expiratory film, the heart appears larger and the lungs appear congested.

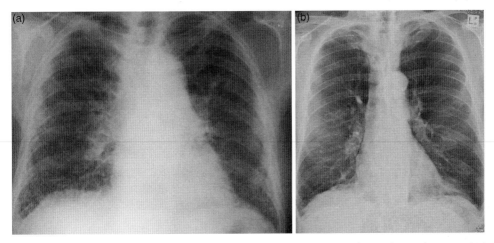

Fig. 4.4. Assessment of lung volumes. (a) Pulmonary fibrosis – low lung volumes from widespread scarring which decreases the volume of lung tissue. (b) Emphysema – much of the normal functioning lung tissue is destroyed and replaced by larger airspaces, which trap air and cause over-expansion of the lungs.

- If a second view such as a lateral film is available, this allows more accurate description of the anatomical location, e.g. "A rounded opacity is projected over the right lower zone; the lateral film shows it to lie anteriorly and thus it is most likely in the right middle lobe."
- The lungs may be divided into upper, middle and lower zones for description, since on a frontal CXR there are many areas of overlap between lobes, so without a lateral view more precise anatomical location of pathology is often impossible.

- An opacity projected over the lungs may lie anywhere along the line of the X-ray beam. This includes outside the patient (e.g. in a pocket!), chest wall (including skin and breast tissue), pleura, and lung.
- An important clue to location is the loss of a normal border, i.e. loss of its silhouette. For example, if the opacity causes loss of the normal outline of the right side of the heart, then it usually lies in the right middle lobe. Similarly, opacity may be projected over a normal structure such as the hilum, but if the normal outlines of that

structure are maintained, the opacity must lie in front of, or behind it.

- An easier way to localize the opacity further is to view a lateral film (Fig. 4.5).

Types of lung opacity

Pulmonary opacities may be divided into three main groups:

Airspace opacity (Fig. 4.6)

- Also referred to as alveolar opacity
- Most often caused by infection, pulmonary edema or hemorrhage
- May be bounded by a pleural surface (Fig. 4.6(a))
- Ill-defined opacity often with air bronchograms (Fig. 4.6(b))

Interstitial opacities

- Irregular lines and nodules
- Causes include interstitial pulmonary edema, atypical infections, pulmonary fibrosis (Fig. 4.7)

Nodules/masses

- round, usually well defined
- granulomatous infections such as TB
- primary or secondary malignancy (Fig. 4.8)

Pulmonary vessels

- The pattern of vascular markings should be uniform in distribution, with regular tapering of vessels toward the periphery. Disorganization of markings may indicate pulmonary pathology, for example, bullous emphysema.
- Pulmonary veins draining the upper lobes become enlarged in the first stages of left ventricular failure and fluid overload.

Pleura and pleural space

- The pleural membranes lie outside the lungs and are mostly invisible. The fissures however may be seen (major fissures on lateral films, minor fissure on frontal and lateral). Air in the pleural space (pneumothorax) is seen as a lucent, usually crescentic area outside the lungs and devoid of any pulmonary markings.
- Fluid in the pleural space may collect between the visceral and parietal layers around the periphery of the thoracic cavity, or between the visceral layers in the fissures.
- In obese patients, extrapleural fat may be seen displacing the parietal pleura centrally and may mimic pleural fluid or pleural tumor

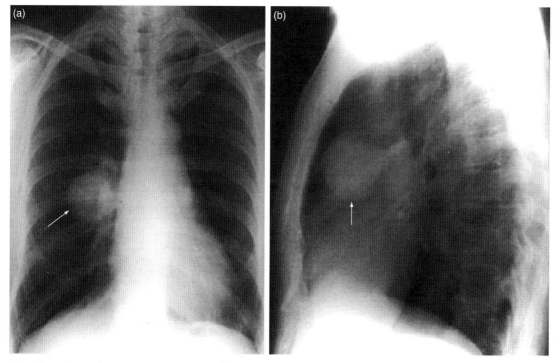

Fig. 4.5. On the PA film (a) a rounded opacity (arrow) is projected over the right hilum. The outlines of the hilar structures can be clearly seen "through it" meaning the opacity must be either in front of or behind the hilum. (b) On the lateral view it lies anteriorly (arrow), probably in the anterior segment of the right upper lobe.

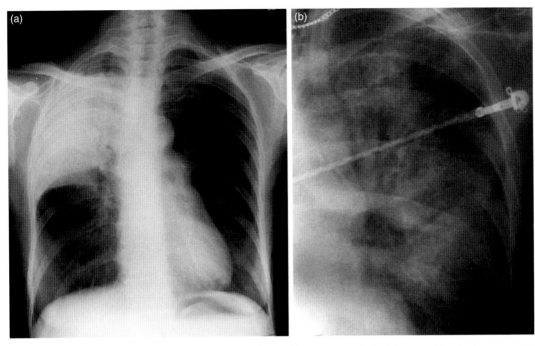

Fig. 4.6. Two examples of airspace opacity both due to infection. (a) airspace opacity in right upper lobe due to pneumonia. (b) airspace opacity in left lung due to pneumonia demonstrating air bronchograms.

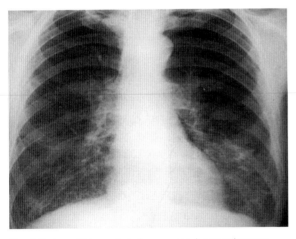

Fig. 4.7. Interstitial opacity in lower zones due to pulmonary fibrosis.

Heart size and position

- Although variable, about one-third of the cardiac outline should lie to the right of the midline and two-thirds to the left.
- The greatest transverse diameter of the heart is compared to the greatest transverse dimension of the bony thorax above the diaphragm (measure from the inner cortex of the ribs).
- If this ratio ("cardiothoracic ratio") is less than 50%, the heart size is likely to be normal (Fig. 4.9).

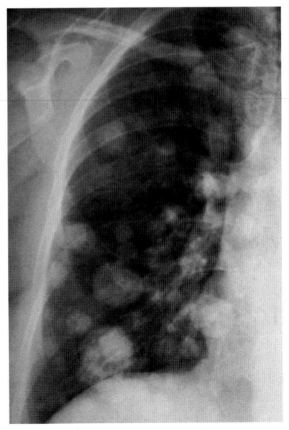

Fig. 4.8. Multiple lung nodules due to metastases.

67

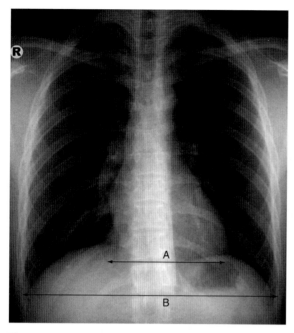

Fig. 4.9. Cardiothoracic ratio is measured as A/B. "A" is the transverse distance between the right and left limits of the cardiac outline. "B" is the maximum transverse distance between the inner margins of the ribs above the costophrenic angles.

Hila

The hila should be the same size and the left should be slightly higher than the right. They should also be of the same density; an abnormally dense hilum may harbor an enlarged lymph node or small lung cancer. Remember that both hila may enlarge symmetrically.

Mediastinal contours

A useful way to remember the structures making up the cardiomediastinal contour is to think of the right side as the "venous" side and the left as "arterial."

Tracing these structures from the upper right side of the mediastinum in an anticlockwise direction:

- The right-sided contour is made up of the right brachiocephalic vein, the superior vena cava, and the right atrium
- The inferior border of the cardiac shadow, going right to left, is made up of the right and left ventricles, and
- Going superiorly from the cardiac apex, the left side is made up of left ventricle, left atrium, pulmonary artery, aortopulmonary window, aorta and left subclavian artery.

Although these structures do not need to be traced out every time you look at a CXR, it is useful to know them to better localize pathological processes.

An abnormal bulge in these contours may indicate a mediastinal mass. In addition, as all these structures normally have air-containing lung next to them, their borders should be sharp. Loss of a normal sharp border indicates abnormality in the adjacent lung or pleural space.

Check areas and traps

At the end of the examination, there are several areas that should be specifically checked as they can hide pathology.

- Lung apices
- Costophrenic recesses
- Retrocardiac area
- Pulmonary hila

Remember normal anatomy and artifacts that may simulate disease. Some common ones are nipple opacities mimicking a pulmonary nodule or skin folds mimicking a pneumothorax.

Additional radiographic views

There are several variations from the standard PA and lateral CXR projections, which can be very helpful in demonstrating pathology in certain situations.

If a pneumothorax is suspected clinically, an expiratory PA film may assist in showing the pneumothorax and indeed may be the only image on which it is evident.

If a pleural effusion is suspected but not conclusively shown (for example, if it is hidden by other pathology such as lower lobe pneumonia), a decubitus image may be of use. In a decubitus image, the patient lies on the side of interest; fluid in the ipsilateral pleural cavity should flow to the most dependent portion of the image, in this case the lateral pleural space, where it should be clearly visible, and separate from other pathology.

An apical lordotic view is useful to display opacities projected in the lung apices, where overlying bony structures obscure detail and where lateral images are of no use. This view is taken by angling the X-ray beam upwards which throws anterior bony markings off the lung apices.

Approach to chest CT

As with all imaging, check the name, age and date on the images. This information is usually in the top left or right corner of each image.

How do you know if intravenous contrast has been given and what phase of the scan you are looking at?

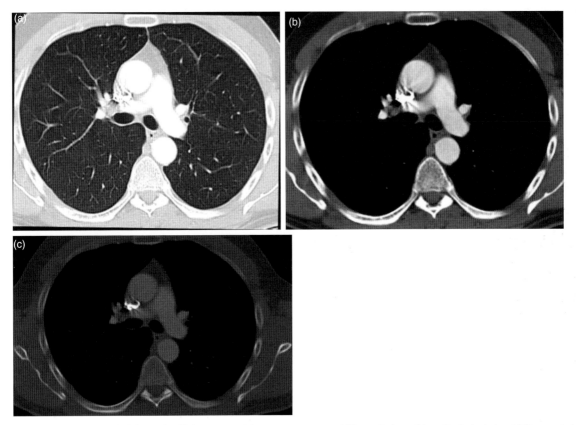

Fig. 4.10. CT at the level of the tracheal bifurcation, with intravenous contrast: (a) lung windows, (b) mediastinal windows, (c) bone windows.

- Sometimes a non-contrast scan only is performed, for example, for high resolution chest CT (HRCT), or if there is contraindication to contrast such as renal failure or previous allergic reaction.
- Contrast-enhanced scan timing can vary according to the clinical question
  - Early scanning will show mainly central veins draining into right side of heart, and pulmonary arteries (e.g. for evaluation of pulmonary embolism)
  - Scanning slightly later will show the aorta and its main branches well.

  Depending on timing therefore some or all of these vessels with appear dense (enhanced).

  What plane are the images in, and how are they displayed?
- Most CT chest is transverse although various planes can be reconstructed, most commonly coronal, as well as special reformats for CT angiography
- Scans vary in thickness mostly from 1 mm to 8 or 10 mm

- High resolution chest CT (HRCT) typically scans with very thin intervals at 8–10 mm intervals, and may be done in both inspiration and expiration, and sometimes with additional prone scans.
- Transverse scans are displayed (as with all transverse CT and MRI) with the right of patient on the left as you view it (the "foot of the bed view")
- If multiple sections are on the screen or film you are looking at, the display is usually with the more superior sections starting top left and proceeding inferiorly like the words on a page, left to right and top to bottom
- As with all CT the "window" and "level" of photography/display can be manipulated to display certain anatomy and pathology to advantage. This explains some of the wide differences you will notice between images of the same anatomical region.
- The common windows used in the chest are (Fig. 4.10)
  - Lung windows
  - Soft tissue or mediastinal windows
  - Bone windows, particularly in trauma.

Terminology

Use the correct terminology when describing the images. When describing CT abnormalities, use terms like high density (hyperdense or high attenuation) when referring to something that is "white." For lesions that are "more black," use terms like low density (hypodense or low attenuation).

Lung fields
- When viewing the lung fields, use the lung windows
- Increased opacity
  - May be the result of airspace disease (consolidation), collapse, lung mass, interstitial disease, pleural disease (pleural effusion, pleural thickening)
- Decreased opacity
  - May be the result of destruction of lung parenchyma (emphysema, bullae, cysts), decreased blood flow (pulmonary embolus), pleural disease (pneumothorax)
- Structural abnormality
  - For example, dilated thick-walled bronchi in bronchiectasis

Mediastinum
- When viewing the mediastinum, use the mediastinal windows
- Increased opacity
  - May be the result of enlarged lymph nodes (greater than 1 cm short axis), mediastinal neoplasm, hematoma, retrosternal goiter
- Decreased opacity
  - e.g. pneumomediastinum
- Structural abnormality
  - e.g. mediastinal shift, cardiac enlargement, aortic dissection or aneurysm

Bones
- When viewing the bones, use bone windows.
  - Check ribs, shoulder girdles, spine (e.g. lytic or sclerotic metastatic lesions, fractures).

Gastrointestinal imaging – approach to the abdominal X-ray
Radiographic technique
- No special patient preparation is required for plain film imaging. The best quality plain films are obtained in the radiology department as opposed to "portable" or "mobile" films.

- Plain films of the abdomen can be obtained in a variety of positions:
  - Supine anteroposterior (less often prone posteroanterior)
  - Erect – useful for detecting air–fluid levels in the bowel and free intraperitoneal gas (although an erect CXR is more sensitive for the latter)
  - Decubitus: the patient lies on their side with a horizontal X-ray beam. Used to look for free intraperitoneal gas when the patient is too unwell for an erect film
  - Oblique – e.g. to help determine position of opacities such as suspected urinary tract calculi

Indications
- Plain films are most often requested for the evaluation of acute abdominal pain including suspected acute bowel obstruction.
- Plain films of the urinary tract are often referred to as KUB films (kidney, ureters, bladder) and may include oblique films.

Viewing the plain abdominal film
Take note of the patient's name, age, the date and projection of the film.

It is important to have a systematic approach to viewing the abdominal film so that all areas are covered and no abnormalities are missed.

Solid "organs"
- Liver and spleen.
- Kidneys – size should not be larger than the height of three vertebral bodies plus two intervertebral disks. Kidney outline is aided by normal perinephric fat plane.
- Psoas muscles – outlines should be visible due to adjacent fat plane

Hollow organs
Assess overall amount of gas
- Gas is normally seen in the stomach, duodenum and large bowel. Small amounts of gas and some air–fluid levels in the small bowel are generally not significant if the small bowel diameter is less than 3 cm. Up to two to three air–fluid levels of 2–3 cm length can be quite normal. Beware of a paucity of bowel gas (the gasless abdomen) which may indicate, for example, a proximal bowel obstruction. (see also "Bowel obstruction" in Chapter 8)

Assess distribution of gas

- Small bowel loops are centrally placed and have visible plicae (circumferential folds which extend across the width of the bowel). Large bowel loops are peripherally placed except for transverse and sigmoid colon which can be more central. Colon has visible haustra (incomplete folds which do not extend across the width of the bowel).
- Displacement of bowel gas by a soft tissue mass or enlarged solid organ (e.g. liver, spleen) can guide further imaging.

Assess distension of bowel loops

- Fluid, gas and, in the large bowel, feces accumulate proximal to the site of an obstruction, resulting in bowel loop distension. This can be assessed if there is enough air in the bowel to outline luminal width. The upper limits of normal for small bowel are 3 cm for jejunum, and 2 cm for ileum.
- With large bowel obstruction or toxic megacolon (a complication of inflammatory bowel disease), there may be extreme dilatation of the colon
- Traditionally, a 9–10 cm diameter caecum is regarded as at high risk of perforation.
- When bowel is distended with fluid but very little air is present, a clue to the obstruction may be the appearance of tiny pockets of air arranged in rows, separated by mucosal folds.

Assess bowel wall

- When the bowel loop is gas filled, gas serves to act as a natural contrast agent allowing important information to be obtained about the bowel wall. Look at the wall thickness (should be only 2–3 mm) and look for regularity of mucosal folds. Mucosal edema may be seen in various conditions including bowel ischemia (classically "thumb printing" pattern) and inflammatory bowel disease.

Assess for bowel obstruction and its possible causes

- Plain films usually can establish the presence and level of an obstruction. Bowel loops proximal to obstruction become distended and distal loops become gasless (after some hours). Air–fluid levels within distended loops are seen on the erect film.
- Plain films are usually limited in providing evidence of the cause of obstruction but in specific cases can provide the answer, such as with
  - Sigmoid or cecal volvulus.
  - Gallstone ileus – sometimes the calcified stone can be detected in the lower abdomen but more often the clue lies with the presence of

gas in the biliary tree (biliary tree gas also seen following sphincterotomy, biliary stenting or biliary–enteric surgical bypass).
  - Gas in a loop of bowel overlying the inguinal/femoral region, which may be a clue to an obstructing hernia.
- Differentiating a paralytic or functional ileus (focal or diffuse distension without obstruction) from mechanical obstruction can be difficult radiologically and clinical history and examination generally is more helpful.

Extraluminal gas

- Free intraperitoneal gas can best be detected on an erect chest film, collecting beneath the diaphragm. If the patient is unable to sit up, the decubitus film (usually left side down) is satisfactory. The supine film can also demonstrate evidence of free gas by showing the smooth external aspect of bowel wall.

Calcifications

- Liver, spleen – hydatid, small granulomas
- Kidney – calculi (80% radio-opaque), nephrocalcinosis, TB
- Ureter – calculi
- Gallbladder – calculi (5%–10% radio-opaque), limey bile, porcelain GB
- Pancreas – chronic pancreatitis
- Vascular
  - Atheroma (aorta, iliac arteries, including aneurysms)
  - Phleboliths (calcifications in veins, usually in the pelvis), which often have a central lucency unlike ureteric calculi
- Female pelvis – ovarian dermoid/teratoma
- Adrenal – old hemorrhage, TB
- Other – e.g. lymph nodes (past TB), old injection sites in buttocks

Bones

- Survey all bones – ribs, vertebrae, pelvis

Gastrointestinal imaging – contrast studies of the gastrointestinal tract

Barium or Gastrograffin – which contrast agent to request?

- Barium sulphate (a liquid emulsion) is a generally safe contrast material and is not absorbed into the body. However, if it should leak into the peritoneal cavity, it can cause peritonitis and create severe adhesions. If there is any suspicion of a gastrointestinal perforation, then barium should not be used and the study should be performed with a water-soluble contrast material (e.g. Gastrograffin).

- Water-soluble contrast agents, however, do not coat the mucosa, and so do not provide adequate detail to exclude ulcers, small masses, or other mucosal abnormalities. These agents are very useful to evaluate mucosal leaks and may be helpful in assessing suspected small bowel obstruction. In addition, agents like Gastrograffin are severe pulmonary irritants and should not be given to patients likely to aspirate or in whom a tracheo-esophageal fistula is likely.

Barium swallow

- The barium swallow study is a simple and non-invasive study of the esophagus. It includes fluoroscopic evaluation of both the structure and function of the esophagus and hypopharynx.
- The single contrast method involves the patient drinking barium and is adequate for assessing intraluminal masses, motility disorders, spasm, and diverticula but does not give good mucosal detail.
- The double contrast method involves swallowing a gas-producing solution immediately followed by high-density barium. This provides more detailed visualization of the mucosa.
- Multiple images are obtained to document the study, including all phases of swallowing. The presence of gastro-esophageal reflux is assessed.
- Videofluoroscopy, in which the barium swallow is recorded and reviewed in real time, is extremely valuable for assessing motility disorders. Barium-soaked bread, or similar semi-solid material, is also used to better assess motility or the functional significance of a minor stricture.
- In some patients, videofluoroscopy involves a speech pathologist who is experienced in evaluating the initiation of swallowing, and assessing tongue, pharyngeal and laryngeal function, using liquid and semi-solid material opacified with barium. This examination is extremely useful in patients with, for example, strokes or bulbar disorders.

Barium meal

- The barium meal is an examination of the esophagus, stomach, and duodenum.

- Oral barium is administered with fluoroscopic monitoring. Double-contrast images are obtained when the mucosa is coated with barium and the stomach distended with gas (using ingestion of a gas producing agent).
- Most of the examination is dedicated to studying the stomach and duodenum but, if clinically indicated, detailed evaluation of the esophagus is performed as well. The patient is studied in erect, supine, prone, and oblique positions. The examination is usually performed on a tilting table.
- Buscopan is sometimes used to paralyze the upper gastrointestinal tract for a short period so that peristaltic motion does not interfere with obtaining detailed images.

Barium small bowel study

- This study is often referred to as a "barium small bowel follow-through" (SBFT). It is performed by having the patient drink a large amount of barium, then following its passage through the small bowel to the cecum, taking multiple abdominal radiographs. Fluoroscopy of any abnormal areas and usually the terminal ileum is performed with additional films of these areas.
- A barium SBFT, in the hands of an experienced examiner, is capable of detecting many diseases of the small bowel but, if further detail is required, enteroclysis (small bowel enema) may be performed.
- The small bowel enteroclysis involves introducing barium directly into the duodenum through a nasoduodenal tube. The small bowel is then distended with water (or water combined with other agents) creating a double contrast study. This provides more mucosal detail than the oral method, but is much more uncomfortable for the patient, and often does not improve diagnostic yield.
- Small bowel enteroclysis is now being combined with CT or MRI.

Barium enema

- The double-contrast barium enema is performed by inserting a self-retaining balloon catheter into the rectum and instilling high-density barium into the rectum and colon to coat the mucosa.
- The excess barium is then removed and air is inserted to distend the colon, creating the double contrast study. The examination is monitored using fluoroscopy and multiple images are obtained in a variety of projections to record the examination.

- The procedure can be performed without using air (single contrast enema). This is relatively easy and requires less patient co-operation. It is generally indicated where detailed mucosal evaluation is not necessary, for example, in the investigation of suspected colon obstruction, volvulus, intussusception, and diverticular disease.
- The barium enema may be a strenuous examination (especially for an elderly patient) requiring a fair degree of patient co-operation and mobility.
- Patient preparation is important in order to achieve a relatively clean colon using a low residue, high fluid intake diet and a cathartic agent.

Gastrointestinal imaging – approach to CT studies of abdomen and pelvis

The following is a guide to assist with reviewing CT scans of the abdomen and pelvis.

What contrast has been given?
- Oral contrast
  Oral contrast is routine for most scans. A dilute water-soluble contrast is given within one hour prior to the scan. Stomach, small bowel and the large bowel will be high density if enough time has elapsed between administration of contrast and scanning (provided there is no bowel obstruction).
- Rectal contrast
  Rectal contrast is given selectively for scanning of the pelvis.
- Intravenous contrast
  - Intravenous contrast is used in most cases.
  - It is administered via an arm vein usually, and delivered by a mechanical injector with scanning commencing during or immediately after the injection.
  - The contrast is the same as used for IVPs and angiograms and is excreted promptly by the kidneys.

How to recognize that intravenous contrast has been given and what phase of the scan you are looking at?
- Sometimes a non-contrast scan only is performed, for example, for suspected renal colic, or if a contraindication to contrast exists (e.g. renal failure, previous allergic reaction).
- Sometimes a non-contrast scan is performed prior to the contrast-enhanced scan.

- Non-contrast scans can be recognized by:
  - Lack of high density in the aorta, other blood vessels, or kidney parenchyma
  - Label on images such as "Non-contrast," "No C," "C–"
- Contrast-enhanced scans can be recognized by:
  - Enhancement of various structures depending on the "phase" of scanning
  - Label on images such as "Contrast," "C," "C+"

Phases of scanning (Figs. 4.11, 4.12)
Most CT scanners now are "helical" or "spiral" and multi-slice. The result is that scanning time is very rapid and it is possible to scan the abdomen (e.g. liver) several times in a few minutes. This results in sequential enhancement of;
- Arteries
- Capillary beds – including renal cortex
- Veins – including portal vein
- Renal collecting system – pelvicalyceal system, ureter, and eventually bladder
- Hence the phases are often referred to (and labelled on scans) as:
  - Arterial phase
  - Portal or venous phase
  - Delayed phase
- Arterial phase scans are especially useful for:
  - Evaluation of aorta and its branches
  - Detection of tumor vascularity such as hepatocellular carcinoma

Oral contrast
- For most scans of the abdomen and pelvis oral contrast is given to opacify the small and large bowel so that it can be readily identified. This is particularly helpful for the small bowel (Fig. 4.13).

What plane are images in, and how are they displayed?
- CT of the abdomen and pelvis is acquired and displayed in transverse planes (Fig. 4.13), although various planes can be reconstructed, most commonly coronal, as well as special reformats for such things as CT angiography.
- Scans vary in thickness mostly from 2 mm to 8–10 mm.
- Transverse scans are displayed (as with all transverse CT and MRI) with the right of patient on the left as you view it (the "foot of bed" view).

73

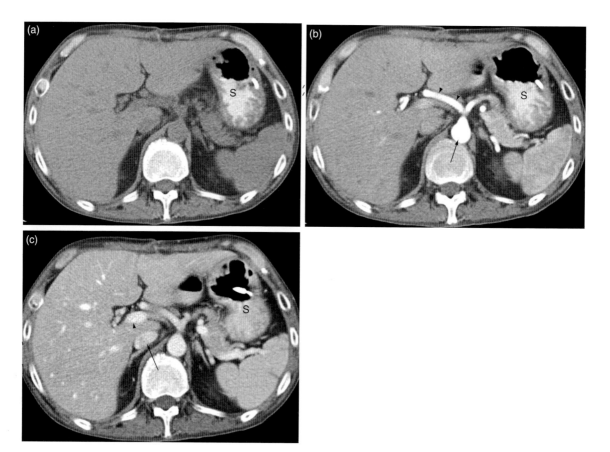

Fig. 4.11. Transverse CT section through upper abdomen. (a) Plain scan. Oral contrast has been given making the stomach (S) lumen dense (a nasogastric tube lies in the stomach). (b) The same level approximately 30 seconds after contrast has been given via an arm vein (arterial phase). The contrast has reached the arteries. Note the aorta (arrow) and hepatic artery (arrowheads). (c) The same level approximately 30 seconds later (portal phase). The contrast has reached the portal veins (arrowheads) and the inferior vena cava (arrow).

- If multiple sections are on the screen or film, the display is usually with the more superior sections starting top left and proceeding inferiorly like the words on a page, left to right and top to bottom).
- As with all CT the "window" and "level" of photography/display can be manipulated to display certain anatomy and pathology to advantage. This explains some of the wide differences you will notice between images of the same anatomical region.

Check list of structures to look at
- Kidneys (a good place to start as it gives you information about contrast usage and phase of scanning)
- Liver
- Spleen
- Pancreas
- Adrenal glands

- Aorta
- Para-aortic and iliac node regions
- Bowel – this is often neglected
- Peritoneal fluid – ascites, blood (high density, check pelvis as this is where small amounts often collect)
- Peritoneal gas – pneumoperitoneum
- Bones – usually the bones are not very well seen unless the images have been manipulated especially to show them

Cholangiography and pancreatography
Endoscopic retrograde cholangiopancreatography (ERCP)
ERCP is used to image the biliary and pancreatic ducts and is performed by a trained endoscopist. A fiberoptic endoscope is passed from the patient's

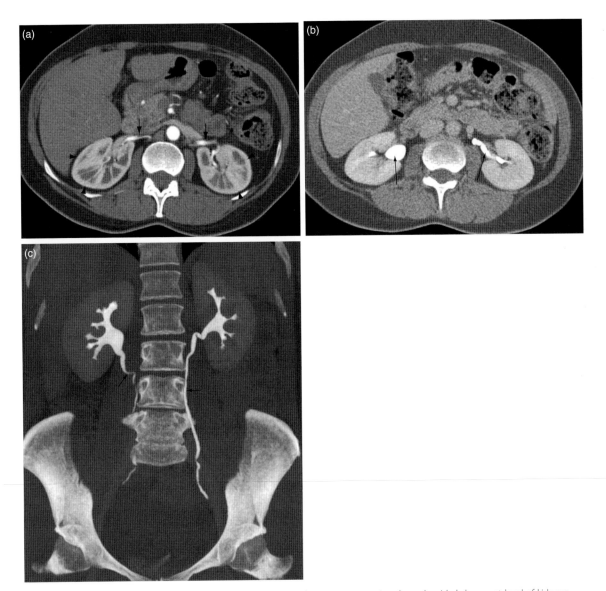

Fig. 4.12. CT showing different phases of urinary tract contrast enhancement – section through mid abdomen at level of kidneys. (a) Transverse section at arterial phase. Contrast enhances the aorta, the renal arteries (arrows) and the renal cortex (arrowheads), but has not yet reached the renal medulla. (b) Transverse section at pyelogram phase – obtained after approximately 5 minutes. Contrast has been excreted into the pelvicalyceal systems (arrows). (c) Coronal reformat performed to demonstrate the pelvicalyceal systems and ureters (arrows).

mouth into the duodenum, under sedation. The ampulla of Vater is visualized and a fine catheter is passed through it into the common bile duct or pancreatic duct. Contrast media is then injected under fluoroscopic control and images of the biliary and pancreatic ducts are obtained.

Indications
ERCP has been used most often for evaluating suspected bile duct obstruction prior to surgical or endoscopic intervention. However, with improvements in ultrasound, CT and especially with the advent of MRCP, it is used much less often as a purely diagnostic tool and more as part of intervention to remove bile duct stones or stent malignant obstructions.

ERCP is useful for investigating pathology involving the pancreatic ducts but this role has also diminished with increased utilization of other modalities in particular multislice CT, MRCP and endoscopic ultrasound (EUS).

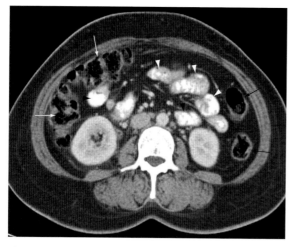

Fig. 4.13. Transverse CT section through mid abdomen. i.v. and oral contrast has been given and the oral contrast opacifies small bowel loops (arrowheads) but has not yet reached the colon (arrows).

Limitations

- ERCP may be technically unsuccessful – less than 5% in experienced hands.
- Complications – the most common is pancreatitis

Percutaneous transhepatic cholangiography (PTC)

PTC is used to opacify the biliary tree and gain access for transhepatic drainage if required. A fine needle is passed percutaneously into the liver under fluoroscopic guidance, either into the right lobe from the right flank or into the left lobe via the epigastrium. Contrast medium is then injected through the needle to opacify the biliary tree.

Indications

It has been used as a diagnostic tool in the past, but is now almost exclusively used as part of percutaneous transhepatic procedures such as insertion of a transhepatic biliary catheter or stent for malignant obstruction.

Limitations

- Invasive – complications include hemorrhage, bile leak and peritonitis
- Technically difficult in patients with non-dilated bile ducts

Magnetic resonance cholangiopancreatography (MRCP)

Magnetic resonance cholangiopancreatography allows imaging of the biliary system and pancreatic ducts without the use of any contrast agents.

MRCP has replaced the majority of diagnostic ERCP in many centers. It is approaching ERCP for accuracy in determining the site and cause of biliary obstruction and is non-invasive.

It can be used in jaundiced patients.

CT intravenous cholangiography (CT–IVC)

CT intravenous cholangiography (CT–IVC) makes use of intravenous contrast agents (e.g. iotroxate, iodipamide) that are selectively excreted into the bile. About 30 minutes after infusion of the contrast agent, a spiral CT is performed and the bile ducts (and anything that communicates with them) will appear as high density. The scans can be viewed in axial or in reformatted modes. There is a small risk of allergic reactions.

Limitations

- Relies on normal or near normal liver excretory function and therefore is of no value in clinically jaundiced patients, or if bilirubin is above two to three times normal.

Intravenous urography

- Intravenous urography (IVU), also called intravenous pyelography (IVP), is an excellent means of imaging the entire renal tract in patients with normal or only slightly impaired renal function.
- When renal function is severely impaired the renal excretion of contrast is inadequate and other methods of imaging are required.
- The contrast agents also can be nephrotoxic so caution is required in considering its use in patients with renal impairment.

Technique

- Various phases of contrast excretion are filmed following intravenous injection of conventional water-soluble iodine-containing contrast media which undergoes renal excretion.
- Prior to contrast injection plain images of the kidneys, ureters and bladder (KUB), often including plain tomograms of the kidneys are performed, mainly to detect opaque calculi.
- An image is taken immediately after injection to record the nephrogram (when the renal parenchyma is opacified due to contrast in the capillary bed and nephrons). After several minutes images are obtained in the pyelogram phase

(when the pelvicalyceal system is opacified with contrast).

- The mid-abdomen is then usually compressed with a belt device to compress the ureters, to improve retention of contrast in the pelvicalyceal system, and further images are obtained to show the pelvicalyceal systems.
- Compression is released and a film is taken immediately to outline the ureters.
- Views of the bladder and a "post-micturition" film conclude the study. Oblique views and further tomograms may be taken during the study.

Patient preparation

- This need not be rigorous in terms of dietary restriction but most centers recommend a mild laxative the night before examination to clear overlying feces and gas. Patients should empty the bladder immediately prior to contrast injection to ensure optimal opacification of the bladder.
- Enquiries should be made prior to examination about renal function, possible pregnancy, use of metformin in diabetics, and history of allergic reaction to contrast medium.
- Patients with renal impairment should not be examined with IVU to avoid the risk of further renal impairment due to the potential nephrotoxic effect of contrast agents.

Indications

- IVU has been the preferred imaging procedure for confirming ureteric stone disease and assessing patients with persistent renal colic in most centers. More recently, plain spiral CT is replacing IVU for this indication and is more accurate.
- For many other diseases of the kidney IVU has been the preferred initial means of investigation unless renal failure is present. It is being replaced in many centers by the CT equivalent of IVU (CT–IVU), which provides more information but does so at higher cost and more radiation so the IVU still has a role.
- When trauma is associated with hematuria an IVU may be obtained to exclude renal injury. Occasionally, a "one shot" IVU, or single film taken soon after contrast injection, is adequate to investigate massive renal injury (fracture, vascular avulsion). Renal trauma is more accurately evaluated, however, with CT.

Head CT – approach to CT brain

- Determine whether you are looking at brain, bone or subdural hematoma windows, as each is designed to best show that relevant structure.
- Determine if i.v. contrast has been given. There is usually a "C," "C+" or "contrast" in the data information on the images. Compare pre-contrast with post-contrast images. Contrast is very commonly, but not routinely, administered in brain imaging. Indications hinge on the suspicion that an abnormality in the blood–brain barrier will be present, or that a hypervascular lesion will be found.
- Look at the ventricles – are they normal in site, size and configuration?
- After the overall morphology of the brain has been assessed, the density (attenuation) of the brain substance should be analysed. When looking at cerebral and cerebellar density, gray matter appears denser (higher attenuation, "more white") than white matter. Normal deep white matter should be well demarcated from the overlying cortex and the basal ganglia (gray matter). The internal and external capsules (also white matter) should also be recognizable (less dense or hypodense compared with the adjacent basal ganglia gray matter).
- Look for something too white
  - Lesions appearing whiter (more dense or hyperdense) relative to brain include calcified lesions or hemorrhage; compare one side with the other.
- Look for something too black
  - Lesions appearing darker (less dense or hypodense) relative to brain include edema. Edema may be reactive (termed vasogenic edema) as seen in areas surrounding a hemorrhage, or may be caused by cellular swelling as with infarction (termed cytotoxic edema). Other hypodense lesions include fat (found in some tumors) and air (which may be related to trauma).
- Look for enhancement
  - Lesions enhance with i.v. contrast medium due to breakdown of the blood–brain barrier (e.g. infarction, inflammation, tumors, infection, abscesses), or because of an increase in size or number of blood vessels (e.g. aneurysms, vascular malformations).

77

- Look for distortion or displacement of normal structures
  - Lesions may exert mass effect, and distort the normal anatomy. Look particularly at the basal cisterns and the cerebral and cerebellar sulci, which give valuable information about mass effect within the cranial cavity.
- Look at bone windows
  - Look at skull, sinuses, orbits and facial bones.

Head MRI – approach to MRI brain

- Determine if it is a T1- or T2-weighted image. The easiest way to do this is by looking at the CSF. T1-weighted images have black CSF and are best for looking at anatomy. T2-weighted images have white CSF and are best for looking at pathology. Most pathology has edema, and edema shows up as white on a T2-weighted image, making the area of pathology easier to recognize.
- Determine the plane of the images that you are viewing: axial, sagittal, coronal.
- Determine if i.v. gadolinium has been given – there is often "gad" or "C+" displayed in the data information on the image.

- Look at the ventricles. Are they normal in site, size and shape?
- Look for distortion or displacement of a normal structure.
- After the overall morphology of the brain has been assessed, the "signal" of the cerebral and cerebellar substance should be analyzed (use the term "signal" when talking about MR images as opposed to density when talking about CT images, and as opposed to echogenicity when talking about ultrasound images).
- Look for something too white (increased signal, hyperintense) or too black (decreased signal, hypointense), comparing one side with the other.
- Look for gadolinium enhancement – compare the contrast-enhanced T1-weighted sequences with the pre-contrast T1-weighted sequences.
- Finally look at the skull, sinuses, orbits, and other facial structures. Note that no signal normally is detected from bone or from air in the sinuses.
- A range of other sequences, apart from the basic T1- and T2-weighted sequences, are used to provide additional information in particular clinical settings (refer to Chapter 10).

Nuclear medicine

Contents

Low level radiation exposure and health

All radiological imaging investigations with the exception of ultrasound and MRI use ionizing radiation, known to damage cells and be carcinogenic at high doses. There is, therefore, a small potential risk from low-level radiation exposure, so care should be taken to minimize exposure, particularly in children. However, in many patients, particularly the elderly and those with reduced life expectancy, the benefits derived from these investigations outweigh the risk.

Doses
- Nuclear medicine doses involve gamma rays that are emitted from the nucleus of unstable radioisotopes. (X-rays come from outside the nucleus.)
- Low-level radiation exposure is measured in millisieverts (mSv).

- The amount of radiation exposure received from a nuclear medicine investigation varies from 3 to 25 mSv, most being around 6 mSv.
- A chest CT dose, by comparison, is around 8 mSv.
- Natural background radiation exposure is approximately 2–3 mSv per year.

Ill effects
- The ill effects of high radiation doses are well documented, e.g. increased cancer rates and death occur in populations exposed to nuclear explosions.
- Exposure of at least 500 mSv is required for any immediate effects or a transient reduction in fertility.
- 200 mSv is required for an increased risk of leukemia.

Risks from low dose
- For low doses of radiation, around 6 mSv, the risks are not completely known and have to be estimated using theoretical models based on high dose data.
- The acknowledged model takes a conservative approach, and suggests that the risk of developing a fatal cancer over a lifetime, after exposure to 1 mSv, is about 1 in 20000.
- There is a delay of at least 10 years between exposure to radiation and increased cancer incidence.
- Compared to other risks in everyday life, this risk is considered minor. The risk of dying from a radiation dose of 1 mSv equals the risk of dying from smoking 80 cigarettes, or travelling 4000 km by car, or travelling 40000 km by commercial aircraft, or rock climbing for 2 hours.

Cancer risk
- Although there is theoretical risk, cancer as a direct result of low-level radiation exposure has not been shown.

79

- Large studies have found no relationship between cancer incidence and varying background radiation levels. An inverse relationship between domestic levels of radon (a naturally occurring alpha emitter) and cancer incidence was found in the USA, and a study of 100 000 female USA radiographers found a lower incidence of breast cancer than in the general population.
- Higher radiation exposure is received from therapy with radioisotopes. Even here, no significant increase in cancer incidence has been shown after treatment for hyperthyroidism with the beta emitter [131]iodine compared to surgically treated patients with follow-up over several decades. The whole body radiation dose received with this treatment is typically 100 mSv.

Minimizing staff exposure

- Simple measures are recommended to minimize exposure to staff caring for patients who have received a diagnostic radiopharmaceutical.
- Minimize time spent close to the patient where practical on the day of the study. An inverse square rule applies in this situation, so that doubling the distance from the patient reduces radiation exposure fourfold.
- If the patient has a bladder catheter in place, the bag should be emptied frequently in the usual way wearing disposable gloves.
- The radiation dose received by staff is very small. For example, after 3 hours spent 1 meter from a patient who has just had a bone scan, the exposure is 0.02 mSv (i.e. 4 days of background exposure).

Nuclear medicine imaging hardware

Gamma cameras and single photon emission computed tomography (SPECT)

The main elements of a gamma camera (Fig. 5.1) are the collimator, the detector crystal, a bank of photomultiplier tubes (PMTs) and the processing electronics.

Following injection of a radiopharmaceutical, gamma ray photons are emitted from the organ of interest in all directions. Only photons travelling parallel to the collimator channels can reach the sodium iodide detector crystal. This reacts by producing photoelectrons, i.e. it scintillates (releases light), which is then amplified by the PMTs, thereby producing an electrical pulse. By combining the

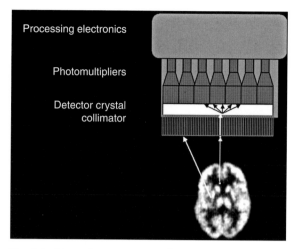

Fig. 5.1. Schematic representation of a gamma camera.

signals from the different PMTs, the position of the scintillation event can be determined.

The collimator is a honeycomb mesh of channels made out of lead or tungsten that only accepts a narrow range of photons. It is the limiting factor in the system efficiency of a gamma camera. The design of a collimator is a compromise between sensitivity and spatial resolution. A typical collimator accepts 0.01% of gamma rays from the object being imaged. Allowing more radiation through the collimator (e.g., with larger holes), increases sensitivity, but degrades spatial resolution.

SPECT uses single photon emitters detected at a range of angles. By imaging over 360°, and using image reconstruction techniques, image "slices" through the patient can be created.

Cyclotrons and isotope production for positron emission tomography (PET)

The stability of nuclei is dictated by the proton/neutron balance. If there is a sufficient excess of protons, then such nuclei are unstable and decay by positron emission in order to reduce the proton excess. The level of instability dictates the decay half-life of the isotope. Low atomic mass nuclei that decay by positron emission are highly unstable and so have relatively short decay half-lives.

Positron-emitting isotopes include: ^{18}F, ^{15}O, ^{13}N, and ^{11}C. These are usually produced in a cyclotron, which operates by circularly accelerating charged particles in a high, static magnetic field, to add protons to a stable isotope. They require extensive shielding against neutron and gamma radiation.

Table 5.1. Common PET isotopes and their clinical uses

Isotope	Half-life (mins)	Common forms	Applications
^{15}O	2	$^{15}O\text{-}H_2O$, $^{15}O\text{-}O_2$	Blood flow, metabolism
^{13}N	10	$^{13}NH_3$	Cardiac viability
^{11}C	20	$^{11}C\text{-}DOPA$	Neuro-receptors
^{18}F	110	$^{18}F\text{-}FDG$, $^{18}F\text{-}FMISO$	Metabolism

Table 5.1 summarizes the common PET isotopes and their clinical uses.

The positron decays by annihilation with an electron and thereby gives rise to two 180° opposing gamma ray photons.

The PET camera consists of a ring of detector crystals coupled to photomultiplier tubes (Fig. 5.2).

PET differs from SPECT in several major regards:

- It requires a cyclotron to produce the isotope.
- The sensitivity of a PET scanner is around 25 times higher than a triple headed SPECT camera.
- PET spatial resolution is depth independent.

Consequently, PET images (Fig. 5.3) are of higher quality than SPECT images. The clinical use of PET is limited by its expense and relatively restricted availability. In contrast, SPECT is widely available and cheaper.

Whilst PET demonstrates exquisite sensitivity in detecting molecular processes, the spatial resolution is limited to approximately 4 mm as compared to CT or MR imaging where sub-millimeter resolution is possible. To overcome this, often the images from PET and CT or MR are "fused" to provide functional anatomical localization. In the latest generation of PET scanners a CT scanner is incorporated, to allow more accurate anatomical localization of the PET imaging data.

Nuclear cardiology
Myocardial perfusion imaging

- Myocardial perfusion imaging (MPI) scans are the second most commonly performed nuclear medicine investigation after bone scans. They are often named according to the radiopharmaceutical used, e.g. stress thallium scan (Fig. 5.4), stress sestamibi scan.
- The technique compares myocardial perfusion during stress (either exercise or pharmacologically induced) when coronary artery blood flow is normally increased, with myocardial perfusion at rest.
- A hemodynamically significant stenosis in a coronary artery (>50%–70%) impairs perfusion to the area of supply, so that less radiopharmaceutical is delivered than to normally perfused areas. This shows as an area of reduced activity.
- At rest, perfusion beyond a stenosis is usually similar to other areas of the heart unless the stenosis is extremely tight. Consequently, a reversible perfusion defect (i.e. present with stress but not at rest) represents coronary ischemia, while a fixed defect (present with stress and at rest) usually means an area of infarction.
- An apparent fixed defect may be artifactual, i.e. if gamma ray photons are absorbed by tissue between the heart and the gamma camera (e.g. breast or diaphragm).

Fig. 5.2. Principle of coincident photon detection used in PET scanner. Photons detected simultaneously by pairs of detectors are recorded and the associated line of origin of the decay is calculated.

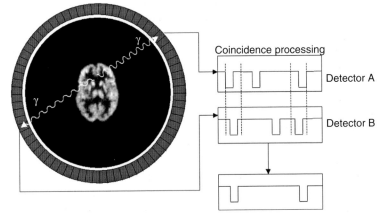

Coincidence processing

Detector A

Detector B

Detector pair AB coincidence output

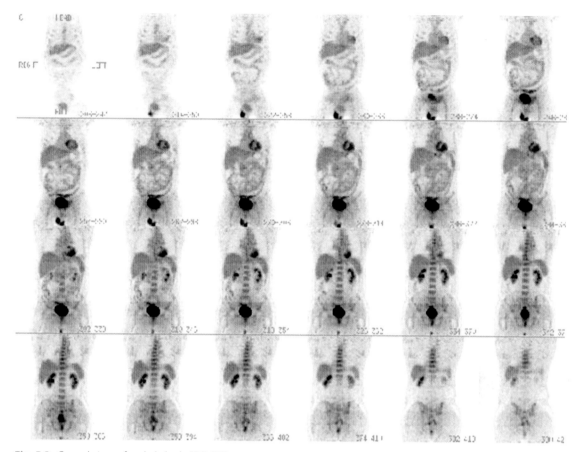

Fig. 5.3. Coronal views of a whole body FDG–PET scan.

- With a technique called "gating," MPI permits measurement of the left ventricular ejection fraction (LVEF) at rest and following stress, and allows regional wall motion to be assessed. Database programs allow comparison of perfusion to the normal range, and automatically quantify any perfusion defect, usually as a percentage of the total left ventricle.

Radiopharmaceuticals for MPI
- Three commonly used agents for MPI are ^{201}thallium, ^{99m}Tc sestamibi (MIBI) and ^{99m}Tc tetrofosmin.
- Thallium behaves as an analog of potassium as it is transported into living cells by the sodium–potassium pump. Imaging is performed very soon after a post-stress injection. Because the agent "redistributes" with time into all areas of viable myocardium, rest images can be obtained after a 4-hour delay.

- ^{99m}Tc (technetium) labeled agents are irreversibly trapped in cells. Therefore, a separate injection of radiopharmaceutical is required at rest. Uptake of the ^{99m}Tc agents at high coronary artery flow rates is less than thallium, but the much shorter radioactive decay half-life of 6 hours for ^{99m}Tc versus 3 days for ^{201}thallium means a much larger dose can be given. This results in better image quality with lower radiation exposure to the patient.

Sensitivity, specificity and predictive value
- Overall sensitivity of MPI for detection of significant coronary artery disease (CAD) is 90% but this increases according to severity of disease, from 85% for single vessel disease, to 95% for three-vessel disease.
- Specificity is 70% with thallium, and more recent studies of gated SPECT and ^{99m}technetium labeled agents report specificity of 90%.

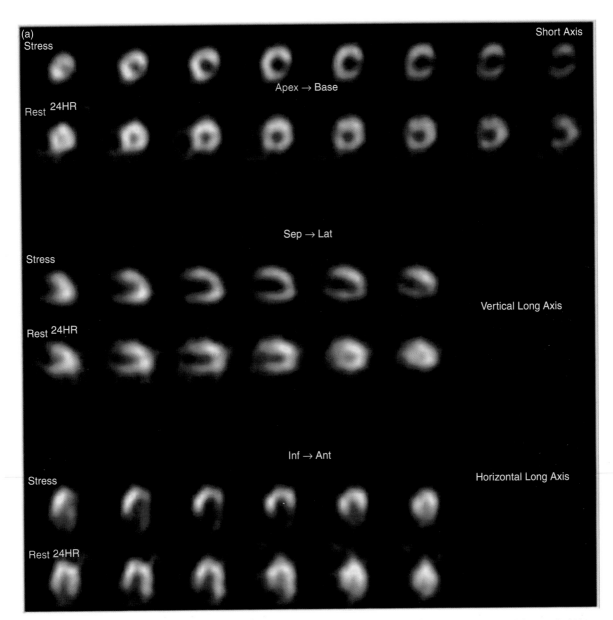

Fig. 5.4. Stress thallium scan. (a) Rows of stress perfusion images are paired with the rest perfusion images. Only the left ventricle (LV) is clearly visible reflecting its thickness and the proportion of coronary blood flow it receives. The top rows are short axis slices, the next two rows are the vertical long axis slices (anterior wall at the top, inferior wall at the bottom). The bottom two rows are horizontal long axis views (septum on the left, lateral wall on the right). The stress images show relatively reduced uptake in the area supplied by the left circumflex artery. (b) The "bull's eye" display shows the entire LV in each circle, apex in the center, base at the outer edge, anterior wall at the top, septum on the left, inferior wall at the bottom and lateral wall on the right. Imagine that you are looking into the LV from the apex and the image you see is squashed flat. There are bull's eyes for the stress images (top row) and rest images (bottom row). Green lines show the usual distribution of the three main coronary arteries. Any areas of statistically reduced activity compared to a database of normal subjects matched by sex and radiopharmaceutical, are displayed as black areas on the third bull's eye. White areas on the bottom right bull's eye represent statistically significant reversible ischemia. The percent of each coronary artery territory and the total LV occupied by a significant perfusion defect is displayed.

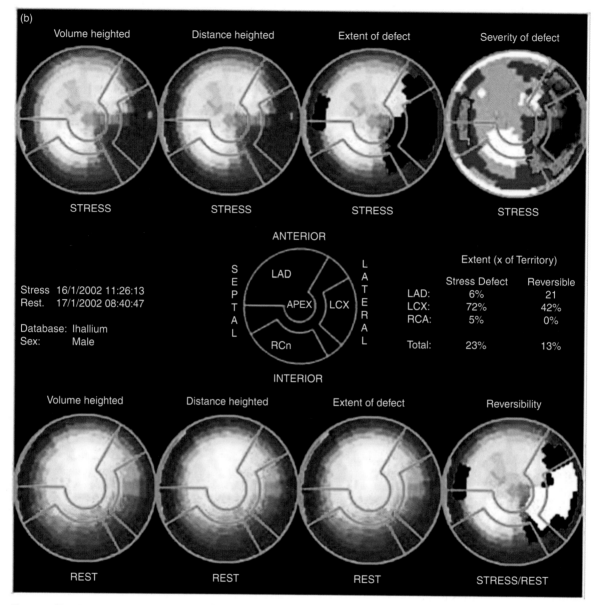

Fig. 5.4. (Cont.)

MPI has an excellent negative predictive value for serious cardiac events such as death or myocardial infarction (MI). In large follow-up studies, the risk of death or MI after a normal stress MPI study is less than 1% per year. If the left ventricular ejection fraction is also normal (LVEF >50%), the serious event risk is 0.5%.

If the scan is mildly abnormal the risk rises to 2%, although the death risk remains less than 1%. If moderately or severely abnormal, the serious event rate is 7%–10% per year.

Potential causes of misleading results

- Reversible perfusion defects may be seen with left bundle branch block (LBBB) or right ventricular pacing, as these cause heart rate dependent septal hypoperfusion. This can be largely avoided by using dipyridamole or adenosine stress as these only minimally elevate heart rate.

- Small vessel disease (commonly present in diabetics), coronary artery spasm, idiopathic cardiomyopathy, and asymmetric septal hypertrophy, may all cause reversible perfusion defects despite normal coronary angiography.

Procedure

Preparation

- The patient should have a light breakfast and wear comfortable clothes and shoes suitable for exercise.
- Caffeine-containing drinks and food must be avoided for 48 hours.
- Stop beta-blockers and calcium antagonists for 48 hours unless contraindicated.
- Stop nitrates on the day of study unless contraindicated.

Exercise

- Exercise is performed on a treadmill or bicycle using standard protocols. Performance is measured by peak heart rate and blood pressure (the rate–pressure product) or by measurement of unit of metabolic equivalent (METs). One MET that is used is the average oxygen consumption at rest.
- When using thallium, the tracer is injected at peak stress and the scan performed almost immediately upon recovery from the exercise. A resting top up dose is then often given after the scan and a rest scan is performed 3–4 hours later. Late images at 24 hours are taken if myocardial viability is an issue.
- When using ^{99m}Tc agents, injection is also given at peak stress, but scanning can be delayed as there is no redistribution of these tracers. A dose is given 3–4 hours later and a scan obtained to image perfusion at rest.

Non-exercise stress

- Pharmacological stress is indicated if the patient cannot exercise, is in left bundle branch block (LBBB), and when elevation of blood pressure and cardiac stress is not desirable, e.g. aortic aneurysm or very recent myocardial infarction. Accuracy is similar to exercise stress MPI but the negative predictive value is less, as patients are less healthy.
- Dipyridamole oradenosine are used to increase coronary blood flow 3–4 fold, similar to exercise, while only slightly elevating heart rate and lowering blood pressure.
- Severe asthma is a contraindication for these agents. In such cases dobutamine is used, but this has less effect on blood flow.

Indications

Diagnosis of coronary artery disease

- Chest pain of uncertain etiology is the most common indication. Unexplained dyspnea on exertion or left ventricular failure are other valid indications. The test is not cost-effective in very low risk individuals. In high-risk patients, coronary angiography is more appropriate. In patients with an intermediate clinical risk of coronary artery disease, stress MPI is often useful.
- An exercise test alone has limitations, including lower sensitivity for CAD (around 70%), reduced specificity in females, poor ability to localize ischemia, and an event rate after a negative test that is relatively high unless the patient is in the low clinical risk category. Exercise testing is particularly unreliable with: LBBB; resting ST abnormality; digoxin effects evident on the resting ECG; and when the patient cannot achieve 85% of maximum predicted heart rate for their age.

Management decisions – medical therapy versus revascularization

- Accurate prognostic information and symptoms are necessary for decision making (medical versus revascularization) in patients with known or suspected coronary artery disease.
- A normal MPI with normal LVEF indicates less than 1% risk of MI or death even with known CAD. The risk of cardiac events is proportional to the extent and severity of perfusion defects. Small defects therefore suggest that medical management is appropriate, while revascularization is considered for large defects or in multi-vessel disease.

Pre-operative cardiac risk assessment before major surgery

- The risk of a cardiac event complicating major surgery is 6% in unselected patients over 40 years of age. With major vascular surgery, the risk increases to 30%.
- Low-risk surgery (e.g. urological, breast, skin) has <1% risk of cardiac events so pre-operative screening is not required. Routine evaluation is not indicated for low risk surgery or low clinical risk patients.
- In higher-risk patients or in patients undergoing high-risk surgery, a moderate or larger reversible perfusion defect implies a 25% event rate versus 4% for a normal scan. Pre-operative MPI should

be considered in patients with poor functional capacity, or previous myocardial infarction, angina, or CCF, or who are to have high risk surgery.

Myocardial viability assessment (hibernating or stunned myocardium)

- Perfusion imaging can determine if an akinetic wall of the left ventricle supplied by a diseased coronary artery will recover function if revascularized. This is best done with thallium images obtained 24 hours after injection. Thallium gradually accumulates in viable myocardium over this time.
- PET scanning using ^{18}F-fluorodeoxyglucose to image myocardial glucose metabolism is slightly more sensitive for assessing viability, but is less widely available.

Cardiac gated blood pool scan

- Cardiac gated blood pool scan (GBPS) gives a reproducible measurement of left ventricular ejection fraction (LVEF) and examines regional wall motion. It is also called a radionuclide ventriculogram (RNVG).
- The patient's blood is labeled with ^{99m}Tc, either in vivo, or in vitro by removing 10 ml of blood and reinjecting the labeled blood. The in vitro method has higher labeling efficiency but involves blood handling and therefore increased risk to staff and patients.
- The gamma camera is placed over the chest, ECG leads are attached and connected to a gating device that recognizes each R wave and triggers acquisition of a series of fast pictures or frames (usually 16) per R–R interval. This process is repeated each R wave and images are summed over several hundred cardiac cycles, resulting in 16 pictures, each at a successive part of the contraction cycle. These pictures are then played in a cine loop, to show cardiac motion.
- The radioactivity in the cardiac blood pool (i.e. in the chambers) is directly proportional to chamber volume. Therefore, by choosing the end-diastole and end-systole frames, and drawing a region around the left ventricular blood pool in these images, the LVEF can be calculated.
- The normal LVEF is greater than 50%.
- The right ventricular EF cannot be calculated as accurately.

Indications

Indications include:

- Detection of cardiotoxicity of drugs (e.g. anthrocycline, a chemotherapeutic agent) before it becomes symptomatic and irreversible.
- Assessment of LV function in patients with dyspnea.
- Prognostic information in cardiomyopathy.

Bone scintigraphy

Bone scintigraphy assesses vascularity and osteoblastic activity of bone.

Radiopharmaceuticals and dose

- ^{99m}Technetium methylene diphosphate (MDP)
- ^{99m}Technetium hydroxymethylene diphosphonate (HDP)
- 800–925 MBq (22–25 mCi)
- Total body radiation = 0.16 rads/25 mCi (or 1.6 mGy/925 MBq)

Patient preparation

- Patients are advised to drink plenty of water between the time of injection and delayed scanning. They also need to void prior to imaging if the pelvis is the region of interest as bladder activity may obscure bony abnormality.

Image acquisition

Early

- Dynamic imaging over the region of interest at the time of tracer injection at 2–3 seconds per frame over the first minute.
- Static imaging performed over the region(s) of interest for 5–10 minutes.

Late

- Whole body or localized static imaging 3–4 hours later.
- Single photon emission computerized tomography (SPECT).
- Delayed imaging of up to 24 hours may be performed.

Interpretation

Knowledge of the clinical/radiographic findings is mandatory for interpretation.

- History of trauma (fracture)
- Fever, pain, swelling, redness, previous treatment (infective vs. inflammatory)

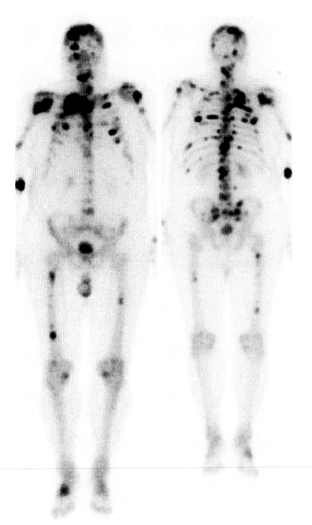

Fig. 5.5. Bone scan (anterior view on left, posterior view on right). Metastatic carcinoma of prostate with increased MDP uptake at multiple sites resulting from bone metastases.

- History of primary carcinoma and subsequent treatment (chemotherapy or radiotherapy)
- Correlative radiology and results
  The pattern of abnormality in each phase of the study leads to the specific diagnosis.

Indications
- Detection of osseous metastases – osteoblastic (Fig. 5.5) and most osteolytic metastases show increased uptake
- Diagnosis of bone/joint or prosthetic joint infection
- Diagnosis of reflex sympathetic dystrophy
- Evaluation of Paget's disease activity

- Diagnosis of occult fracture and investigation of unexplained bone pain
- Evaluation of benign and malignant bone lesion

Positron emission tomography (PET) imaging

- ^{18}F-fluorodeoxyglucose (FDG) is the most commonly used radiopharmaceutical in PET. It allows imaging of glucose metabolism and has a short radiation half-life of 110 minutes.
- FDG is transported into cells by the GLUT1 glucose transporter. It is then phosphorylated intracellularly to ^{18}F-FDG-6-phosphate. ^{18}F-FDG-6-phosphate cannot be further metabolized, resulting in accumulation within glucose avid cells.
- In cancer cells there is reduced glucose-6-phosphatase, so that dephosphorylation is slowed, further enhancing accumulation of ^{18}F-FDG.
- Malignant tumors, in general, are associated with an increase in glucose transporters and a high glycolytic rate, and uptake of ^{18}F-FDG into cells reflects disease metabolic activity.

Applications
Over 90% of PET studies are performed for cancer. The remainder are for epilepsy and neurodegenerative conditions and a few are for cardiac indications.

Oncology
- Most tumors avidly take up ^{18}F-FDG.
- This is especially the case for non-small cell lung cancer (NSCLC).
- Prostate cancer and well-differentiated thyroid cancer are much less FDG avid.

Pre-operative staging – e.g. non-small cell lung cancer (NSCLC)
- ^{18}F-FDG–PET scanning is more accurate than CT in mediastinal staging and in the detection of distant metastases.
- Adrenal masses are common in patients with NSCLC and up to 60% are incidental benign lesions. ^{18}F-FDG–PET is highly accurate (96%) in differentiating between a benign adrenal adenoma and a metastasis.

Assessment of a solitary pulmonary nodule
- An asymptomatic solitary pulmonary nodule is a common finding on chest X-rays. CT guided fine needle aspiration for cytology is the preferred method for precise diagnosis. However, when

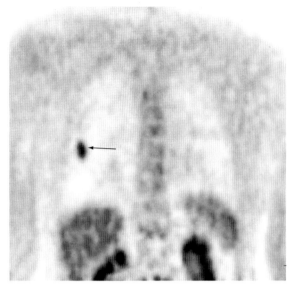

Fig. 5.6. Coronal PET scan. A 1 cm nodule was detected on chest X-ray. Chest CT was not diagnostic. PET demonstrates increased FDG uptake (arrow) strongly suggesting the nodule is malignant. NSCLC was confirmed at resection.

needle biopsy fails or is contraindicated, FDG–PET can show if it is metabolically active or not (Fig. 5.6).

Differentiation between post-therapy scar and residual tumor
- After treatment of many cancers, there is often a residual mass on CT that may be scar, or residual or recurrent cancer. FDG–PET can accurately distinguish between scar and residual disease.

Show response to therapy and detect tumor recurrences
- FDG–PET shows the metabolic response of a tumor to therapy prior to any change in size, and therefore can give the earliest feedback on efficacy of therapy. It is also sensitive for detection of recurrent cancer.

Neurological applications
Evaluation prior to surgery for epilepsy
- FDG–PET is a useful non-invasive method that assists localization of the seizure focus in patients with intractable focal epilepsy being considered for surgical treatment. In patients with temporal lobe epilepsy, hypometabolism is present in the epileptogenic temporal lobe in 85%.
- Imaging of ictal metabolism during a seizure is not practical, but ictal blood flow imaging is possible with SPECT blood flow tracers. This provides very useful complementary information

that further improves the accuracy of seizure localization.

Identification of dementia types
- Hypometabolism in the medial temporal lobe, parietotemporal regions, and posterior cingulate cortex is seen in early Alzheimer's disease.

Cardiology
- The main role is in assessment of myocardial viability. However, PET use is generally limited as low-dose dobutamine stress echocardiography, and nitrate augmented 24-hour delayed thallium imaging usually provide sufficient information for clinical decision making.

Lung scans
Ventilation perfusion lung scan (VQ scan)
Indications
- Diagnosis ± follow-up of patients with pulmonary embolism (PE)
- Assessment prior to surgical resection (tumor, lung volume reduction, lung transplant)
- Assessment of activity of pneumonitis

Method
- Ventilation: ^{99m}technetium Technegas and ^{99m}TC-DTPA aerosol are most commonly used. The patient inhales the radioactive "gas," and eight standard views are acquired.
- Perfusion: Same set of images are acquired following i.v. administration of ^{99m}Tc labeled macroaggregated albumin (MAA) or similar substance.

Interpretation of scan
Normal
- Uniform ventilation and perfusion
- Likelihood of pulmonary embolism is almost zero

Low probability of pulmonary embolism
- Small areas of either matched VQ defects, or ventilation abnormality > perfusion abnormality (reverse mismatch)
- Probability of abnormality due to PE is <5%.

Intermediate probability of pulmonary embolism
- 20%–30%

High probability of pulmonary embolism
- Multiple subsegmental or segmental VQ mismatch (Fig. 5.7)

Posterior   Left Post. obl.   Lt Ant obliq

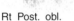

Anterior   Rt Post. obl.   Rt Ant oblique

Fig. 5.7. Multiple pulmonary emboli on ventilation/perfusion lung scan. Multiple segments of ventilation–perfusion mismatch. The first and third rows are ventilation scans with the corresponding view from the perfusion scans below each.

- Probability of patients having PE is 80%–100%

Clinical information is important for scan interpretation. VQ mismatch may result from pulmonary hypertension or tumor obstruction of a pulmonary artery. And single small subsegmental VQ mismatch in the setting of known DVT may be highly suspicious of pulmonary embolism (PE). An intermediate probability study does not alter the pre-test likelihood of PE.

Follow-up VQ scans
- These may be performed following extensive PE, 4–7 days into therapy, to assess for resolution or recurrent event. It also provides baseline information prior to discharge. Ideally, all patients should have a repeat study prior to cessation of Warfarin to assess resolution and act as a baseline for future reference.

Thyroid imaging
Indications
- To distinguish between autoimmune thyroid disease (Graves' disease) and other causes of a hyperthyroid state, e.g. toxic multinodular goiter, factitious thyroiditis or thyroiditis.
- To evaluate the functional state of a thyroid nodule (Fig. 5.8).
- To determine if a retrosternal mass is a goiter.
- To evaluate a possible congenital thyroid abnormality.

Radiopharmaceuticals
- ^{99m}Tc pertechnetate – most commonly used tracer due to lower radiation, and more readily available.
- ^{131}I and ^{123}I – mainly used for assessment prior to ^{131}I therapy for either hyperthyroidism or thyroid carcinoma.
- ^{99m}Tc dimercaptosuccinic acid (DMSA) V: for suspected medullary carcinoma of the thyroid.

Principles
- ^{99m}Tc pertechnetate is transported actively into the follicular cells (trapped) but not organified. Uptake can be used to evaluate trapping capacity of the thyroid gland.

89

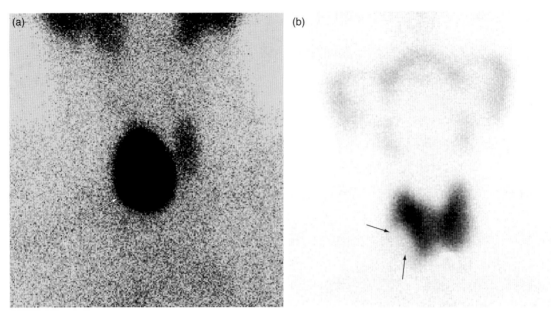

Fig. 5.8. Thyroid scans (a) autonomous "hot" thyroid nodule (arrow) with incomplete suppression of remaining thyroid tissue. (b) "Cold" nodule (hypofunctioning) in lower pole of right lobe (arrows).

Parathyroid imaging

- Main application is to localize parathyroid adenoma(s) in primary hyperthyroidism.

Radiopharmaceutical

Dual isotope technique

- ^{99m}Technetium pertechnetate
  - Tracer taken up by thyroid tissues but not parathyroid tissues
  - Helps differentiate parathyroid from thyroid tissues
- ^{99m}Technetium sestamibi
  - Taken up by both thyroid and parathyroid tissues
  - Concentrates in parathyroid adenoma
  - Classically shows preferential retention in parathyroid adenoma and washout in thyroid adenoma

Renal scintigraphy

- Renal scintigraphy consists of a series of images of the kidney as a radionuclide tracer passes through the kidney, is removed from the blood, enters the urine and ultimately the bladder.
- Quantitative analysis provides a measure of the relative renal function.

Radiopharmaceuticals

- ^{99m}Technetium-mercaptoacetyltriglycerine (MAG$_3$)
  - 40%–50% extraction by the proximal tubules at each pass through the kidneys. ^{99m}Tc-MAG$_3$ is then secreted by the proximal tubules. Clearance is highly correlated with the effective renal plasma flow (ERPF).
- ^{99m}Technetium-diethylenetriaminepentaacetic acid (DTPA)
  - Filtered by the glomerulus and may be used to measure glomerular filtration rate (GFR). Extraction fraction is only about 20%.

Patient preparation

The patient should be hydrated orally prior to injection. Images may be acquired supine or sitting.

Renovascular hypertension – renal artery stenosis

Principles

- Renal hypoperfusion and subsequent activation of the renin–angiotensin–aldosterone system results in renovascular hypertension. This is usually due to renal artery stenosis (RAS).
- RAS is an uncommon (1%–5% cases) yet important cause of hypertension because of its

associated cardiovascular and renal morbidity and potential curability with surgery or angioplasty. It is often suspected in middle-aged, previously normotensive patients or in young adults, and results from atherosclerosis or fibromuscular dysplasia, respectively.

- ACE inhibitors reduce angiotensin II dependent constriction of the efferent arterioles, decrease the resistance to flow, and thereby lower the transcapillary pressure gradient maintaining GFR. This results in a relative change in function or tracer retention in the renal tubules due to decreased GFR.

Patient preparation
- ACE inhibitors or angiotensin II receptor antagonists should be withheld 3–7 days prior to the study.

Results
- A positive captopril (an ACE inhibitor) challenge predicts good response following therapeutic intervention.

Renal scintigraphy with diuretic challenge
- A non-invasive method to evaluate renal function and urodynamics when there is evidence of dilatation of the collecting system. The aim is to exclude significant obstruction as the cause of dilatation.
- When there is pooling of urinary activity in the pelvicalyceal system, 10–20 mg of frusemide is administered intravenously, followed by dynamic imaging of the kidneys for a further 20–30 minutes.

Hepatobiliary imaging – cholescintigraphy
Cholescintigraphy (often referred to as a HIDA scan because they use agents like iminodiacetic acid) aims to delineate the biliary tree, assess function and demonstrate patency of the cystic duct and common bile duct.

Indications
- Acute or chronic cholecystitis
- Bile leak post-op
- Biliary colic without cholelithiasis on US

Radiopharmaceutical and dose
- ^{99m}Tc DISIDA (disofenin) – an analog of ^{99m}Tc-iminodiacetic acid (IDA) 185 MBq

Patient preparation
- Fasting for 4 hours prior to scan
  - Many normal subjects do not show gall bladder visualization in non-fasted state because of the effects of endogenous cholecystokinin (CCK) which induces gallbladder contraction and reduces net bile and isotope entry into the gallbladder, and similarly, prolonged fasting may cause non-visualization of the gallbladder.
- Avoid morphine prior to test

Procedure
- Acquire a series of dynamic images upon injection of the radiopharmaceutical
- ± Pharmacological interventions, e.g. morphine, CCK (or Sincalide, a synthetic CCK), oral milk

Common patterns observed
- Normal
  - Gallbladder seen within 30 minutes post-injection, which indicates patent cystic duct, and effectively excludes acute cholecystitis
  - Negative predictive value of normal cholescintigram in excluding acute cholecystitis >99%
  - 85%–90% of patients with chronic cholecystitis have normal pattern
- Persistent gallbladder non-visualization (despite delayed images ± morphine)
  - Consistent with acute cholecystitis (Fig. 5.9)
  - Other causes: chronic cholecystitis, non-fasting, prolonged fasting, intercurrent severe illness, acute pancreatitis, severe liver disease, hyperalimentation
- Delayed gallbladder visualization
  - Gallbladder visualized between 1 and 4 hours or within 30 minutes post-morphine infusion
  - Most commonly seen in chronic cholecystitis
  - Other causes:
    - Hepatocellular dysfunction – delayed tracer transit from liver to bowel with delayed peak of common bile duct activity (normal less than 50 minutes)
    - Partial CBD obstruction
    - Acalculous or calculous cholecystitis
- Obstructive
  - No biliary tree seen within 1 hour despite good hepatic uptake

91

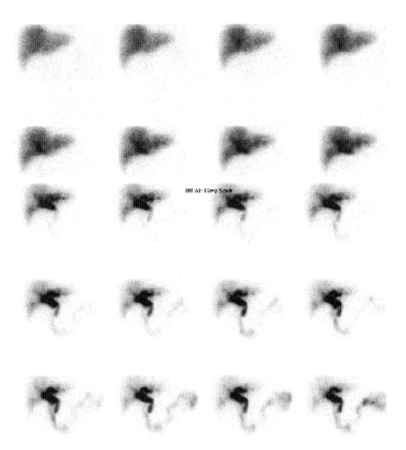

Fig. 5.9. HIDA scan in acute cholecystitis which is diagnosed by absence of gallbladder filling. Bile ducts and small bowel show progressive accumulation of activity.

- Usually indicates acute CBD obstruction
- Other causes: cholestatic jaundice, hepatocellular disease
  - Extrahepatic and enteric activity
    - Bile leak – post-traumatic or post-operative

Gastrointestinal imaging
Gastrointestinal motility studies
Esophageal transit study
- Demonstrates movement of a swallowed bolus through the esophagus, into the stomach
- Assesses esophageal motility and reflux quantitatively
- Radiopharmaceutical
  - ^{99m}Technetium sulphur colloid in water
- Patient preparation
  - Overnight fast
- Image acquisition
  - Dynamic imaging in supine and erect position
  - Delayed images may be required to detect reflux or aspiration

Gastric emptying
- Demonstrates movement of ingested material from the stomach into the small intestine
- Diagnosis of functional gastric dysmotility ± gastro-esophageal reflux.
- Radiopharmaceuticals
  - Solid: 40 MBq ^{99m}Technetium sulphur colloid in solid food (e.g. sandwich of standard caloric contents)
  - Liquid: ^{99m}Technetium DTPA in standard amount of water
- Patient preparation
  - Overnight fast
- Image acquisition
  - Dynamic or static abdominal images in supine position acquired over 120 minutes

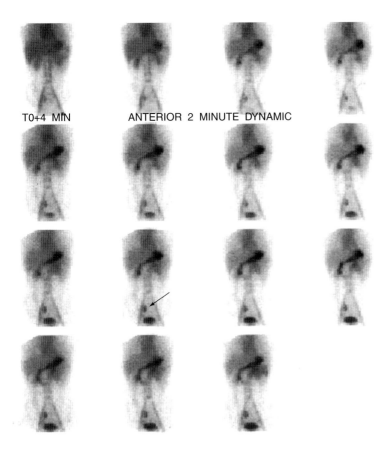

T0+4 MIN   ANTERIOR 2 MINUTE DYNAMIC

Fig. 5.10. Meckel's diverticulum in right iliac fossa (arrow) shown by uptake of ^{99m}Technetium pertechnetate.

Small bowel transit and colonic transit
- Transit of ingested liquid tracer (^{67}gallium citrate) is studied over 1 week
- Patient preparation
  - Overnight fast on day 1 only
  - Aperients should be avoided before and during the study period.
- Static images of the abdomen are performed at 2, 4 and 6 hours on day 1, and then at 24, 48, 72, and 96 hours

Gastrointestinal bleeding
Identification of site of bleeding
- Only active bleeding (>0.05–0.1 ml/min) can be detected
- Radiopharmaceutical
  - ^{99m}Technetium labeled autologous red cells
  - Dose: ~ 1000 MBq
- Patient preparation: nil
- Imaging: dynamic acquisition is performed for as long as required

Meckel's diverticulum scan
- Ectopic gastric mucosa present in only 10%–30% of all Meckel's cases, but in 98% of those that bleed
- Radiopharmaceuticals
  - ^{99m}Technetium pertechnetate (localizes in gastric mucosa) (Fig. 5.10)
  - Dose: 400 Mbq
- Patient preparation: fast for 6–8 hours. Pre-treatment with H_2 antagonist is required for 2 days prior and 1 hour before injection.

^{14}Carbon breath test
Recovery of $^{14}CO_2$ in the breath after oral administration of ^{14}C labeled substrates indicates that metabolism of the compound has occurred within the body. By estimating the amount and rate of $^{14}CO_2$ excretion, deductions about metabolism may be made.

This test is used for the following indications:
- ^{14}C Glycocholic acid for bile acid malabsorption and/or for bacterial overgrowth
- ^{14}C Urea for *Helicobacter pylori* infection

93

- ^{14}C Triglyceride (e.g. triolein) for fat malabsorption
- ^{14}C D-xylose for small intestinal bacterial overgrowth
- ^{14}C Lactose for lactose malabsorption

^{14}C urea breath test

Principle

- *Helicobacter pylori* (HP) produces large amounts of urease, an enzyme not present in mammalian cells or normal human gastric mucosa. In infection with HP, increased urease activity results in the rapid hydrolysis of urea in gastric juice, producing ammonia and carbon dioxide. ^{14}C urea produces $^{14}CO_2$, which is excreted in the breath.
- Ingested urea passes unaltered into the urine or may be hydrolyzed by bacteria. In HP positive patients about 40% of ^{14}C dose is excreted in the urine. In HP negative patients about 70% of the administered isotope is excreted in the urine, therefore, the dose to the bladder is about 70 uGy.
- Sensitivity = 93%; Specificity = 95%.

Procedure

- Fasting – overnight or at least 6 hours
- Post-eradication therapy – the patient should not have antibiotics, or bismuth-containing products for at least 28 days before the test.
- Dose: 400 kBq (or a 40 kBq dose can be administered in a capsule).
- Route of administration: orally.
- Most patients with positive results peak at between 10 and 20 minutes.

Infection imaging

Bone scintigraphy

A three-phase bone scan (e.g. using ^{99m}technetium-MDP) is often used to diagnose skeletal infections, which cause increase in vascularity (blood flow phase), increase in early bony uptake (blood pool phase), in-crease in osteoblastic activity (delayed phase). Three patterns may be observed:

- Osteomyelitis – concordant abnormalities in all three phases.
- Septic arthritis – concordant abnormalities in all three phases, but joint based.
- Soft tissue infection/inflammation – abnormal vascularity and early blood pool activity

but relatively normal bony uptake on delayed phase.

^{67}Gallium citrate

- ^{67}Gallium citrate shows uptake in non-microbial inflammation, tumors and infection
- Gallium binds to circulating transferrin after i.v. injection. A high level of lactoferrin in neutrophils and abscess fluid is thought to be an important factor in gallium accumulation in infections.
- In chronic soft tissue infection and osteomyelitis, it is more sensitive but less specific than radiolabeled leukocytes. Correlation with bone scans is important in the interpretation of gallium images as gallium normally localizes in bone.

Radiolabeled autologous white blood cells

- ^{111}Indium – not readily available and expensive
- ^{99m}Technetium – HMPAO (hexamethylpropy-leneamine oxime) – relatively cheap but labor intensive in preparation
- ^{99m}Technetium nanocolloid – cheap, but more prominent marrow uptake

Clinical indications

- Intra-abdominal abscess
- Osteomyelitis
- Prosthetic vascular graft infection
- Inflammatory bowel disease
- Infected orthopedic prostheses (Fig. 5.11)
- Occult fever

Limitations

- Normal shedding of leukocytes from bowel.
- Labeling requires handling of patient's blood which is reinjected back into the patient. Meticulous care has to be taken to ensure aseptic techniques are used.
- May be difficult in neutropenic patients (white cell count <2000 cells/ml and neutrophils <1000 cells/ml).
- Non-infective inflammatory process may cause false-positive results, e.g. inflammatory bowel disease, rheumatoid arthritis.

Other isotopes

- ^{18}F-FDG PET – commonly seen at site of infection/inflammation.
  - Not widely available

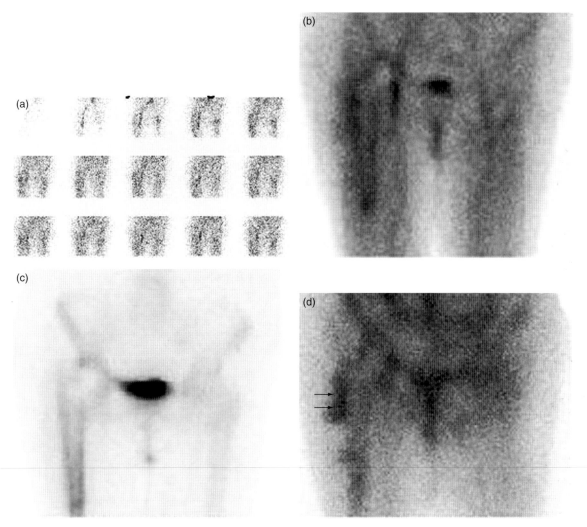

Fig. 5.11. 80-year-old with right hip replacement and right hip pain. Abnormal three-phase bone scan, (a) with vascular changes and (b) early blood pool activity (c) more prominent than the delayed bony uptake. (d) Discordant degree of uptake between bone scan and gallium scan (arrows) suggests prosthetic joint infection.

- Expensive
- [99m]Technetium Leukoscan® (monoclonal antibodies directed against cell membrane antigen)
  - Expensive
  - No need for blood handling

Nuclear medicine in human immunodeficiency virus (HIV)
Type of scintigraphy
(see HIV section for further details)
- Gallium scan
- Thallium scan
- Thallium–gallium scan

- Other scans may be useful for:
  - Possible AIDS dementia – SPECT
  - Bone and soft tissue infections – bone scan
  - AIDS-related cholecystitis from cholangiopathy – HIDA scan
  - Depressed cardiac function – gated blood pool scan
  - Autologous white cell scan

Brain SPECT – cerebral blood flow imaging
- Ceretec (^{99m}Tc-HMPAO) or Neurolyte (^{99m}Tc ECD) are highly lipophilic radiopharmaceuticals

95

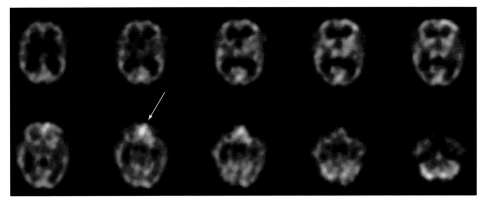

Fig. 5.12. Ictal SPECT demonstrating a seizure focus (increased uptake) anteriorly in the inferior left frontal lobe just to the left of the midline (arrow).

that freely cross the blood–brain barrier and are trapped within brain cells largely on first pass. The uptake therefore reflects regional cerebral blood flow (CBF). This is imaged with SPECT. The images are basically of gray matter as it has three times the perfusion of white matter. Regional CBF is coupled to metabolic activity that, in turn, is linked to synaptic activity. Therefore, brain SPECT imaging of CBF indirectly gives images of regional brain activity.

- This is useful in conditions that have functional change but little structural change, e.g. epilepsy and Alzheimer's disease.

Seizures

- In seizure focus investigation:
  - Brain SPECT can help localize the seizure focus in patients with medically resistant epilepsy being considered for surgical treatment.
  - Between seizures (interictal SPECT), regional CBF is reduced at the seizure focus in about 50% of patients with intractable temporal lobe epilepsy (TLE).

- PET imaging of regional cerebral glucose metabolism is more accurate, demonstrating reduced F-18 fluorodeoxyglucose uptake in 85% of patients.
- Ceretec and Neurolyte can be injected during a seizure (ictal SPECT). During seizures regional CBF increases markedly at the seizure focus (Fig. 5.12). Ictal SPECT shows the focus in 90% of TLE patients.

SPECT in Alzheimer's Disease

- A characteristic pattern of regional hypoperfusion and hypometabolism is seen in Alzheimer's Disease (AD).
- This involves parietal and temporal lobes, sparing the primary sensorimotor and occipital cortex.
- SPECT is abnormal in 90% of those with severe dementia, but in only 50% of those with mild dementia.
- PET imaging is more sensitive and therefore more useful in early diagnosis of AD.
- The same pattern may be seen in diffuse Lewy body dementia, Parkinson's disease with dementia, and cortico-basal degeneration.

Cardiorespiratory system

Contents

Cardiac failure, pulmonary edema, and pulmonary hypertension

Imaging modalities

- The chest radiograph (preferably with posteroanterior as well as lateral views) is the first and simplest imaging modality for suspected cardiac disease, including suspected cardiac failure. In unwell patients an anteroposterior frontal radiograph is used.
- Echocardiography is extremely valuable in assessment of cardiac structure and function.
  - Uses a combination of real-time ultrasound, Doppler techniques, and M-mode (motion mode).
  - Used to assess cardiac anatomy and function, including ventricular function, congenital heart disease, valvular disease, intracardiac shunts, and pericardial disease.
  - Ultrasound contrast agents (microbubbles) are now frequently used to improve interpretation of structure and function and may provide some information about myocardial perfusion.
  - Usually performed percutaneously as with most ultrasound, but transesophageal probes also can be used to gain more detailed information in some situations.
  - Can be combined with stress studies.
- Radioisotope techniques are used to assess function as well as myocardial perfusion (see Chapter 5).
  - Ventricular function can be examined with gated blood pool scans (e.g. to derive left ventricular ejection fraction).
  - Myocardial perfusion and global assessment of coronary artery disease can be performed with different agents (e.g. thallium) and can be performed at rest and as stress studies to improve sensitivity. Cardiac PET studies are used less widely and provide information about myocardial perfusion and function.
- Coronary artery anatomy and disease is best assessed with coronary angiography, although CT angiography is improving in quality and replacing catheter angiography for some indications.
- In the future it is likely that many anatomical and functional cardiac studies will be performed using MRI, with no ionizing radiation and minimal invasiveness.

Chest radiograph

Characteristic findings of cardiac failure are (Figs. 6.1–6.3):

- Enlarged heart – sometimes absent, e.g. in acute myocardial infarction when ventricular function has previously been good.
- Upper zone pulmonary vascular prominence (often difficult to diagnose confidently). The upper zone vessels should normally be smaller than the lower zone vessels.
- Pleural effusions – often larger on right or, if unilateral, usually on the right

97

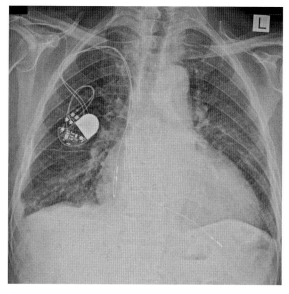

Fig. 6.1. Left heart failure. Cardiomegaly with pulmonary congestion (upper zone vessels are more prominent than usual), interstitial pulmonary edema evidenced by indistinctness of the perihilar vessels, and a small right pleural effusion. A dual chamber pacemaker is in place.

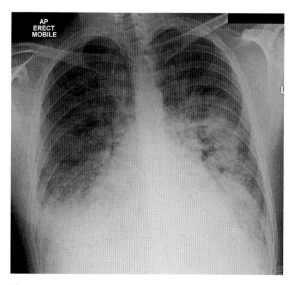

Fig. 6.2. Acute pulmonary edema as evidenced by mid and lower zone air space opacity, more prominent on the left. A small right, and probably a smaller left, pleural effusion are present.

- Pulmonary edema. Pulmonary edema, which has many other causes apart from the commonest one of cardiac failure, appears as
  - Alveolar edema (air space opacity) and/or
  - Interstitial edema

Pericardial effusion
- Can cause apparent gross cardiac enlargement, with a "globular" heart shape due to bulging of the lower cardiac margins
- Echocardiography is the most sensitive test

Cardiac valvular disease
- Aortic and mitral valves are the most commonly involved
- Best assessed by echocardiography (structural and functional information), and nuclear medicine (functional information)
- Chest radiograph may show
  - Chamber enlargement – valvular incompetence produces more chamber enlargement than stenosis, e.g. aortic incompetence causes more left ventricular dilatation than aortic stenosis
  - Valve calcification – does not necessarily indicate functional valve disease
  - Signs of left heart failure

Mitral valve disease
- Valve may be stenotic or incompetent (or combination)
- Causes include mitral valve prolapse, papillary muscle rupture, rheumatic fever, and bacterial endocarditis

Radiological findings
- Heart size normal initially
- Cardiac enlargement with enlarged left atrium (Fig. 6.4)
- Signs of pulmonary venous hypertension (left heart failure)
- Changes of secondary pulmonary arterial hypertension (see Pulmonary hypertension section)
- Occasionally, valve calcification (this does not necessarily indicate functional abnormality)

Aortic valve disease
Radiological findings
- Cardiac enlargement, especially left ventricle
- Dilatation of ascending aorta in aortic incompetence
- May see calcification of aortic valves
- Signs of pulmonary venous hypertension (left heart failure)

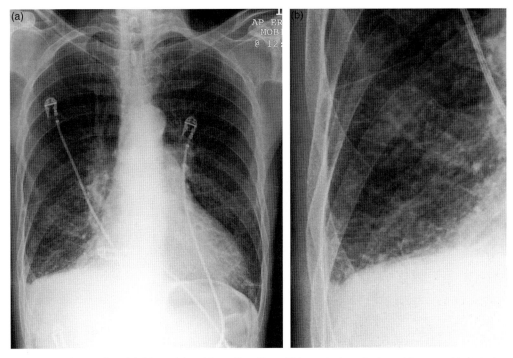

Fig. 6.3. Cardiomegally with left heart failure. Bilateral basal interstitial septal edema (horizontal linear opacities), also known as Kerley B lines. (b) Magnified view of right lung base.

Non-cardiogenic pulmonary edema

Pulmonary edema may result from causes other than cardiac disease. These include:

- Fluid overload in renal failure
- Over-hydration
- Acute respiratory distress syndrome (ARDS) or shock lung syndrome – leaking from capillary membranes and exudation into the alveolar spaces. It can be caused by any major lung inflammation or injury.
- Raised intracranial pressure
- Drug overdose
- Inhalation of toxic substances
- Near-drowning

Pulmonary hypertension

- The pulmonary vascular system has much lower resistance than the systemic system, with much lower arterial and venous pressures.
- Systolic pulmonary arterial pressure is usually 30 mm Hg or below, and the mean is around 18 mm Hg. Pulmonary venous pressure is usually below 12 mm Hg.

- Pulmonary hypertension is defined as measurements above these levels, and is divided into pulmonary venous and pulmonary arterial hypertension.
- The term "pulmonary hypertension" is often used to mean pulmonary arterial hypertension.

Pulmonary venous hypertension (PVHT)
Causes

- Left ventricular failure is the commonest cause, usually related to coronary artery disease. The dysfunctional left ventricle (LV) fails to pump the required blood volume, leading to an increase in pressure within the ventricle during diastole (increased LV end-diastolic pressure), which is transmitted directly to the left atrium and the pulmonary veins.
- Mitral valve disease (including mitral stenosis and incompetence) is the next most common cause.

Radiographic signs

Mild PVHT shows as upper lobe venous diversion (or vascular redistribution):

- Upper lobe veins, normally of smaller caliber than their lower lobe counterparts, increase in size (Fig. 6.1)

99

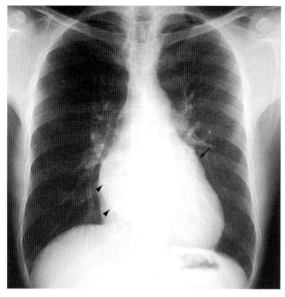

Fig. 6.4. Mitral valve disease with mild enlargement of overall heart size with more pronounced enlargement of left atrium, the left margin of which bulges the left heart border (arrow), and the right margin of which can be seen as a second density on the right side (arrowheads).

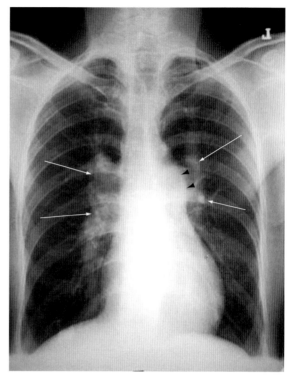

Fig. 6.5. Pulmonary arterial hypertension due to COAD. Note markedly enlarged main pulmonary artery (arrowheads) and right and left pulmonary arteries (arrows). The lungs are hyper-inflated indicating emphysema.

- By convention, veins are measured in the first anterior intercostal space, and should be less than 3 mm in diameter.

Moderately severe PVHT causes interstitial edema (Figs. 6.1, 6.3) shown as:

- Thickening of bronchial walls (peribronchial cuffing)
- Poor definition of bronchial and vascular walls (normally sharply defined)
- Thickening of the lung fissures, and septal (Kerley's) lines, which represent dilated lymphatic channels
- Kerley B lines occur in the periphery in the lower zones as discrete 1–2 cm long horizontal lines extending to the pleura
- Kerley A lines are longer (up to 4 cm) and occur in the mid to upper zones, radiating out from the hila

Severe PVHT results in alveolar edema (Fig. 6.2) seen as:

- Air-space opacity (ill-defined, "fluffy," with air bronchograms)
- Classically perihilar (in a "bat's-wing" appearance) or bi-basal
- Differential diagnosis includes other causes of air-space disease, e.g. non-cardiogenic pulmonary edema, infection or pulmonary hemorrhage

Pulmonary arterial hypertension (PAHT)

Causes

- Severe chronic PVHT is commonest, with the increased venous pressure transmitted via the capillaries to the arterial system
- Increased pulmonary arterial blood flow – congenital heart disease with a left-to-right shunt (e.g. atrial septal defect, ventricular septal defect, patent ductus arteriosus)
- Increased pulmonary vascular resistance – most often secondary to chronic obstructive airways disease or pulmonary fibrosis (where normal vessels are destroyed)
- Unknown cause, i.e. idiopathic or primary pulmonary hypertension

Radiographic signs

- Increased size of central pulmonary arteries (Fig. 6.5)
- Rapid tapering of vessels in the mid and distal portions of the lung ("peripheral pruning")
- In the early stages of high flow PAHT (e.g. due to a left to right shunt such as atrial septal

defect), both pulmonary arteries and veins enlarge, an appearance known as pulmonary plethora

- Right ventricular enlargement which results in elevation of the cardiac apex on the frontal film, and "filling in" of the retro-sternal air space on the lateral view.

Acute chest pain and aortic dissection

Causes of acute chest pain can be considered by anatomical origin (see other sections for further discussion):

- Cardiac
  - Ischemia/infarction
  - Pericarditis
- Pleural – inflammation associated with
  - Underlying lung infection
  - Pulmonary embolus
- Thoracic aorta
  - Aortic dissection (see below)
- Esophageal
  - Reflux esophagitis
  - Motility disorder – spasm
  - Esophageal perforation–spontaneous or associated with vomiting (Mallory–Weiss)
- Chest wall
  - Musculoskeletal

Aortic dissection

- Aortic dissection is life-threatening and about half of untreated patients die within 48 hours.
- An intramural tear extends along a variable length of the aortic wall, creating a false lumen within the wall. This communicates with the true lumen via an intimal tear in at least one site. Blood flow in the true lumen and to branches of the affected aorta can be severely compromised.
- The vast majority involve the ascending aorta or aortic arch.
- Most patients are >50 years.
- The typical presentation is sudden onset of severe chest pain, which may radiate elsewhere, e.g. interscapular region. Other symptoms and signs reflect the presence of aortic branch occlusion/stenosis.
- Dissection should not be confused with traumatic rupture of the thoracic aorta.

Classification

- Type A involves ascending aorta and usually requires surgery.
- Type B does not involve ascending aorta, and is usually managed by endovascular stenting or medically.

Complications

- As dissections can involve the aortic arch and the abdominal aorta, there is potential for major ischemic injury to brain, spine, and abdominal organs
- If the dissection extends proximally, it can result in:
  - Pericardial tamponade if it extends into the pericardium
  - Coronary artery occlusion
  - Acute aortic valve incompetence

Predisposing conditions

- Atherosclerosis
- Hypertension
- Connective tissue disorders, e.g. Marfan's syndrome (cystic medial necrosis)

Imaging modalities

- Chest X-ray
- Trans-esophageal echo (TOE)
- Contrast-enhanced CT angiography
- Conventional angiography – if others are inconclusive

In general, the current approach is to perform CT angiography or, in some centers, TOE. Angiography is now used mainly as part of endovascular stenting.

Chest X-ray
Findings include:

- Widened aortic arch (Fig. 6.6)
- Left pleural effusion – suggests rupture of dissection into left hemithorax (unusual on right side)
- Cardiomegaly
- *Note*: A normal chest X-ray does not exclude dissection

Trans-esophageal echocardiography (TOE)

- Sensitive
- Minimally invasive
- Mobile – can be used at bedside in emergency department

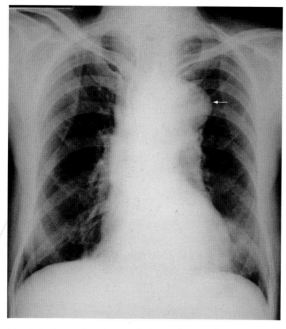

Fig. 6.6. Aortic dissection producing widening of the aortic arch (arrow).

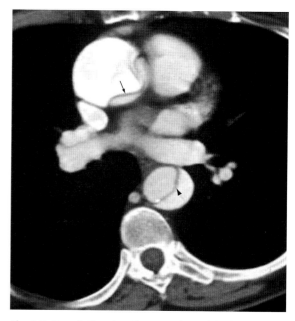

Fig. 6.7. Type A dissection. Contrast-enhanced CT shows intimal flap in ascending aorta (arrow) and descending aorta (arrowhead). The false lumen is likely to be the more faintly opacified one.

- Can assess pericardium, aortic valve
- Cannot assess abdominal aorta or involvement of carotid vessels

CT angiography (CTA) (Fig. 6.7)
- Readily available
- Can assess complete thoracic and abdominal aorta
- Good visualization of head and neck vessels
- Can detect pericardial hematoma

Conventional angiography
- More invasive than CTA or TOE
- Can be followed by endovascular stenting in selected patients

Pulmonary embolism
Imaging modalities
- Ventilation perfusion lung scan (V/Q scan)
- CT pulmonary angiogram (CTPA)
- DSA angiography

Chest radiographs
- Low sensitivity and specificity for diagnosis of PE
- A normal radiograph does not exclude PE
  Non-specific abnormal findings include:

- Alveolar consolidation, especially lower zones (which may subsequently cavitate)
- Pleural effusion
- Reduced lung vascular markings in region of embolus

Ventilation perfusion lung scan (V/Q scan)
- Performed in two parts with ventilation phase (patient inhales radioisotope), and perfusion phase (radioisotope injected intravenously) (Fig. 6.8)
- The key sign of PE on V/Q scans is normal ventilation in an area of a perfusion defect, so-called mismatch (Fig. 6.9)
  Advantages of V/Q scan:
- Minimally invasive
- Readily available
- Relatively low dose of ionizing radiation
  Limitations of V/Q scan:
- May be indeterminate, particularly in patients with chronic obstructive lung disease or other lung pathology

CT Pulmonary angiogram (CTPA)
- CTPA is performed with spiral CT and a bolus intravenous injection of contrast agent

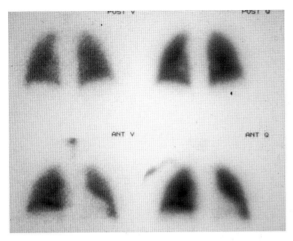

Fig. 6.8. Normal V/Q scan. Anterior views below and posterior views above. There is normal distribution of isotope in both the ventilatory (on left) and perfusion parts (on right) of the study.

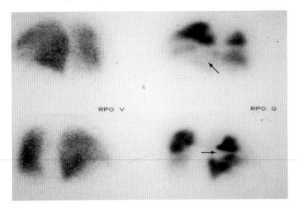

Fig. 6.9. V/Q scan images from left posterior view (above) and right posterior view (below). Ventilation scans on left and perfusion scans on right. Note areas of normal ventilation with decreased perfusion (arrows). This indicates a high probability of PE.

- Pulmonary emboli are recognized as unopacified filling defects within pulmonary arteries (Fig. 6.10).
  Advantages of CTPA:
- High accuracy for central and proximal branch emboli (to segmental level).
- Able to evaluate lung parenchyma and airways – may provide alternative diagnosis.
- Readily available.
  Disadvantages of CTPA:
- Lower sensitivity for subsegmental small peripheral emboli.
- Intravenous contrast agent required.

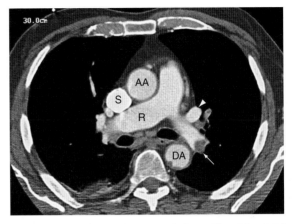

Fig. 6.10. CTPA shows pulmonary embolus as filling defect in left lower lobe pulmonary artery (arrow). Arrowhead = left upper lobe pulmonary artery, R = right pulmonary artery, AA = ascending aorta. DA = descending aorta. S = superior vena cava.

- Relatively high radiation dose
- Moderately expensive

Pulmonary angiography (DSA)
- PE appears as filling defects in arteries or as "amputated" arterial branches
- In the past has been regarded as the "gold standard" for diagnosis of PE, but is seldom used now because of its invasiveness and the acceptably high accuracy of V/Q scans or CTPA
  Disadvantages of Pulmonary DSA:
- Invasive
- Large volume contrast material
- High radiation dose
- Risk of arrhythmias
- Expensive

Lobar pulmonary processes
Collapse and consolidation are two important pathological processes that occur in a lobar distribution.

Lobar collapse
- Collapse (or atelectasis) may involve a lobe (in part or as a whole), multiple lobes, or an entire lung.
- Its cause is usually obstruction of a major bronchus.
- The likely obstructing lesion differs according to age. In children, pneumonia, mucus plugging and foreign body inhalation are common causes. In adults, cancer or mucus plugging are the most common.

103

The two most important radiographic signs of collapse on plain radiographs are opacity and loss of volume. Signs of collapse include:

Direct signs
- Opaque collapsed lobe.
- Altered position of bronchi or blood vessels due to loss of volume.
- "Silhouette" sign – This refers to loss of the normal "silhouette" of a mediastinal or diaphragmatic border. The normal silhouette is caused by air-containing lung lying immediately next to the border of the mediastinum or hemidiaphragm. The "silhouette sign" occurs when a pathological pulmonary process replaces that air-containing lung, so the mediastinal or diaphragmatic contour is no longer normal.

Indirect signs
- Altered position of other structures to compensate for the loss of volume.
- Compensatory over-expansion of unaffected lung (on both the same and opposite sides).
- Elevation of the hemidiaphragm and ipsilateral mediastinal shift (movement of the mediastinal structures to the same side as the collapse).

Lower lobe collapse
- Appearances are similar for both left and right sides
- Lower lobes collapse posteriorly and medially

Direct signs
- Characteristic triangular opacity (Fig. 6.11)
- Hemidiaphragm may be obscured
- Inferior displacement of ipsilateral hilum
- On the lateral film, increasing density of each lower thoracic vertebral body in relation to the one above it (normal is opposite of this)

Right upper lobe collapse
The right upper lobe collapses superomedially to lie against the mediastinum and lung apex (Fig. 6.12). The signs are:
- Right para-mediastinal opacity causing loss of the normal right superior mediastinal border
- Elevation of ipsilateral hemidiaphragm
- Upward and outward displacement of the lower lobe arteries

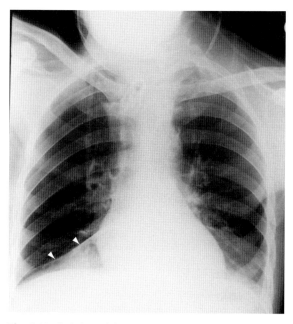

Fig. 6.11. Right lower lobe collapse. Characteristic medial triangular opacity. Upper border of the opacity (arrowheads) represents the major pleural fissure. Right hemidiaphragm outline (silhouette) is not obscured in this case as the dome of the diaphragm lies anteriorly and the collapsed lower lobe lies posteriorly.

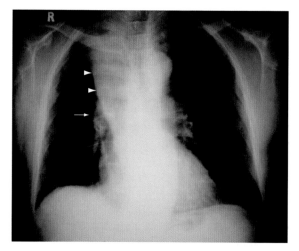

Fig. 6.12. Right upper lobe collapse. Opaque lobe with loss of normal right superior mediastinal border, well-defined lateral margin (arrowheads) and right hilar elevation (arrow).

Left upper lobe collapse
Absence of a minor fissure on the left makes this appear very different from right upper lobe collapse. This lobe collapses anteriorly to lie against the anterior chest wall.

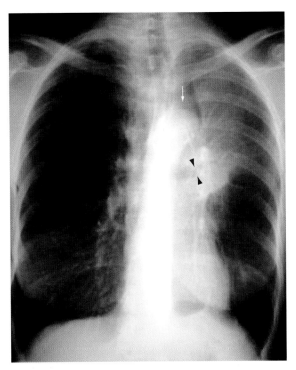

Fig. 6.13. Left upper lobe collapse with central cancer causing obstruction of the left upper lobe bronchus (arrowheads). Ill-defined lateral border is due to lack of a minor fissure; the major fissure is not tangential to the X-ray beam and therefore does not create a sharp border. Note the lucency outlining the aortic knob (arrow).

Radiographic signs – frontal film (Fig. 6.13)
- Hazy opacity, most dense at the left hilum, fading peripherally, particularly inferiorly and laterally.
- Left mediastinal borders obscured.
- Left hilar elevation.
- Greatly expanded superior segment of left lower lobe may lie postero-superiorly and medially, causing a left para-mediastinal lucency that sharply outlines the aortic knob.

Radiographic signs – lateral film
- A wedge of tissue seen anteriorly against the chest wall (less reliable than frontal signs).

Right middle lobe (RML) collapse

Major and minor fissures collapse towards each other creating a wedge of tissue that is thickest anteriorly and medially, tapering superiorly and laterally.

Radiographic signs (Fig. 6.14):
- Frontal film – loss of right heart border silhouette (in severe RML collapse this is easy to miss!)
- Lateral film (more useful than frontal) – curved wedge opacity as described above.

Whole lung collapse

The entire hemithorax becomes opaque, with severe ipsilateral loss of volume and marked compensatory shift into the affected hemithorax (including herniation of contralateral lung).

Other types of atelectasis

Cicatrization atelectasis
- Related to scarring/local fibrosis

Round atelectasis
- A chronic atelectasis, most common in asbestos-related pleural disease
- Peripheral rounded opacity
- Easily mistaken for neoplasm

Linear (plate or discoid) atelectasis
- Due to under-ventilation rather than obstruction
- Very common in lower lobes of hospitalized patients

Compressive atelectasis
- Simple mechanical compression of lung adjacent to a large pleural effusion or mass

Lobar consolidation

Consolidation is also described as airspace or alveolar opacity.

Radiological signs (Figs. 6.15, 6.16):
- Opacity with ill-defined edges (except when adjacent to the pleura).
- Air bronchograms – patent, air-filled bronchi within the opacity stand out as dark, linear, and/or branching structures within the opacified lung.
- Consolidation may involve almost any volume of lung tissue, from a few pulmonary lobules to an entire lung.
- Involvement of a single lobe is relatively common, as the pleural fissures limit the pathological process.

Causes
- The most common causes for lobar consolidation are pneumonia and neoplasm. Pulmonary embolus may result in segmental lobar opacities (see below).
- Chest radiographs are important for diagnosis, assessing complications and for assessing response to treatment.
- Lobar pneumonia is usually bacterial. The infection begins in the periphery of a lobe and

105

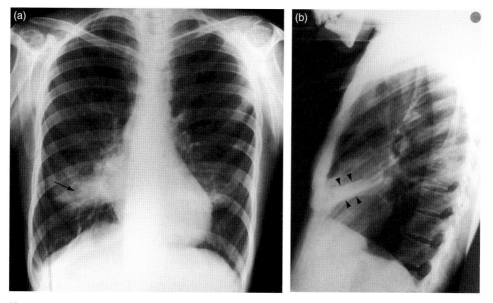

Fig. 6.14. Right middle lobe – (a) PA view – the collapsed lobe (arrow) obscures part of the right heart border, (b) lateral view – the collapsed lobe is bounded by the minor and major pleural fissures (arrowheads).

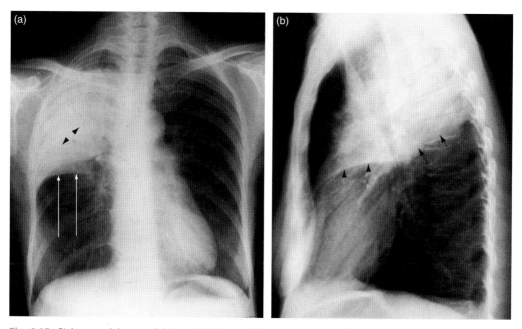

Fig. 6.15. Right upper lobe consolidation. (a) PA image of airspace opacity involving virtually the entire right upper lobe. Note: ill-defined margins of the opacity superiorly, and sharp margin inferiorly where the minor fissure limits the spread of infection (arrow). Air bronchograms can just be made out as more lucent structures (arrowheads). (b) Lateral film shows limitation of the infective process by the major (arrows) and minor (arrowheads) fissures.

spreads freely through the airspaces, limited by the fissures (Fig. 6.15)

- The most common organism is *Streptococcus pneumoniae* ("pneumococcal pneumonia").

- Less common organisms include *Klebsiella pneumoniae*, *Staphylococcus aureus*, *Mycobacterium tuberculosis* and *Legionella pneumophila*.

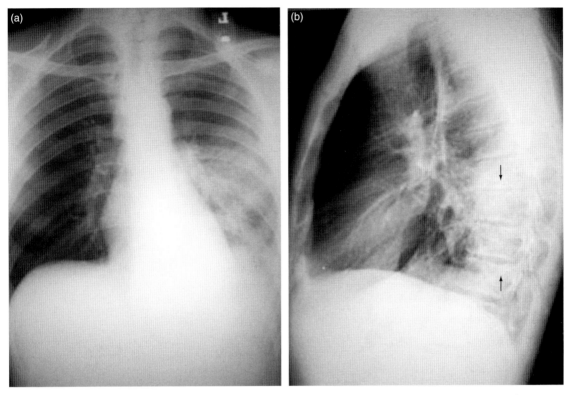

Fig. 6.16. Left lower lobe consolidation due to infection. (a) PA film with loss of normal left hemidiaphragm contour and preservation of outline of left side of heart, localizing the process in the left lower lobe. (b) Lateral film confirms lower lobe position. Note increased density of the lower thoracic vertebral bodies (arrows) which should normally be "darker" than the upper thoracic vertebral bodies.

- *Streptococcus* and *Klebsiella* may cause bulging of fissures due to the volume of pus formed.
- Anerobic and/or gram-negative organisms are more frequent in aspiration pneumonia.

Complications of pneumonia

Complications include cavitation (Fig. 6.17), pleural effusion and empyema (infected pleural effusion). Radiographs and often CT are needed for diagnosis and monitoring of treatment. CT can show gas locules within a pleural effusion suggesting empyema.

Neoplasm and pulmonary embolism

Occasionally, neoplasms such as broncho-alveolar carcinoma and lymphoma (and Kaposi's sarcoma in HIV/AIDS) can cause lobar airspace opacity.

Pulmonary embolus may cause lobar consolidation via infarction and hemorrhage of the affected lung. It rarely accounts for consolidation of a whole lobe, wedge-shaped segmental opacities being more common.

Pulmonary infections
Tuberculosis (TB)
Primary TB
- Primary TB occurs in those with no prior TB infection.
- Primary TB usually appears as an area of consolidation, anywhere in the lungs, often associated with marked hilar and mediastinal lymphadenopathy.
- With healing, the primary consolidation may completely resolve or form a small calcified (Ghon's) focus.
- The mediastinal nodes may heal completely, but often heal with calcification.

Secondary TB
- Secondary TB represents reactivation in patients who have had a primary tuberculous episode.
- Characteristically involves upper lobe and apical segments of the lower lobes.

107

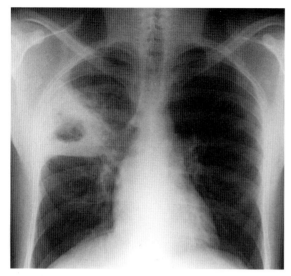

Fig. 6.17. Cavitating right upper lobe pneumonia.

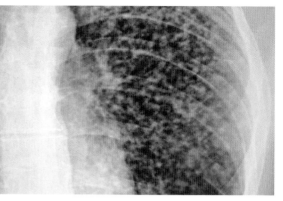

Fig. 6.19. Miliary TB. Multiple small nodules are dispersed through the left upper lobe.

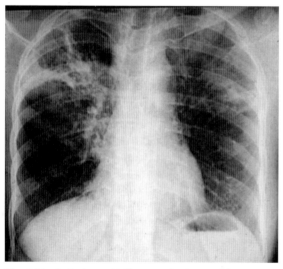

Fig. 6.18. Cavitation and infiltration in both upper lobes. This represents reactivation TB.

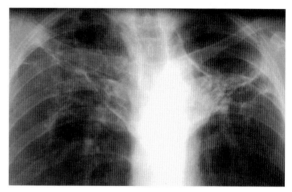

Fig. 6.20. Bilateral upper lobe fibrosis from previous TB.

- Radiographic appearance varies from areas of discrete nodules, an ill-defined single opacity or multiple areas of cavitation. It may be unilateral or bilateral (Fig. 6.18).
- Hilar and mediastinal nodes are rarely involved in secondary TB.
- Upper lobe TB may be difficult to see on standard radiographs, and apical lordotic views that specifically show the lung apices, may better demonstrate pathology.
- CT can also be used to assess the lung parenchyma.

Miliary TB
- This is hematogenous dissemination of TB throughout both lungs fields from rupture of a lung focus into blood vessels.
- There are multiple small nodules (<3 mm) evenly distributed through both lungs (Fig. 6.19).
- Similar appearances may be due to sarcoidosis and occasionally metastases.

Healing of secondary TB
- Complete resolution may occur but, more commonly, as TB heals it leaves areas of fibrous scarring.
- Fibrosis/scarring may be very marked, resulting in significant loss of volume of one or both upper lobes (Fig. 6.20).

Mycetomas
- Cavities may develop in association with fibrosis.
- These may then be colonized by fungi, most commonly, aspergillus, resulting in a mycetoma

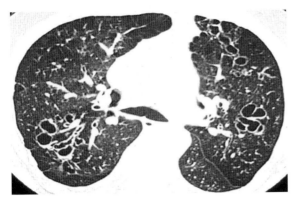

Fig. 6.21. Bilateral bronchiectasis. CT shows multiple cyst-like expansions of the bronchi.

in an upper lobe cavity (mycetomas can develop in any lung cavity).

- Mycetomas can cause repeated hemoptysis.
- Chest radiographs and CT typically show a soft tissue density within a lung cavity. This represents the "fungus ball" caused by secondary infection with aspergillus.

Lung abscess

Abscesses can complicate bacterial pneumonia, and are usually recognized when they contain gas (i.e. a cavity within the lung), often surrounded by consolidation.

Other causes of lung cavitation include:
- TB
- Pyogenic abscess
- Necrotic tumor (primary or secondary)
- Bronchiectasis (usually multiple cavities)
- Septic emboli (e.g. in i.v. drug users)
- Cavitating infarct
- Hydatid

Bronchiectasis
- Bronchiectasis is often visible on chest films but is more reliably detected and its extent better determined by CT (Fig. 6.21).

Atypical infections
- Viral infections, mycoplasma, fungi and other atypical organisms often cause an interstitial pattern of opacity, rather than air space consolidation, sometimes with lymphadenopathy.
- They are important to consider in immuno-compromised patients.

Asthma and chronic obstructive pulmonary disease

Asthma
On chest radiographs, the commonest finding is lung hyperinflation.

Radiology is mainly used to diagnose complications, including:
- Areas of consolidation (infection) and collapse, secondary to mucus plugging
- Pneumomediastinum – air in the mediastinum tracking into the neck
- Pneumothorax – uncommon
- Pulmonary eosinophilia – areas of patchy alveolar consolidation, often changing in size and location on serial radiographs

In suspected asthma, CT can sometimes be helpful to:
- Diagnose mucous plugging and secondary collapse
- Detect bronchiectasis
- Diagnose interstitial lung disease, which may mimic asthma clinically

CT in this setting, and for most diffuse lung diseases, is usually performed using a high resolution CT (HRCT) technique.

Chronic obstructive pulmonary disease (COPD)
A characteristic pathological abnormality in COPD (or chronic obstructive airways disease – COAD) is emphysema, defined as the presence of enlarged air spaces secondary to destruction of alveolar walls.

Chest radiographs in COPD show:
- Increased lung volume (Fig. 6.22)
  - Increase in lung height with flattened diaphragmatic domes
  - Increase in anteroposterior lung dimension – increased retrosternal air space (the area between the ascending aorta and the sternum)
- Bullae, single or multiple, usually with thin walls (Fig. 6.23)
- Enlargement of central pulmonary vessels with sparse peripheral vasculature
- Bronchial wall thickening

109

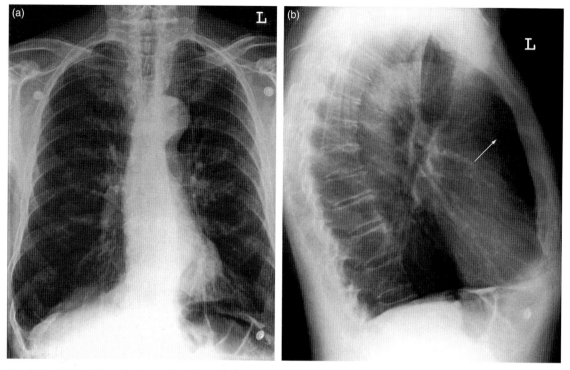

Fig. 6.22. COPD. (a) Note the hyper-inflated lungs with flattened hemidiaphragms, narrow "elongated" mediastinum and, in the lateral view (b), increased retrosternal airspace (arrow).

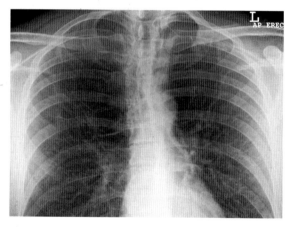

Fig. 6.23. COPD with bullous changes in both upper zones, more obvious on the right, resulting in reduction and displacement of pulmonary vessels.

CT in COPD

HRCT is used to demonstrate areas of emphysema in both lungs. Bullae are well seen, and their size and extent are better appreciated than on radiographs

Nuclear medicine in COPD

- Isotope lung scans have little role in evaluation of COPD.

- When ventilation/perfusion (V/Q) scans are performed for possible pulmonary embolism in patients with COPD, ventilation abnormalities frequently make interpretation difficult.
- The ventilatory phase reflects the emphysema, with accumulation of isotope within the destroyed airspaces, usually matched by corresponding areas of abnormal perfusion (as opposed to mismatched areas seen in pulmonary embolism).

Interstitial lung disease

Chronic interstitial lung processes are usually due to:
- Fibrosis, of which there are many causes
- Lymphangitis carcinomatosis
  Acute interstitial lung processes are usually due to:
- Interstitial edema
- Atypical infections

Radiology of chronic interstitial lung disease

- Most imaging is by chest X-ray and high resolution CT (HRCT).

- The basic radiological finding is an "interstitial pattern" of opacity which is linear, nodular or a combination.
- Associated findings, depending on cause, include:
  - Reduced lung volume in pulmonary fibrosis
  - Pleural plaques and calcification in asbestos-related disease
  - An alveolar component of opacity in acute phases of some types of pulmonary fibrosis, best appreciated on HRCT.

Role of CT in pulmonary fibrosis
- Early changes best assessed with HRCT
- Alveolitis best seen on HRCT
- Monitor progress and response to treatment
- Identify suitable area for biopsy

Causes of pulmonary fibrosis
These include:
- Connective tissue diseases, e.g. scleroderma, rheumatoid arthritis
- Asbestosis
- Idiopathic
- Post-radiotherapy
- Healed tuberculosis
- Healed sarcoidosis
- Ankylosing spondylitis
- Drug-related

The cause may be apparent from the history (drug or industrial exposure) or other clinical features, but biopsy may be required.

Pattern of distribution of pulmonary fibrosis
The distribution of changes may provide clues about the cause:

Predominantly lower lung zones (Fig. 6.24)
- Asbestosis – history of asbestos exposure, pleural plaques or calcification
- Connective tissue diseases
- Idiopathic
  - No systemic condition or predisposing factors
  - Eventually becomes diffuse pattern with loss of lung volume
  - Alveolitis occurs in the active phase

Predominantly upper zone lung fibrosis
- Healed TB (Fig. 6.20)
- Healed sarcoidosis (Fig. 6.25)
- Prior radiotherapy

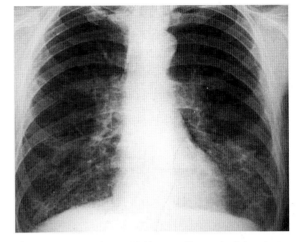

Fig. 6.24. Increased interstitial lung markings at both lung bases due to fibrosis in this case caused by connective tissue disease.

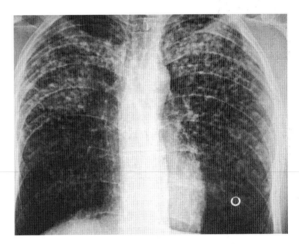

Fig. 6.25. Sarcoidosis with a nodular pattern in mid to upper zones.

- Silicosis
- Ankylosing spondylitis

Pneumoconioses
- These usually result from chronic exposure to certain categories of dust particles, generally occupation related.
- Dust maybe fibrogenic or non-fibrogenic. Silica and asbestos are fibrogenic. Silica and asbestos characteristically lead to symptoms and disability; non-fibrogenic dusts do not.
- Silicosis (often referred to as coal-miner's pneumoconiosis) is lung fibrosis caused by

111

inhalation of silicon dioxide. It occurs in mining, quarrying and tunneling occupations. Some masonry and foundry workers are also at risk. The characteristic radiological appearance includes multiple lung nodules and interstitial fibrosis.

- Pleural plaques and calcifications, fibrosis, and mesothelioma are complications of asbestos exposure.

Lymphangitis carcinomatosis

- Seen most commonly with breast and lung carcinoma
- Usually starts with unilateral involvement
- Associated with poor prognosis, with poor response to chemotherapy

Pleural disease

Pleural fluid may be:

- Effusion
- Blood (hemothorax)
- Pus (empyema)

Pleural effusions

Causes include (*more common causes):

- *Cardiac failure – usually bilateral often larger on right; usually on right if unilateral
- *Infection
- Tumor
    - *Primary lung or metastatic disease
    - Mesothelioma
    - Lymphoma
- Pulmonary embolism
- Subphrenic pathology
    - Subphrenic abscess
    - Pancreatitis
- Esophageal rupture
- Connective tissue disease

Role of radiology

- Confirm suspected effusion.
- Help determine cause, e.g. confirm cardiac failure, detect associated infective consolidation or tumor.
- Provide guidance for diagnostic aspiration or biopsy (usually ultrasound for fluid; occasionally CT for biopsy of suspected pleural tumor).
- Therapeutic drainage for relief of dyspnea, usually under ultrasound guidance.

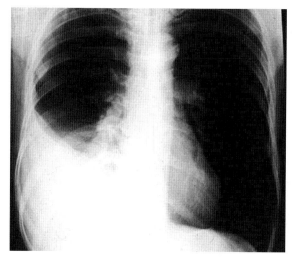

Fig. 6.26. Typical appearance of a moderately large pleural effusion on the right. The upper border of the opacity has a concave upper border.

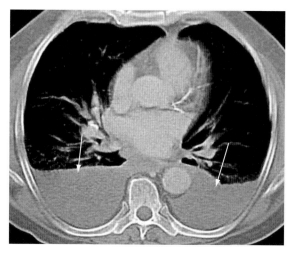

Fig. 6.27. CT with large bilateral pleural effusions (arrows).

Chest radiographs

- An effusion needs to be at least 100 ml in volume before it is seen on a conventional frontal chest radiograph, as the posterior costophrenic angles are more inferior than the lateral costophrenic angles, and fluid usually accumulates in the most dependent posterior portion of the pleural space.
- It typically produces a basal opacity with a concave upper border (meniscus) (Fig. 6.26).

CT and ultrasound

- Both CT and ultrasound can display small pleural effusions (Fig. 6.27), of smaller size than seen on

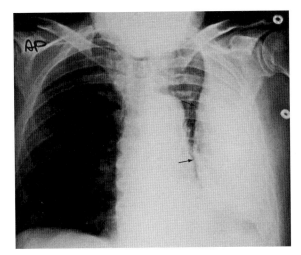

Fig. 6.28. Large left pleural effusion, loculated laterally (arrows).

conventional CXR. Both may be used for guiding aspiration but usually this is easier with ultrasound.

- CT may show the cause of the effusion (e.g. tumor). Ultrasound rarely helps determine the cause.
- If a connective tissue disease is suspected, then high resolution CT can assess the lung for alveolitis and interstitial fibrosis.

Loculated pleural effusions and empyemas

- Loculated pleural collections (Fig. 6.28) may be simple effusions or may be infected (empyema). If aspiration is required, ultrasound guidance is often needed.

Hemothorax

- This is usually from blunt, penetrating trauma, or occasionally iatrogenic trauma (e.g. thoracotomy and central venous catheterization). Occasionally it is spontaneous (e.g. aortic dissection).
- The hemorrhagic nature of pleural fluid may be presumed in trauma, and can be recognized on CT as blood density (higher density than clear fluid)

Pleural tumors

- These are usually malignant, either metastatic or primary mesothelioma. Carcinomas of breast and bronchus are the most common pleural infiltrations.
- Mesothelioma is usually in a background of asbestos exposure. There may, therefore, be changes of asbestos exposure, with pleural

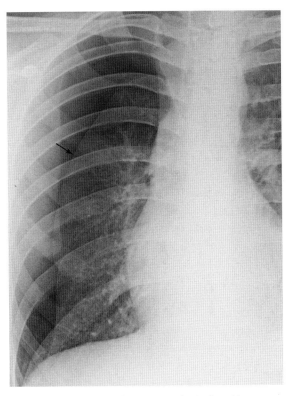

Fig. 6.29. Right pneumothorax. Lung edge indicated by arrow.

calcification and pulmonary fibrosis. Radiographs and CT show irregular solid tissue involving the pleural surfaces.

Pneumothorax

Pneumothorax is the presence of air in the pleural cavity. Common causes include:

- Spontaneous – especially in COPD, asthma
- Trauma
- Following chest procedures, e.g. lung biopsy, pleural aspirations and central venous catheterization.
- Following thoracic surgery.

Chest radiographs

- Most are diagnosed on standard inspiratory chest radiographs. In cases of doubt, expiratory views increase the sensitivity, as there is improved contrast between lung parenchyma and air in the pleural space (Fig. 6.29).

CT

- More sensitive for small pneumothoraces but not often required (Fig. 6.30).

113

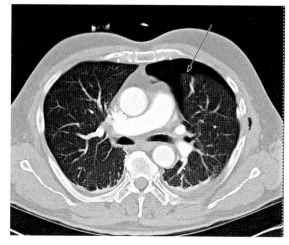

Fig. 6.30. Small left pneumothorax on CT (arrow).

- Most clinically important pneumothoraces are visible on chest radiographs.
- Can be useful in the presence of severe bullous emphysema, where lung markings are very sparse and may mimic a pneumothorax.

Tension pneumothorax
- Occurs when the pneumothorax develops unusually high pressure.
- Can result in almost complete collapse of the entire lung, mediastinal shift away from the side of the pneumothorax, and inferior displacement of the ipsilateral hemidiaphragm (Fig. 6.31).
- Can compress vital mediastinal structures as well as the other lung
- Potentially life-threatening and requires urgent intercostal catheterization

Hydropneumothorax
If pleural fluid is present in addition to a pneumo-thorax, a horizontal straight air fluid level is seen (Fig. 6.32). This is called:
- Hydropneumothorax – if pleural effusion
- Hemopneumothorax – if blood
- Pyopneumothorax – if pus

Pneumothorax and surgical emphysema
- Sometimes air accumulates in the soft tissues of the chest wall and mediastinum, so-called surgical emphysema (Fig. 6.33).

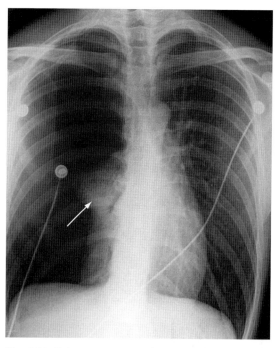

Fig. 6.31. Right tension pneumothorax requiring urgent treatment. The left lung is almost completely collapsed (arrow). The mediastinum is displaced toward the left.

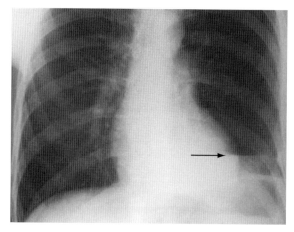

Fig. 6.32. Left hydropneumothorax – note the air fluid level (arrow).

- Usually this occurs following trauma or post-thoracotomy.
- It can make a pneumothorax difficult to see on a chest film.

Lung tumors
Primary lung cancer
- Modes of presentation include pneumonia, cough, hemoptysis, chest pain, symptoms, or

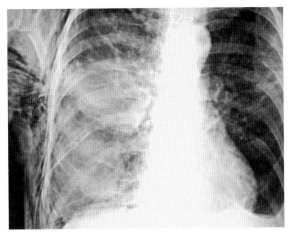

Fig. 6.33. Extensive subcutaneous surgical emphysema, particularly on the right, following a thoracotomy. A right intercostal catheter has been inserted to reinflate the lung. The surgical emphysema obscures a small pneumothorax.

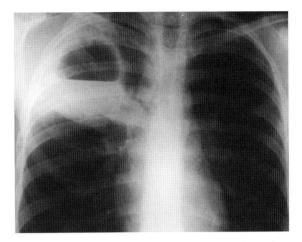

Fig. 6.35. Cavitating squamous cell primary lung cancer. This type is more prone to cavitation and can mimic an abscess.

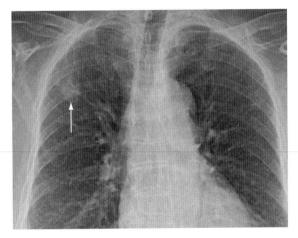

Fig. 6.34. Small right upper lobe primary lung cancer (arrow).

signs of metastatic disease, paraneoplastic syndromes
- Common histological types are small cell, squamous, and adenocarcinoma

Imaging manifestations
- Mass
  - Well-defined or spiculated edges (Fig. 6.34)
  - May cavitate (Fig. 6.35)
  - 7%–10% contain calcification
  - Usually increase in size on serial films, although volume doubling time varies and can be slow
  - Most cancers are initially discovered on chest radiographs

- Pneumonia – it is important to follow up pneumonia with chest films, after infection is resolved, to ensure there is no underlying tumor.
- Lobar collapse
- Pleural effusion
- Hilar and mediastinal lymphadenopathy
- Distant metastases, e.g. bone, adrenal, liver, brain

Staging lung cancer
The TNM classification is routinely used. Useful staging imaging modalities are:
- Chest radiographs – may show, for example, lymphadenopathy or bone metastases
- CT thorax and upper abdomen to assess lungs, mediastinum, chest wall, liver and adrenal glands
- Isotope bone scan for bone metastases
- PET/CT scanning – this has become standard of care

Metastatic tumor and lymphoma
- Metastases and lymphoma typically appear as round/ovoid nodules although lymphoma can have a more varied appearance (Figs. 6.36, 6.37)

Hilar and mediastinal lymphadenopathy
- Hilar and mediastinal lymphadenopathy is most commonly caused by lung cancer spread, lymphoma, or metastases from a distant site.
- Other important causes of lymphadenopathy are primary TB and sarcoidosis (Fig. 6.38)

115

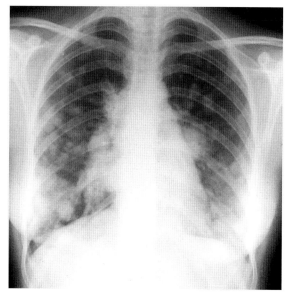

Fig. 6.36. Multiple metastases in both lungs appearing as round soft tissue opacities of varying size.

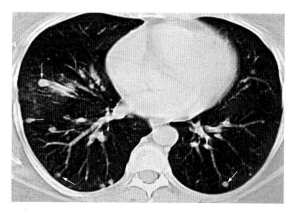

Fig. 6.37. CT shows several small metastases in both lungs (arrows).

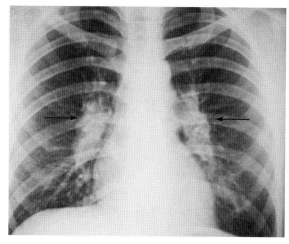

Fig. 6.38. Sarcoidosis with bilateral hilar lymphadenopathy (arrows).

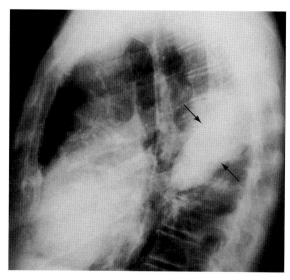

Fig. 6.39. Pleural fluid loculated in posterior oblique fissure (arrows) mimics a mass.

Lymphangitis carcinomatosis
- Occurs with a variety of tumors: commonly lung and breast cancer and appears as a combination of linear and small nodular opacities

Tumor mimickers
- A number of pathologies can mimic tumors on imaging. Some are of no clinical importance; others are important because they require treatment. The more common causes are marked*:
  - Infections
    - Abscesses*

- Atypical infections – including fungal, TB*
- Hydatid
- Loculated pleural fluid* (Fig. 6.39)
- Granulomas*
- Arteriovenous malformations
- Hamartomas
- Round atelectasis
- Pulmonary infarction
- Comparison with old films is often the best way of determining that an opacity is not a progressive tumor (even if the precise nature is not determined).

- CT can be helpful, and sometimes biopsy is required, particularly if old films do not help.

Interventional radiology in the chest
Lung biopsy
- This is usually carried out under CT guidance in patients with a lung mass.
- May be the first attempt to obtain tissue for cytology, histology or microbiology, or be performed if bronchoscopy or sputum cytology have not been diagnostic.

Biopsy of mediastinal masses
- These can also be carried out under CT guidance, to obtain tissue for pathological evaluation. If lung is traversed there is a risk of pneumothorax.
- Occasionally ultrasound may be used for an anterior or superior mediastinal mass.

Aspiration of pleural effusions
- Best performed under ultrasound guidance.
- Pus in the pleural space (empyema) can be drained using either CT or ultrasound.

Complications following chest biopsy and pleural aspiration
The main complications are pneumothorax and hemo-thorax. Hemothorax is quite rare.

Pneumothorax
- Occurs mainly with lung or mediastinal biopsies if lung is traversed, and is uncommon following simple pleural aspirations.
- Occurs in approximately 20% of lung biopsies, but less than 5% require treatment.

- As most lung biopsies are performed with CT guidance, pneumothorax is often immediately visible.
- Occurs more commonly following biopsy of small central lesions than biopsy of peripheral subpleural lesions.
- Higher incidence after multiple passes of the biopsy needle and in patients with COPD (in whom they are also more likely to compromise respiratory function).
- Treated immediately if large or symptomatic, but otherwise observe with follow-up chest radiographs.

Aspiration of pericardial fluid
- This can be performed using CT or ultrasound to drain effusions, pus or hemorrhage from the pericardial sac.

Vascular intervention
Superior vena caval stenting
- Superior vena cava occlusion, stenosis or compression can occur following radiotherapy, chemotherapy with in-dwelling catheters, or from compression by mediastinal nodes.
- It can be managed either by placement of a metallic stent in the case of stenosis, or dissolution of thrombus.
- If acute clot is present on the diagnostic study, thrombolysis can be performed.

Stenting of aortic dissection
- Thoracic aortic dissections (type B) can be managed percutaneously with a prosthetic stent, particularly in patients unfit or unsuitable for open surgical repair.

Trauma and musculoskeletal system

Contents

Fractures – general principles

Evaluating fractures and dislocations

- Initially obtain radiographs in at least two projections, which are usually orthogonal (at right angles to each other). Complex structures may require additional oblique views, or other imaging modalities (e.g. CT).
- For a long bone, the joints on either side of the injury should be included to assess for dislocation and subluxation.
- Traumatic forces applied to a bone are often applied to adjacent joints, thus it is often necessary to include the joints above and below a fracture on radiographs (especially in children).
- Indirect signs (e.g. joint effusion) are useful "flags" for hidden injuries.
- Do not stop looking after finding one injury, as there may be a second, and a third, or more.

How to describe fractures

- Site
  - e.g. diaphysis, metaphysis, intra-articular

- Type
  - Incomplete: e.g. greenstick fracture in children
  - Complete
    - Simple – oblique, spiral, transverse fracture lines
    - Comminuted – more than two fragments
  - Closed – intact skin
  - Open (or compound) – injury in contact with air (may see soft tissue gas or foreign bodies)
  - Avulsion – when the tensile strength of the tendon or ligament exceeds that of adjacent bone
  - Wedge/compression – from axial loading of vertebral bodies (especially in osteoporosis)
- Special types
  - Stress:
    - In normal bone from prolonged or unaccustomed activity; or
    - In weakened (e.g. osteoporotic) bone
    - Plain X-rays are often normal; often diagnosed on isotope bone scan
  - Pathological: occur in abnormal bone (e.g. Paget's, metastasis). Often oriented transversely in long bones
- Degree of deformity
  - The proximal fragment, regardless of size, is the point of reference
  - Displacement – the linear movement of the distal fragment relative to the proximal fragment (medial, lateral, anterior, or posterior)
  - Angulation – the shifting of long axis direction of the distal fragment relative to the proximal-medial, lateral, anterior (ventral) or posterior (dorsal)
  - Rotation – internal or external rotation of the distal fragment
  - Distraction – bone ends are separated
  - Impaction – bone ends are pressed together
  - Overriding – bone ends overlap without impaction

- Involvement of the growth plate (see Figs. 15.14, 15.15, 15.16)
  - Fractures involving the growth plate ("physis" or epiphyseal plate) are classified into five groups (Salter–Harris I–V) that reflect increasing severity and likelihood of longer term complications. Complications include fusion of part or all of the growth plate leading to angulation or shortening.
- Involvement of the adjacent joint (intra-articular extension) – affects treatment and prognosis

"Indirect" signs of fractures
- Soft tissue swelling
- Joint effusion/hemarthrosis
- Intracapsular fat–fluid level
- Obliteration of fat stripes
- Periosteal and endosteal reaction
- Double cortical line
- Cortical buckling

Complications
- Delayed union: no union within a reasonable time
- Non-union: failure to unite
- Mal-union: union in an unacceptable position
- Reflex sympathetic dystrophy: painful osteoporosis with autonomic changes
- Avascular necrosis: death of bone secondary to disrupted blood supply

Stress fractures
- A bone's initial response to repeated mechanical stress is an osteoclastic resorption followed by periosteal and endosteal proliferation that produces new bone, attempting to buttress the weakened cortex. When new bone formation is not rapid enough, there may be bone weakness and "micro-fractures" occur resulting in a stress fracture.
- Initial X-rays are often normal, and follow-up X-rays are diagnostic in only 50% of cases.
- Visible changes include subtle loss of cortical definition, periosteal reaction and a transverse lucent fracture line (Fig. 7.1).
- Radionuclide bone scan and MRI are the most sensitive imaging modalities for detection.

Upper limb fracture and dislocations
Clavicle
- Common in childhood and adolescence
- Most in mid-shaft (80%) or lateral third (15%)

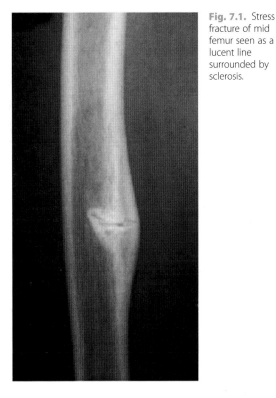

Fig. 7.1. Stress fracture of mid femur seen as a lucent line surrounded by sclerosis.

Scapula
- Described according to anatomic location, e.g. glenoid, body
- Frequently complex
- May require CT for detection or detailed evaluation

Proximal humerus
- Common in the elderly
- Anatomical neck (at articular margin of humeral head)
- Surgical neck (at junction between head and shaft of humerus) (Fig. 7.2)
- Avulsion of the greater or lesser tuberosities also occurs.

Shoulder dislocations
Anterior dislocation
- More than 95% of gleno-humeral dislocations. The humeral head is displaced anteriorly and inferiorly (Fig. 7.3)
- Associated injuries include:
  - Hill–Sacks lesion: compression fracture of the postero-lateral humeral head
  - Bankart lesion: fracture of the anterior aspect of the inferior glenoid rim

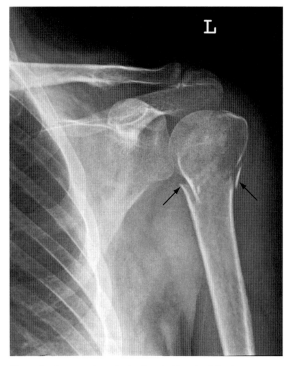

Fig. 7.2. Fracture through the "surgical" neck of the humerus (arrows).

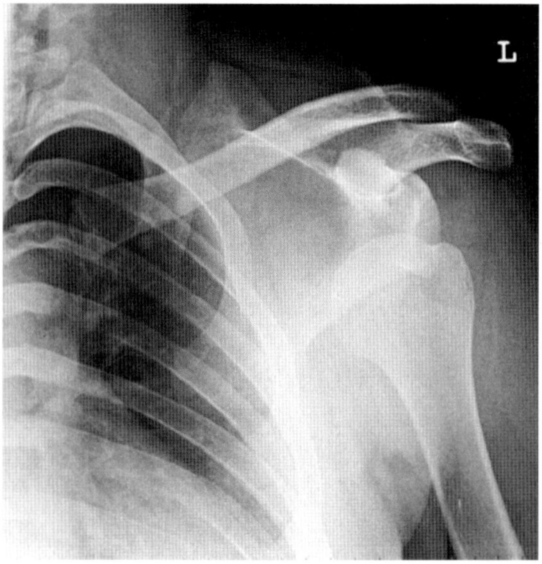

Fig. 7.3. Anterior–inferior dislocation of humeral head (AP view).

Posterior dislocation

- 2%–3% of gleno-humeral dislocations. It usually occurs after direct force to the anterior aspect of the shoulder, or secondary to seizures or electric shock.
- Difficult to diagnose on AP shoulder views, but obvious on tangential or axillary views.
- Compression of the anteromedial humeral head occurs as it impacts on the posterior glenoid rim.

Elbow fractures

- Extra-articular: supracondylar; avulsion of medial and/or lateral epicondyle.
- Intra-articular: trochlear or capitellum, bicondylar fracture, comminuted fracture.
- Between 3 and 10 years of age supracondylar fractures are the most common elbow fracture, and 95% have posterior displacement (hyperextension). In children, knowledge of the normal position and age of appearance of the epiphyses is vital. Comparison views of opposite elbow are helpful.
- Indirect signs such as the "fat pad" sign are important. Because an intra-articular fracture invariably causes an effusion/hemarthrosis, the anterior (initially) and posterior fat pads are displaced away from the bone (Fig. 7.4).

Head of radius

- Usually results from fall onto outstretched arm.
- If there is suspicion of a fracture (e.g. "fat pad" sign) but none is seen, oblique views may help (Fig. 7.4).

Olecranon process

Results from a direct fall onto flexed elbow.

Elbow dislocations
Simple dislocations

- Posterior and postero-lateral dislocations of both radius and ulna account for 80%–90%.
- Radiographs for a suspected ulna fracture should always include views of the elbow to exclude unsuspected elbow dislocation.

Monteggia fracture–dislocation

- Ulna fracture and dislocation of the radial head. This illustrates the importance of imaging wrist and elbow joints in forearm fractures.
- Most have anteriorly angulated ulna shaft fracture, with anterior dislocation of the radial head (Fig. 7.5).

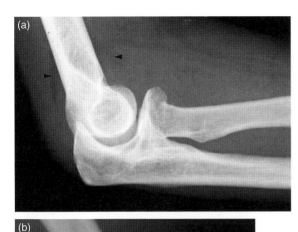

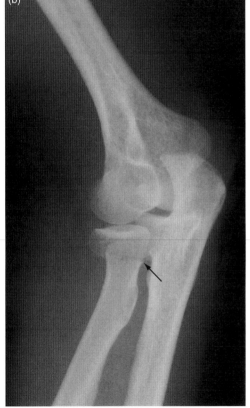

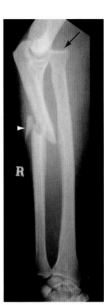

Fig. 7.5. Monteggia fracture. Fracture of ulnar shaft (arrowhead) with dislocation of radial head (arrow).

Fig. 7.4. Elbow (a) Lateral view. Anterior and posterior fat pads are displaced away from the humerus (arrowheads). (b) Oblique view. Non-displaced radial head fracture (arrow).

Forearm, wrist, and hand fractures
Colles fracture
- Usually from a fall onto an outstretched hand. Most common in women over 50 years
- Transverse dorsally angulated distal radius fracture, 2–3 cm from the articular margin (Fig. 7.6)
- Often associated with ulna styloid process fracture.

Smith fracture
Less common than Colles fracture, with volar (anterior) angulation.

Galeazzi fracture–dislocation
Fracture of the distal one-third of the radius, which may involve the articular surface, with dislocation of the distal radio-ulnar joint.

Scaphoid fracture
- Common: 50%–60% of carpal fractures (Fig. 7.7).
- Age range: commonest 5–30 years; after falls onto outstretched hand.
- 70%–80% occur in the scaphoid waist; 15%–20% in the proximal pole.
- As the scaphoid blood supply enters distally, displaced scaphoid fractures have a high risk of subsequent proximal pole avascular necrosis.
- Because of this, and because non-displaced fractures are hard to identify, whenever there is clinical suspicion of a fracture, but no fracture is seen on X-ray, further imaging must be performed, either a repeat X-ray in 10 days (with intervening immobilization), radioisotope bone scan, or MRI.

Carpal bone fractures and dislocations
- Other carpal bones may be fractured or displaced and these injuries may be missed due to bony overlap. CT is useful in complex injuries.

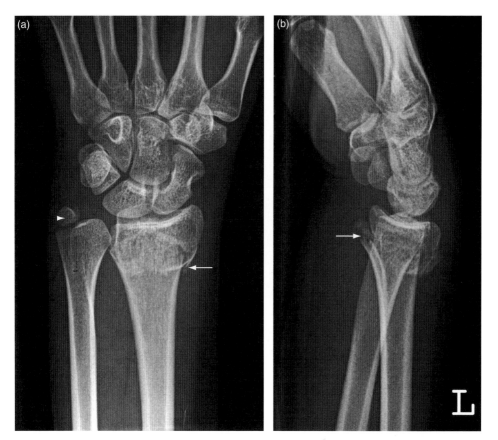

Fig. 7.6. Colles fracture (arrow) of distal radial metaphysis (a) AP and (b) lateral views. Note dorsal angulation of distal radial bony fragment and associated fracture of the styloid process of the ulna (arrowhead).

Bennett fractures
- At base of thumb, with intra-articular component (Fig. 7.8).

Boxer's fracture
- Fracture of metacarpal neck with volar angulation. Commonest in the fifth metacarpal (Fig. 7.9).

Pelvis and lower limb fractures and dislocations

Pelvic fractures
- As the pelvis is a rigid bony ring, if one pelvic fracture is present, a second fracture, or sacroiliac joint disruption, is likely.
- Soft tissue injuries are often associated (e.g. bladder and urethral injuries, and potentially large intra-pelvic hemorrhages).

- Plain radiographs are often supplemented by CT, including 3D reconstructions.
- Isolated fractures of the superior and inferior pubic rami are a relatively common fall injury in the elderly.

Acetabular fractures
- Often require CT for assessment, and to detect intra-articular loose bodies.

Avulsion fractures
Stable fractures which commonly occur in athletes:
- Anterosuperior iliac spine (ASIS): sartorius muscle origin avulsion
- Anteroinferior iliac spine (AIIS): rectus femoris muscle origin avulsion
- Ischial tuberosity – hamstring origin avulsion

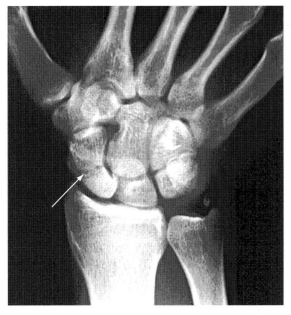

Fig. 7.7. Non-displaced fracture (arrow) of the waist of the scaphoid (AP view).

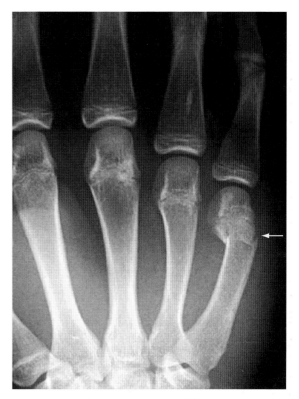

Fig. 7.9. Boxer's fracture through neck of fifth metacarpal (arrow).

Proximal femur fractures

- AP and lateral views are usually adequate, but subtle and/or impacted fractures often require other modalities, e.g. bone scan, CT, or MRI.
- It is important to distinguish:
  - Intracapsular fracture (femoral head or neck) – capital, subcapital, transcervical (Fig. 7.10), or basicervical
  - Extracapsular fracture – intertrochanteric (Fig. 7.11) or subtrochanteric.
- 15%–35% of intracapsular fractures develop avascular necrosis because the femoral head is supplied from the circumflex vessels at the base of the femoral neck. Any intracapsular fracture may disrupt blood supply. Avascular necrosis causes femoral head sclerosis and destruction. With time, the femoral head collapses, causing osteoarthritis and the potential long-term need for joint replacement (Fig. 7.12).

Hip dislocations

- An uncommon injury, often accompanied by other injuries. A high-energy impact is required because the hip is a stable joint.

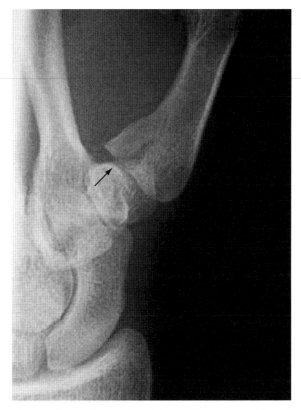

Fig. 7.8. Bennett fracture through base of first metacarpal (arrow) extending into proximal articular surface.

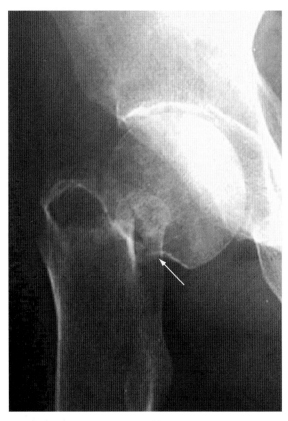

Fig. 7.10. Transcervical fracture of femoral neck (arrow). Note external rotation of femur below fracture.

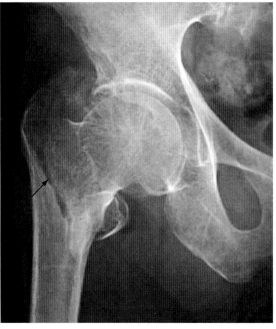

Fig. 7.11. Intertrochanteric fracture of femur (arrow).

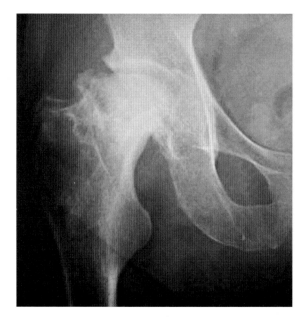

Fig. 7.12. Avascular necrosis (loss of volume and sclerosis) of femoral head and secondary osteoarthritis following femoral neck fracture.

- Posterior: more common than anterior; often associated with fracture of the posterior acetabulum
- Anterior: 5%–20% of dislocations
- Central: medial displacement of femoral head; always associated with fractures (Fig. 7.13)
- The major complications are avascular necrosis and osteoarthritis.

Knee
Distal femur
- Fractures types: supracondylar, condylar or intercondylar

Proximal tibia
- Fractures across the medial and lateral tibial plateaus are commonest, often with rotational displacement or depressed fracture of a tibial plateau (Fig. 7.14).
- CT is often very useful, especially with 2D and 3D reconstructions.
- These fractures are intra-articular. An important indirect sign of such a fracture is a fat blood/fluid interface (lipohemarthrosis) in the supra-patellar pouch (Fig. 7.15).

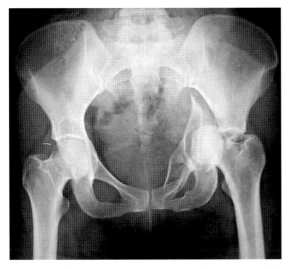

Fig. 7.13. Left acetabular fracture with central displacement of the femoral head.

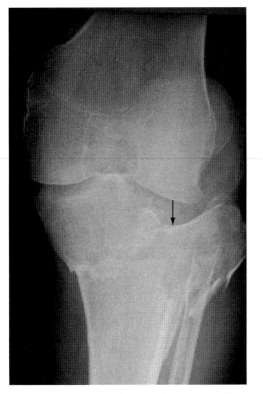

Fig. 7.14. Proximal tibial fracture with depression of lateral tibial plateau fragment (arrow).

Knee dislocation

Significant force is required for complete knee dislocation.

The soft tissue supporting structures are disrupted, with a high incidence of associated fractures.

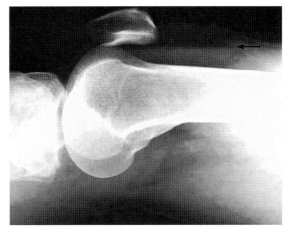

Fig. 7.15. Horizontal shoot-through lateral X-ray knee, which shows a fluid–fluid view (arrow) representing a lipohemarthrosis.

Patella fracture and dislocation

- Fractures are most often transverse or slightly oblique (differential diagnosis is a congenital bipartite or multipartite patella).
- Patella dislocations are usually lateral.

Tibia and fibula

- Mid-shaft tibial fractures are often spiral unless due to a direct blow.
- Associated fibular fracture is common, as the tibia and fibula form a "ring" completed by the proximal and distal tibiofibular articulations. Thus the disruption of one part of this ring commonly leads to fracture or disruption to another component.

Ankle

- Unimalleolar: medial or lateral malleolus (Fig. 7.16)
- Bimalleolar: both malleoli
- Trimalleolar: medial, lateral malleoli and posterior lip of the distal tibia (Fig. 7.17)
- Complex fracture: comminuted fractures of distal tibia and fibula
- Potts fracture: Fracture of distal fibula above the distal tibiofibular joint (syndesmosis)

Foot fractures
Calcaneus

- Relatively common (60% of all major tarsal injuries); 10% are bilateral.
- Often associated with a fall from a height, so associated with vertebral fractures.

125

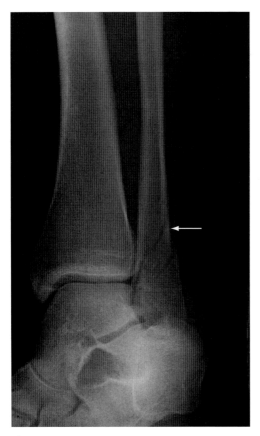

Fig. 7.16. Isolated fracture of lateral malleolus below the distal tibiofibular joint (arrow).

- CT is very useful to assess subtalar joint involvement and the degree of posterior calcaneal articular surface depression.

Talus
- The second most common tarsal fracture
- Often through the talar neck
- Commonly associated with sub-talar and talonavicular joint dislocations

Fracture fifth metatarsal
- Transverse fracture at base of the fifth metatarsal (Fig. 7.18).
- In children/adolescents, do not mistake the longitudinally oriented normal epiphyseal plate at the base of the fifth metatarsal for a fracture.

Dislocations of the ankle and foot
Ankle joint
- Significant force is required to either disrupt the medial or lateral ankle ligaments and the joint

capsule, or fracture across either the medial or lateral malleolus.

Tarso-metatarsal dislocation (Lisfranc fracture–dislocation)
- The most common foot dislocation, often associated with fractures

Head trauma
Radiological modalities of most value are:
- Non-contrast CT: the initial imaging test of choice. There is no role for plain skull X-rays in acute trauma. If a skull fracture is suspected a CT should be performed, as this will detect any relevant complications.
- MRI and angiography – sometimes used in the early subacute setting for suspected arterial dissection, or for prognostic information in diffuse axonal injury.

Extradural hematoma
- This is a surgical emergency
- 95% have an associated skull fracture
- Types:
  - Arterial 90% (middle meningeal artery)
  - Venous 10% (sinus laceration, meningeal vein)
    Posterior fossa: transverse or sigmoid sinus laceration
    Parasagittal: tear of superior sagittal sinus

Radiological features
- 95% unilateral and temporoparietal
- Biconvex, lenticular shape (Fig. 7.19)
- Does not cross suture lines
- May cross dural reflections (falx tentorium) unlike subdural hematoma
- A venous extradural hematoma is more variable in shape and often associated with delayed onset of bleeding.

Subdural hematoma (SDH)
- Caused by traumatic tear of bridging veins
- Not related to skull fractures
  Common in:
- Infants (child abuse; 80% are interhemispheric)
- Elderly patients

Radiological features
- 90% supratentorial
- Crescentic shape along brain surface (Fig. 7.20)

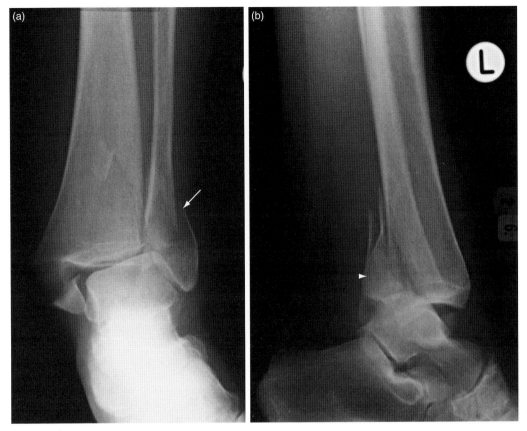

Fig. 7.17. (a) AP and (b) lateral ankle. Trimalleolar fracture involving medial, lateral (arrow) and posterior (arrowhead) malleoli.

- Crosses suture lines
- Does not cross dural reflections
- May see fluid level in subacute and early chronic hematomas
- Acute SDH are hyperdense (<1 week)
- Subacute SDH are isodense (1–2 weeks) and may be difficult to see
- Chronic SDH are hypodense (3–4 weeks), but may have mixed density with rebleeds (Fig. 7.21)

Subdural hygroma
- Acute accumulation of CSF in subdural space after traumatic arachnoid tear

Radiological features
- Crescentic collections of CSF (water) density.
- Does not extend into sulci.
- Vessels cross through lesion.
- Differential diagnosis includes chronic subdural hematoma or atrophy.

Cortical contusions
- Focal brain hemorrhages and edema, secondary to brain impacting on bone, or to rotational forces.
- Lesions evolve with time with delayed hemorrhage occurring in 20%
- Location
  - Anterior temporal lobes 50%
  - Inferior frontal lobes 30% (Fig. 7.22)
  - Parasagittal hemisphere
  - Brainstem

Cerebral herniation
- Mechanical displacement of brain, secondary to swelling, leading to neurological dysfunction and vascular compromise.

Subfalcine herniation
- Cingulate gyrus is pushed under free margin of falx cerebri
- Also described as "midline shift"

127

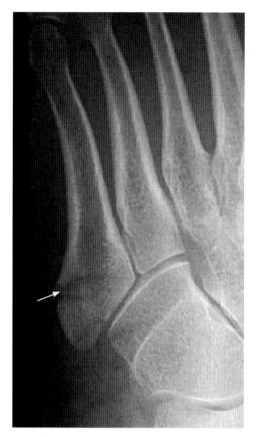

Fig. 7.18. Transverse fracture at base of the fifth metatarsal (arrow).

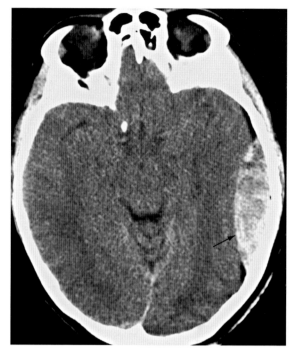

Fig. 7.19. Left temporoparietal extradural hematoma (arrow). Note the biconvex contour of the high density hematoma.

- May result in obstructive hydrocephalus of contralateral lateral ventricle (Fig. 7.20).
- Can cause anterior cerebral artery territory ischemia.

Trans-tentorial herniation
- Uncus/parahippocampal gyrus displaced medially over tentorium
- Duret hemorrhage (anterior midbrain)
- Kernohan's notch (mass effect on peduncle)
- May cause posterior cerebral artery ischemia
- Ascending trans-tentorial herniation occurs from posterior fossa lesions

Tonsillar herniation
- Cerebellar tonsils pushed inferiorly

Diffuse axonal injury
- Axonal disruption from shearing forces of acceleration or deceleration.
- Most commonly in severe head injury, with loss of consciousness at time of injury.

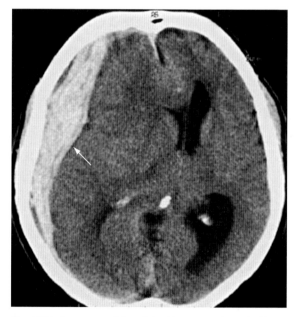

Fig. 7.20. Large acute right subdural hematoma (arrow) with extensive mass effect. Note the subfalcine herniation (midline shift to left), sulcal effacement and compression of right lateral ventricle with contralateral hydrocephalus.

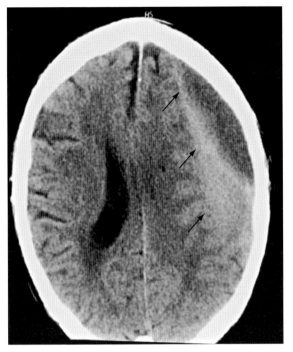

Fig. 7.21. Large left frontoparietal subdural hematoma (arrows) of mixed density indicating acute on chronic hemorrhage.

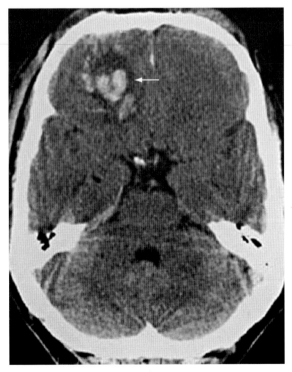

Fig. 7.22. Right frontal parenchymal contusion (arrow) with surrounding edema.

- Initial CT is often normal
- Petechial hemorrhages develop later especially at gray–white matter junction, in corpus callosum and brainstem

Traumatic arterial dissection
- The media of the artery wall splits, creating a false lumen that dissects along arterial wall.
- May be spontaneous or occur after minimal trauma, e.g. sports, spinal manipulations.
- In major trauma it occurs with skull base fractures and shearing injuries, but may be unrecognized until the development of cerebral ischemic complications.
- Sites
  - Extra-cranial internal carotid artery (ICA) – most common
  - ICA within petrous canal
  - Vertebral
- Radiological investigation
  - DSA – rapid, accurate, but invasive
  - MRI – accurate, and detects complications (e.g. acute cerebral infarction), but can be time consuming and difficult in unwell or unco-operative patients
- Complications of dissection – thrombosis, emboli and infarction, false aneurysm

Traumatic carotico-cavernous fistula (CCF)
- Abnormal connection between the internal carotid artery and venous cavernous sinus
- Presents with an ocular bruit, proptosis and chemosis (conjunctival congestion)
- Those caused by trauma are high flow fistulae
- CT may suggest diagnosis. Angiography required for diagnosis and treated via embolization

Facial fractures
- Nasal bone and zygoma are the two most common sites of fractures

Imaging of facial fractures
- Appropriate plain film series depending on suspected site.
- CT used to further characterize fractures (and replaces plain films in major trauma) and for pre-operative assessment (Fig. 7.23). CT can then be used to create reformats including 3D if needed.

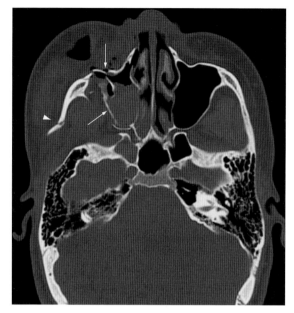

Fig. 7.23. Fractures (arrows) of the anterior and lateral walls of the right maxillary antrum which contains blood, and of the right zygomatic arch (arrowhead). Air is seen in the soft tissues.

- Several different radiographic projections can be obtained.
- Cervical spine must be cleared of injury before obtaining any views that require neck flexion/extension.
- Look for direct signs of fracture such as cortical disruption, bony overlap, and/or displacement.
- Also look for indirect signs, e.g. asymmetry, soft tissue swelling, orbital emphysema, opacity, and air–fluid levels within the paranasal sinuses.

Orbital blow-out fracture
- A direct blow causes sudden increase in intra-orbital pressure, fracturing the orbital floor or, occasionally, the medial orbital wall.
- May present with enophthalmos, diplopia on upward gaze (secondary to inferior rectus entrapment) or paresthesia of the cheek (secondary to infraorbital nerve injury).
- Imaging signs
  - Irregularity of the orbital floor with displaced bony fragments in the maxillary sinus but with intact anterior orbital rim
  - Opacification/air-fluid level in ipsilateral maxillary sinus
  - Intraorbital air

Mandibular fractures
- Most are multiple and bilateral.
- Most occur through body of mandible ipsilateral to the side of injury, with a contralateral fracture of the angle or subcondylar region.
- Can involve the inferior alveolar nerve in its canal.

Zygoma fractures
- Usually at multiple points, often with associated bony depression.
- "Tripod" fracture involves diastasis of zygomatico-frontal suture, posterior zygomatic arch fracture, fracture of inferior orbital rim and lateral maxillary wall.

Maxillary fractures
Dento-alveolar fracture
- Fracture of alveolar process of maxilla secondary to a direct blow.
- May present as loose teeth.
- Managed as an open fracture.

Le Fort fractures
- Occur after severe force, along lines of weakness
- All involve the pterygoid plates of the sphenoid
- CT required for accurate assessment
- Classified as Le Fort Types I–III

Spinal trauma
Plain films are the basic examinations for assessment of spinal trauma. In many centers; however, these now are replaced or supplemented by CT depending on the degree of trauma and imaging resources.

Cervical spine trauma
Plain X-rays
- The most commonly performed screening examination for cervical injury.
- Radiographic evaluation consists of a three- or five-view examination (varies between centers). Anteroposterior, lateral and open mouth dens views are routine, with optional bilateral oblique views to further assess the articular facets.
- A cervical film series is indicated in
  - The presence of cervical pain or tenderness after trauma
  - Patients with neurological signs or symptoms, an altered conscious state, or other injury that may mask a cervical spine injury.

- Trauma patients who are fully alert, with no other injuries, no neurological symptoms, and no cervical pain or tenderness do not require cervical imaging.

Flexion and extension plain films

- Flexion and extension views of the cervical spine are used in limited circumstances. In trauma patients, they are usually only performed when there is a low clinical likelihood of instability, after unstable fractures or serious ligamentous damage have been excluded.
- Movement should be performed actively by the patient under medical supervision, and under no circumstance should the spine be manipulated passively or when the patient is unconscious.
- They are of little use in the acute setting as muscle spasm prevents adequate flexion or extension. The compliant patient is usually discharged in a cervical collar and asked to return 7–10 days after the injury for these views.

Approach to cervical radiographs (refer to Figs. 3.20–3.23)

Lateral views

(1) Count the cervical vertebrae to ensure that the cervicothoracic junction is included. In patients with large shoulders this may be obscured, and a modified view called a swimmer's view is performed (or CT).

(2) Assess the prevertebral soft tissues. They may be widened in cervical injury due to hematoma. This is a useful sign if present, but it is often absent, even when fractures are present, so it should not be relied upon to exclude serious injury.

  - Above C4, the prevertebral soft tissues should measure less than one-third of the anteroposterior width of a vertebral body. Below C4 they can normally measure up to a vertebral body in width.

(3) Assess the three lines of alignment (Fig. 7.24). These are the:

  - Anterior vertebral body line
  - Posterior vertebral body line
  - Spinolaminar line – the line drawn through the base (anterior aspect) of the spinous processes.

    Loss of alignment in any of these lines may be the result of injury and is usually further imaged with CT.

(4) Assess all components of each vertebra individually for evidence of fracture.

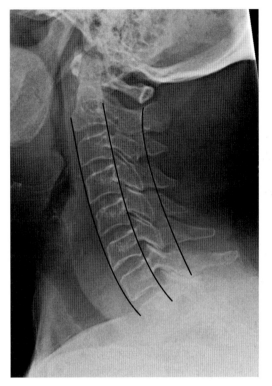

Fig. 7.24. Lateral cervical spine. Three lines should be smooth without a step. Anterior vertebral body line (the most anterior), posterior vertebral body line (middle line), and the spinolaminar line – the line drawn through the base (anterior aspect) of the spinous processes (the most posterior line).

Anteroposterior views

- Assess the individual vertebral bodies, and the alignment of the spinous processes. Unilateral facet dislocation should be suspected if a spinous process deviates abruptly from normal alignment.
- AP "open-mouth" dens view: The dens and the lateral C1–2 facet joints should be visible. This view may be difficult to obtain in intubated patients or patients with facial fractures, and CT may be necessary if the dens and C1–2 facets are poorly seen.
- The dens should be equidistant from the lateral masses of C1 and C2, although allowance must be made for head rotation. Most importantly, the articular surfaces of the C1 and C2 facets must be aligned.
- Finally, the dens should be scrutinized for a fracture.

Oblique views

These are used to assess the laminae. These are projected end-on in the oblique views and should overlap like tiles on a roof.

Computed tomography (CT)

- CT is more sensitive at detecting fractures than radiographs, but is more expensive and has a higher radiation dose. Thus, it has not traditionally been used as a screening investigation.
- In patients at high risk of cervical injury (e.g. high-speed motor vehicle accident), or with associated injuries (e.g. closed head injury and facial fractures) CT is now often performed routinely as the first test.
- CT is also used where needed to assess regions poorly visualized on plain radiographs (e.g. atlanto-axial region or cervicothoracic junction) and to further characterize injuries detected on radiographs.

Magnetic resonance imaging (MRI)

MRI is indicated in all patients with neurological signs following cervical injury.

- Shows soft tissue damage better than CT, e.g. traumatic disk protrusions, ligamentous rupture, extradural hematoma.
- Helpful with prognosis of cord damage. Hemorrhage within the cord indicates a poor chance of neurological recovery.

Cervical injuries

A detailed description of all cervical fractures is beyond the scope of this text. Most commonly, classification is based on a combination of the level and mechanism of injury.

Below is a list of common fractures:

- Jefferson fracture – unstable burst fracture of the atlas (C1) from an axial force (e.g. fall or blow on top of cranium)
- Dens fracture – high or low
- "Hangman's" fracture of C2 – unstable fracture through pedicles and/or posterior body of C2 caused by hyperextension (e.g. forehead hits dashboard) (Fig. 7.25)
- Unilateral facet dislocation – caused by flexion and rotation
- Bilateral facet dislocation – flexion injury
- Vertebral body fractures (Fig. 7.26)
- Articular facet and laminar fractures – hyperextension and rotation injury

Thoracic spine trauma

- AP and lateral radiographs are performed for initial assessment. CT can further characterize

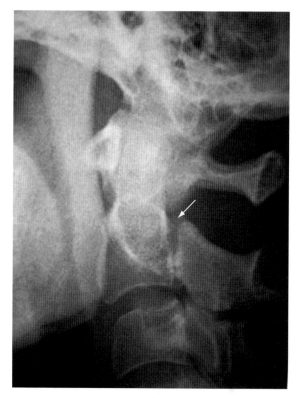

Fig. 7.25. "Hangman" fracture. Defect through the pedicles of C2 (arrow).

detected injuries and better show poorly visualized regions (e.g. upper thoracic spine).

- Fractures of the thoracic spine are less common than cervical or lumbar fractures.
- Because of the stabilizing influence of the thoracic cage, more force is required to cause thoracic fractures. This results in a higher incidence of associated neurological deficit and of fracture dislocations than in the cervical or lumbar regions.
- The presence of a thoracic fracture should prompt a search for further spinal injuries and imaging of the whole spine.

Lumbar spine trauma

- AP and lateral radiographs are performed for initial assessment, supplemented by CT if required.
- Fractures typically involve the upper lumbar or thoracolumbar region.

Injuries are usually classified into four groups:

(1) Wedge compression fractures
   – stable fractures of the anterior vertebral body only.

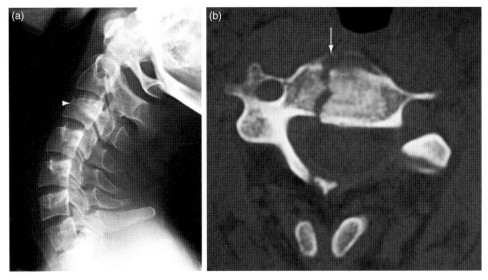

Fig. 7.26. Flexion injury with C3 vertebral body fracture. (a) Lateral view with loss of height of vertebral body anteriorly (arrowhead). Note the absence of significant prevertebral soft tissue swelling. (b) CT shows sagittal fracture line (arrow).

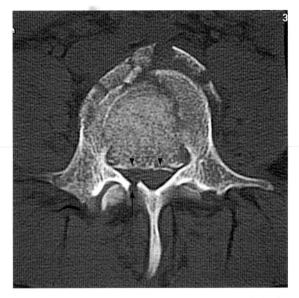

Fig. 7.27. Fracture of body and posterior arch (arrow) of a lumbar vertebra on CT with posterior displacement of a vertebral body fragment (arrowheads) causing central canal stenosis.

(2) Burst fractures
Unstable fractures of the anterior and posterior vertebral body. Fragments can be displaced posteriorly (retropulsed) into the lumbar canal causing neural compression (Fig. 7.27).

(3) Chance fractures
Horizontal fractures typically caused by a lap-belt injury. It is an unstable injury of the vertebral body and the posterior elements. It may be bony or involve only the soft tissues (disk and ligaments). It typically passes horizontally through the vertebral body, and extends posteriorly through the pedicles and spinous process or the interspinous ligament.

(4) Fracture–dislocations
Severe unstable injury with vertebral body and facet joint dislocation.

Chest trauma
Chest trauma can be blunt (e.g. crush injuries), penetrating (e.g. knife wounds) and includes sudden deceleration injuries (e.g. "head on" car accidents).

Chest radiograph
• Plain chest radiographs are used for basic initial imaging assessment and are supplemented by CT depending on the degree of trauma and imaging resources.
• Initial films are performed supine as patients are unwell, and the extent of injury is unknown. They are usually performed on the emergency trolley, sometimes through a spinal board, with clothing, foreign bodies, neck braces and other material on and about the patient. The initial films are often not optimal, but they are necessary to rapidly establish the extent of injuries. May be performed with a mobile X-ray machine or, in some centers, with fixed equipment in emergency department resuscitation bays.

133

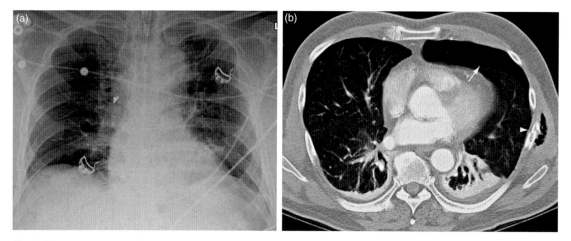

Fig. 7.28. (a) Supine CXR with no detectable pneumothorax. Note the superior mediastinum appears wider on supine films (there was no aortic injury or mediastinal hematoma in this patient). (b) CT in same patient shows left pneumothorax (arrow) and a rib fracture (arrowhead) with overlying localized surgical emphysema.

- Impact of supine films on interpretation – films in major trauma are always supine. A supine projection causes apparent cardiac and superior mediastinal widening, and distends the upper lobe lung veins. The resulting superior mediastinal widening may mimic mediastinal hematoma caused by example by aortic rupture. Small pneumothoraces are difficult to detect in supine films (Fig. 7.28).
- Mechanism of injury, clinical findings and the chest X-ray determine further imaging.

Tubes, catheters, wires
- Patients may require resuscitation with insertion of endotracheal tubes, central lines, and chest tubes before any imaging can be performed, and the position of these should be checked as soon as possible, and to ensure there are no complications, e.g. pneumothorax, hemothorax.

Nasogastric tube (NGI)
- The tip should lie in the stomach, but may coil in the pharynx or esophagus, or pass into a bronchus or even lung parenchyma (Fig. 7.29).

Endotracheal tube (ETT)
- The tip should be approximately 3 cm proximal to the carina (Fig. 7.30).
- If too high, the inflated cuff may damage the vocal chords. If too low, the tube may enter one of the major bronchi and may obstruct bronchial

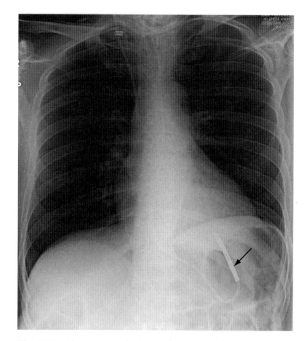

Fig. 7.29. Nasogastric tube in good position with tip in stomach (arrow).

branches and cause partial or complete lobar or contralateral lung collapse (Fig. 7.31).
- Beware of esophageal intubation.

Central venous catheters
- Usually introduced via the subclavian vein or internal jugular vein, with the tip in the superior vena cava close to the junction with the right atrium (overlying the right main bronchus is a useful reference point) (Fig. 7.30).

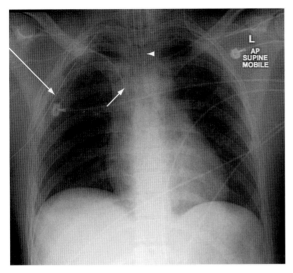

Fig. 7.30. CXR shows ETT tip (arrowhead) in good position above the carina, right subclavian central venous catheter tip (short arrow) in superior vena cava, and right intercostal catheter in the upper hemithorax (long arrow).

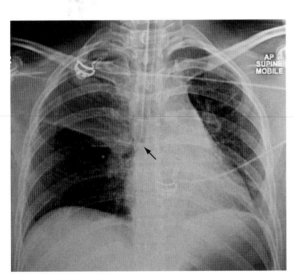

Fig. 7.31. Tip of ETT (arrow) lies in right bronchus causing partial collapse of right upper lobe.

- Introducing a central line in the subclavian or low jugular position may puncture the pleura creating a pneumothorax.

Chest tubes (intercostal catheter)
- Used to drain pneumothoraces.
- Can be placed at the apex (Fig. 7.30) or base of the hemithorax (basal if fluid needs draining). The tubes have an end hole and side holes.

- If a pneumothorax is not draining, it may indicate malposition of the tube, an air leak or ruptured bronchus.

Foreign bodies
- Look for foreign bodies in the lungs, e.g. aspirated teeth. There may be secondary signs such as lung collapse beyond the obstruction.

Bony trauma
Rib fractures
- Common in moderate to severe chest trauma, and best demonstrated by frontal chest film and rib views (obliques), or by CT.
- Fractures of first or second ribs suggest more significant trauma and are associated with mediastinal injury (e.g. ruptured aorta).
- Fractures at two sites in a rib or ribs cause a flail segment, recognized clinically as paradoxical respiratory chest wall movement.

Sternal fracture
- Best seen on lateral chest or sternal X-rays, or on CT. May be associated with cardiac injury/contusion as the force can be transmitted to the heart, and other mediastinal injury (e.g. aortic rupture).

Pleural space
Pneumothorax
- More common with penetrating injuries, or blunt injuries producing rib fractures. Expiratory films may be needed to confirm small pneumothoraces. A small pneumothorax can be difficult to detect on a supine film.

Tension pneumothorax
- After injuring the pleura, a valve effect can occur leading to air being "pumped" from the lung into the pleural space, with resulting high pressure within the pneumothorax.
- Signs of a tension pneumothorax include increased lucency on the side of the pneumothorax, depression of the hemidiaphragm and shift of the mediastinum to the contralateral side.
- Requires urgent insertion of a chest tube.

Hemothorax
- Occurs if there is an associated vascular injury (e.g. trauma to intercostal vessels).
- If there is also a pneumothorax, an air fluid level is visible on horizontal beam X-rays or CT (hemopneumothorax).

135

Lung injuries
Aspiration
- Unconscious patients have an unprotected airway, and vomitus can be inhaled with subsequent radiological changes. These occur relatively rapidly, with fast onset of patchy alveolar opacity, particularly in the lung bases, sometimes with lung collapse.

Pulmonary contusion
- Sometimes associated with rib fracture or pneumothorax.
- Seen on initial imaging in the lung parenchyma appearing as airspace opacity caused by hemorrhage.

Mediastinal injuries
These are life-threatening and include:
- Ruptured aorta
- Ruptured bronchus
- Esophageal injury
- Cardiac injury

Aortic rupture
The aortic arch is anchored at the level of the aortic valve, and distally at the ligamentous arteries. In high velocity deceleration injuries, the arch can flex forward causing a shearing force, leading to partial or complete rupture of the aorta, usually at the junction of the arch and descending aorta. Intima and media are torn but the adventitia remains intact. Signs on chest X-ray are:
- Widened mediastinum (ideally requires an erect film, but usually not possible in severe trauma) (Fig. 7.32).
- Loss of normal silhouette of aorta.
- Associated fractures – first or second ribs, sternum.
- Left pleural fluid.

If there is widening of the superior mediastinum in the setting of major chest trauma, then aortic imaging (usually CT angiography now, rather than conventional angiography) is required (Fig. 7.33).

Diaphragmatic rupture
- Results in apparent elevation of the hemidiaphragm, often with rib fractures, and sometimes with stomach or bowel herniation into the chest (Fig. 7.34).
- CT can be helpful in further assessing diaphragm injuries.

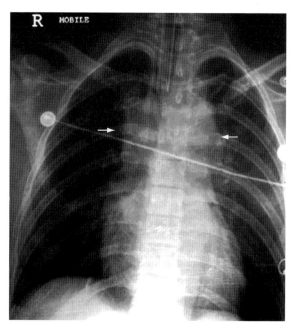

Fig. 7.32. Supine chest film shows widening of the superior mediastinum (arrows) caused by ruptured aorta. ETT is in place.

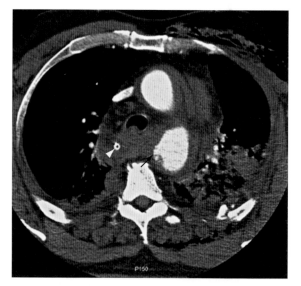

Fig. 7.33. CT angiography (transverse section). Rupture of distal aortic arch (arrow). The esophagus which is marked by a nasogastric tube (arrowhead) is displaced by mediastinal hematoma to the right. Note left lung contusion and left surgical emphysema.

Bronchial and esophageal injuries
- Less common injuries that can both lead to gas within the mediastinum (pneumomediastinum).

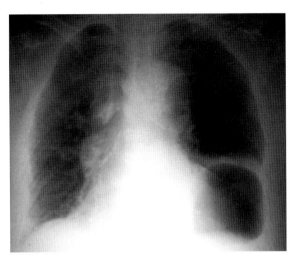

Fig. 7.34. Rupture of left hemidiaphragm. Stomach has herniated through a ruptured left hemidiaphragm producing apparent diaphragmatic elevation.

Abdominal trauma

- Approximately 10% of trauma deaths are from abdominal trauma.
- CT has reduced the morbidity and mortality from abdominal injuries, and markedly reduced the rate of non-therapeutic laparotomy as it allows rapid, accurate assessment of solid organ and hollow viscus injury.
- CT accurately detects hemoperitoneum and free gas, and assesses injuries of the spleen, liver, gallbladder, kidneys, pancreas, bowel, diaphragm, abdominal vessels, spine, and bony pelvis.
- CT has largely replaced abdominal X-rays and IVP in trauma. It may be modified to diagnose bladder injury, although a urethrogram and cystogram are preferred in many centers. Pelvic X-ray is still performed in the initial radiographic survey along with a supine lateral cervical spine and chest X-ray.

CT procedure

- In hemodynamically stable abdominal injuries, abdominal CT is routine. Modern technology has reduced scan times, resulting in a greater proportion of patients deemed stable enough for CT.
- Bowel contrast is often administered orally or via NGT shortly before the scan to improve detection of bowel injury.
- Intravenous contrast is given routinely. Active bleeding is seen as dense contrast extravasation around an organ or vascular structure. It may

occur from spleen, liver, kidneys, bowel, mesentery and pelvic fractures, and is an indication for urgent laparotomy or angiographic arterial embolization.
- In major trauma, the head, spine, and chest may also be scanned during the same examination, if clinically appropriate.

Portable ultrasound

- Unstable patients who cannot be transferred may undergo portable ultrasound in the emergency department. This is frequently referred to as Focused abdominal sonography in trauma (FAST) ultrasound. Its main aim is to detect free intraperitoneal blood.
- It accurately detects hemoperitoneum (indirect evidence of organ injury), but is very much less accurate than CT in demonstrating the actual organ injury. It does not reliably detect free gas. The accuracy of ultrasound is greatly influenced by operator experience.
- Hemodynamically unstable patients may undergo laparotomy without CT if the source of bleeding is thought to be intra-abdominal and if CT cannot be performed quickly.

Splenic injury

- The most commonly injured abdominal organ.
- Should be suspected in trauma to the left upper quadrant and in patients with left-sided rib fractures.
- Injuries include subcapsular hematoma, contusion, laceration, fragmentation and major vascular injuries (Fig. 7.35).
- CT is highly accurate
- Hemoperitoneum is often but not always present, which represents a potential shortcoming of ultrasound.
- The size of hemoperitoneum, age of the patient, and type of injury affect the decision to conserve the spleen, which is now preferred to splenectomy. Patients with massive splenic lacerations, active bleeding and a large hemoperitoneum, and elderly patients, are all more likely to require splenectomy.

Liver injury

- The second most commonly injured abdominal organ.
- Injuries are described in the same way as splenic injuries but in addition, the biliary tree, and the

137

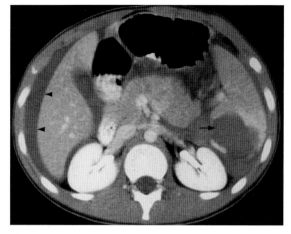

Fig. 7.35. CT with i.v. and oral contrast. Splenic laceration (arrow) is associated with a hemoperitoneum seen around the spleen and liver (arrowheads). Note the normal enhancement of the kidneys.

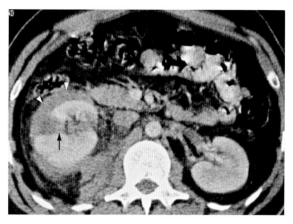

Fig. 7.36. Right renal laceration (arrow) associated with a small perinephric hematoma (arrowheads). The renal parenchyma enhances normally (intravenous and oral contrast have been given).

hepatic arteries and veins may be injured. Associated hemoperitoneum and active bleeding are common.

- Right-sided liver injuries are associated with right chest, right kidney, and spinal column injuries.
- Left-sided liver injuries result from midline trauma, which may also cause pancreatic, small bowel, duodenal and transverse colonic injuries.

Gallbladder injury
- Uncommon and usually from penetrating trauma or severe blunt trauma.
- Gallbladder may perforate or be partly or completely avulsed from the gallbladder fossa or biliary tree.

Bowel and mesenteric injury
- Relatively uncommon, but important to recognize because of the risk of intra-abdominal hemorrhage and peritonitis if untreated.
- The commonest sites include jejunum near its attachment at the ligament of Treitz, duodenum and colon.
- Large mesenteric tears can cause devascularization and bowel ischemia.
- Usually evident on CT and most commonly manifests as free fluid. Free gas and extravasated oral contrast are very specific, but are not always present.
- Usually a result of blunt force to the midline (commonly the steering column of a car) causing

a "blow-out" rupture of the bowel, or a shearing injury to the mesentery or bowel wall from a seat or lap-belt. The latter is also associated with Chance fractures of the lumbar spine.

Renal injury
- Renal injuries are common and are usually contusions or lacerations (Fig. 7.36).
- Most injuries, including rupture of the collecting system, are managed conservatively. Active bleeding and renal artery injury are usually evident on CT and can be treated angiographically or surgically.
- If CT is unavailable, an intravenous pyelogram (IVP) can confirm the presence of functioning (and hence perfused) kidneys, and demonstrate integrity of the renal parenchyma and collecting system. IVP should only be performed in centers with no access to CT.

Bladder and urethral injury
- Bladder rupture may be extraperitoneal (90%) or intraperitoneal (10%).
- Extraperitoneal rupture into the perivesical tissues usually results from laceration by the bony fragments of a pelvic fracture. This is usually managed conservatively.
- Intraperitoneal rupture occurs following a sudden increase of intraperitoneal pressure on a full bladder. The bladder wall usually fails at the dome, and the defect is repaired surgically.

- Diagnosed either by conventional cystography (radio-opaque contrast is introduced retrogradely via the urethra), or with a CT cystogram, where the bladder is filled with contrast prior to the examination.
- Urethral injuries are more common in males, and are usually associated with pelvic fractures.
- Blood is present at the external urethral meatus and the prostate may be displaced superiorly by the hematoma.
- If there is high likelihood of urethral injury an in-dwelling catheter should not be passed until injury has been ruled out with a retrograde urethrogram. This may be performed in the emergency department or in the fluoroscopy room, in conjunction with a cystogram (X-rays are performed whilst radio-opaque contrast is passed into the urethra via a catheter in the external meatus).

Pancreatic injury

- Pancreatic injuries are uncommon.
- Usually the injury is anterior to the lumber spine and results from severe midline blunt trauma that also causes injuries to other organs, e.g. liver, spleen, duodenum, and may be associated with lumbar spine injury.
- Transection of the pancreatic duct is treated surgically, as are severe pancreatic lacerations.
- Duct injury can be difficult to recognize on CT and may be confirmed with MRCP or ERCP.
- If unrecognized, recurrent pancreatitis, pseudocyst, and abscess may result.

Bone tumors

Bone tumors can be classified into benign or malignant depending upon:

- Differentiation/anaplasia
- Growth rate
- Local invasion
- Metastases

Malignant tumors are sub-classified into:

- Primary – tumors of local tissue origin
- Secondary – malignant transformation of benign processes, e.g. Paget's disease
- Metastatic – tumors that have spread from an adjacent or distant source

Both "benign" and "malignant" tumors are categorised according to cell of origin:

- Bone origin (osteogenic)
- Cartilaginous origin (chondrogenic)
- Fibrous origin (fibrogenic)
- Miscellaneous bone tumors

Radiologically, the site, margins, matrix, presence of additional lesions, and age of patient are important in distinguishing between aggressive and non-aggressive tumors.

The most important distinction is the difference between benign and malignant lesions. In general, if a lesion is well defined with a sharp sclerotic margin, it is likely to be "benign." If it is less well defined, particularly if there is a permeative moth-eaten appearance, malignancy is likely.

Some tumors have a specific appearance, and with appropriate imaging, a specific diagnosis can be made. If a lesion is typically benign on X-ray, a tissue diagnosis is not necessary. Others appear less characteristic and require biopsy.

Some tumors are not easily characterized by either radiology or pathology, and require correlation between both for a diagnosis.

Detailed review of the many types of bone tumors is beyond the scope of this text. Several specific tumors and tumor-like conditions are discussed below.

Benign bone lesions – osteogenic
Osteoma

- Slow-growing
- Common sites: outer table of skull vault, frontal and ethmoidal sinuses
- Age: fourth–fifth decades
- Dense ivory-like, sharply demarcated
- Usually asymptomatic, incidental finding

Osteoid osteoma

- 75% have nocturnal localized pain relieved by aspirin
- Age: 10–35 years, especially long bones (femur, tibia)
- Central lucent nidus <1 cm in size, with surrounding reactive bone formation (sclerosis) (Fig. 7.37)
- Seen on X-rays but more obvious on CT
- Marked radioisotope uptake on bone scan
- Treatment: excision of nidus

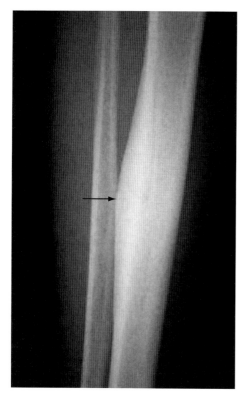

Fig. 7.37. Osteoid osteoma of tibial shaft. Note localized pronounced thickening of cortex (arrow). A central lucent nidus is not apparent in this case.

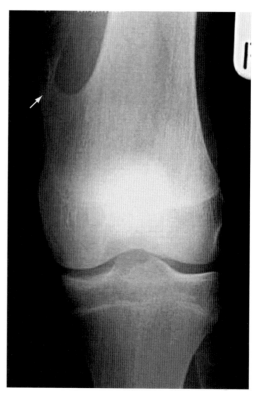

Fig. 7.38. Osteochondroma of distal femur (arrow).

Benign bone lesions – chondrogenic
Enchondroma (chondroma)
- 10% of benign tumors
- Within medullary cavity, mostly in phalanges and metacarpal bones
- Age: second–fourth decades
- Often asymptomatic until pathological fracture occurs
- Lucent, with scalloping of the inner cortical margins
- May contain calcification

Osteochondroma (osteocartilaginous exostosis)
- Commonest benign bone lesion
- Age: under 30 years
- A cartilage capped bony extension from the bone surface
- Mostly at metaphyses of long bones, around knee and proximal humerus (Fig. 7.38)
- Often pedunculated

Other benign bone tumors
Fibrous cortical defect/non-ossifying fibroma (NOF)
- Common
- 30% of all children and adolescents; males > females
- Especially long bones: femur, tibia
- Usually asymptomatic
- Most require no treatment
- Lucent, elliptical, within cortex near growth plate, sclerotic margin

Simple bone cyst (unicameral bone cyst)
- Tumor-like lesion of unknown aetiology
- Mostly in males
- Age: first and second decades
- Majority in proximal diaphysis of humerus and femur
- Usually treated by curettage and bone graft
- Lucent, centrally located, well-circumscribed, sclerotic margins
- May present with pathological fracture (Fig. 7.39)

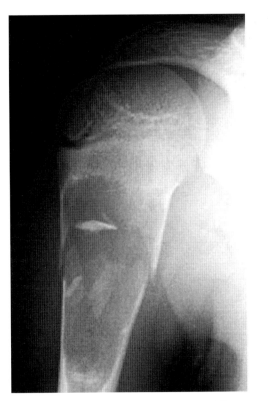

Fig. 7.39. Pathological fracture through a simple bone cyst in proximal humerus.

Medullary bone infarct
- Irregular calcifications surrounded by a sclerotic margin
- In medulla of long bones

Myositis ossificans
- Post-traumatic heterotopic bone formation in soft tissues
- Can mimic osteosarcoma on both X-rays and histology

Brown tumor of hyperparathyroidism
- Contains decomposing blood, and is "brown" in color when cut
- Occurs in secondary hyperparathyroidism
- Single or multiple
- Often poorly defined; mimic aggressive tumors.

Associated imaging findings of hyperparathyroidism:
- Osteopenia (decreased bone density)
- Sub-periosteal bone resorption (especially radial aspect of the second and third fingers)
- Granular "salt and pepper" appearance of skull vault
- Re-absorption of acromial ends of clavicles
- Soft tissue calcification

Hemangioma
- Uncommon and treatment generally not required
- Incidence increases with age: occurs mostly in elderly, with female preponderance (2:1)
- Mostly vertebral body appearing as coarse vertical striations (often incidental)

Non-neoplastic lesions simulating tumors
Langerhans cell histiocytosis (eosinophilic granuloma)
- A disorder of immune regulation (a reticuloendotheliosis)
- Mostly children aged 5–10 years
- Appearance mimics more aggressive tumors
- Single or multiple
- Common sites: skull, ribs, pelvis, spine, long bones
- "Punched-out" appearance, well-defined margins (skull)
- Radiolucent, often with periosteal reaction in long bones, similar to malignant bone tumors, e.g. Ewing's sarcoma.

Malignant bone tumors – osteogenic
Osteosarcoma
- 20% of primary malignant bone tumors.
- May arise de novo (most are in this category) or secondary to other pathology such as Paget's disease, fibrous dysplasia, radiation exposure.

Conventional (de novo) osteosarcoma
- Most frequent type
- Age predominance: second decade
- Males more often than females
- Predilection for knee region (distal femur, proximal tibia), and proximal humerus (Fig. 7.40)
- Presents with pain and a soft-tissue mass
- Cortical and medullary bone destruction with aggressive periosteal reaction
- Abnormal new bone formation
- Most have combined lucency and sclerosis, with an indistinct border

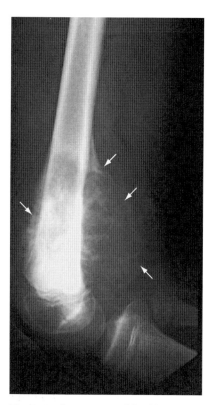

Fig. 7.40. Osteosarcoma of distal femur (lateral view). There is bone destruction and new bone formation within the femoral shaft, as well as new bone formation in the tumor mass extending outside of the femur (arrows).

Malignant bone tumors – chondrosarcoma
- As with osteosarcoma these can arise de novo or be secondary to other pathology.

Primary chondrosarcoma
- Slow growing
- Age: after third decade, M:F = 2:1
- Pelvis, long bones (femur and humerus)

Miscellaneous malignant bone tumors
Fibrosarcoma and malignant fibrous histiocytoma
- Age: third–sixth decades
- Femur, humerus, tibia

Ewing sarcoma
- Highly malignant
- Mostly children, male predominance
- Pelvis, long bones (femur and humerus)
- Diaphysis of long bones, ribs, scapula, pelvis

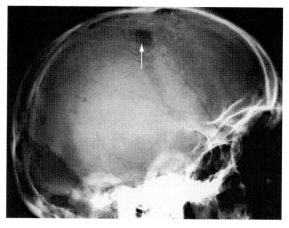

Fig. 7.41. "Punched out" lesions of skull in myeloma. Large lesion in occiput and smaller lesion in parietal bone (arrow).

- Poorly defined, permeative (moth-eaten) pattern
- Aggressive periosteal reaction ("onion-skin" or "sunburst"-like)

Myeloma (multiple myeloma or plasmacytoma)
- Originates in bone marrow
- The most common primary malignant bone tumor
- Age: fifth–seventh decades, males more often than females
- Axial skeleton (skull, spine, ribs and pelvis) most common but can affect any bone
- May be solitary (plasmacytoma), but more often widespread at presentation
- Lytic lesions, usually without sclerosis or periosteal reaction
- Diffuse osteopenia (loss of bony density) or multiple fractures in vertebral bodies
- "Punched out" lesions in the skull (Fig. 7.41)
- "Lace-like" lesions in ribs
- Medullary bone destruction in flat bones

Metastatic bone disease
- Metastases represent the most frequent malignant tumor found in bone, so always consider this diagnosis when assessing an aggressive-appearing bone lesion, especially in the elderly
- Predominantly in axial skeleton (skull, spine and pelvis) and proximal long bones
- Spread to bone is usually hematogenous
- Common primary sources include:

- Breast, lung, prostate (kidney, bowel, stomach, and thyroid)
- Prostate carcinoma – comprises 60% of bony metastases in males
- Breast carcinoma – comprises 70% of bony metastases in females
- Osteolytic (radiolucent) – kidney, breast, lung, thyroid, stomach, colon (Fig. 7.42)
- Sclerotic (radiodense) (Fig. 7.43)
  - Males – prostate, seminoma, neurogenic, carcinoid, osteosarcoma
  - Females – breast, uterus, ovary, neurogenic, carcinoid, osteosarcoma

Paget's disease

- Paget's disease is of unknown etiology. It affects the middle-aged and elderly, more often males and Caucasians.
- Any bone can be involved.
- There are two phases:
  - Hyperemic: increased blood flow and active bone removal, causes radiolucency (e.g. "flame-shaped" lucency in long bones).
  - Sclerotic: disorganized new bone formation causes bone enlargement, increased density, trabecular prominence, and loss of cortico-medullary definition.

Long bones

- In long bones, Paget's typically commences in a subarticular position
- With time, as bones become softer, deformities and bowing occur (Fig. 7.44).
- New bone formation is disorganized, so bones become brittle, with increased risk of pathological fractures (Fig. 7.45). The abnormal bone can delay fracture healing and cause non-union.
- Increased tensile stresses in long bones can lead to incremental (stress) fractures.

Skull

- Lytic and sclerotic phases may co-exist (Fig. 7.46).
- Increasing head circumference is typical.
- Facial bones are rarely involved.
- Involvement of the skull base can cause softening and "basilar invagination" (upwards indentation of the skull base). With the bony thickening, this may produce neurological changes including cranial nerve palsies.

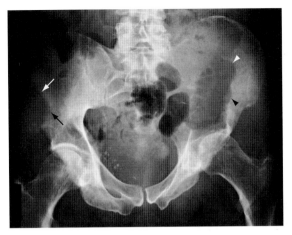

Fig. 7.42. Osteolytic (radiolucent) metastases in left pelvis (arrowheads) and right pelvis (arrows).

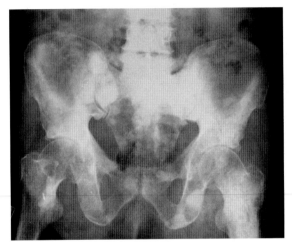

Fig. 7.43. Osteoblastic (radiodense) metastases from prostatic carcinoma. Note multiple sclerotic (dense) lesions in pelvic bones, sacrum, upper femora, and lumbar vertebral bodies.

Spine and pelvis

- Paget's disease involves any part of a vertebra. The vertebral body becomes enlarged and sclerotic with prominent trabeculae. This can result in vertebral canal stenosis
- The pelvis is commonly involved (Fig. 7.47).

Complications of Paget's disease

- Bone softening and deformity
- Pathological fractures
- Osteoarthritis secondary to deformed articular surfaces.
- Sarcomatous change – osteosarcomas occur in 1%.
- High output cardiac failure – may occur with severe widespread involvement causing bone hyperemia.

143

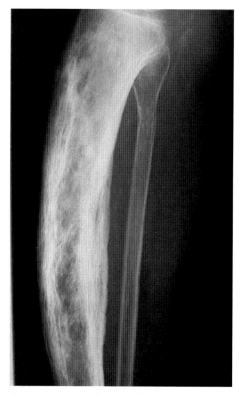

Fig. 7.44. Advanced Paget's of tibia (lateral view) with "saber shin" bowing deformity.

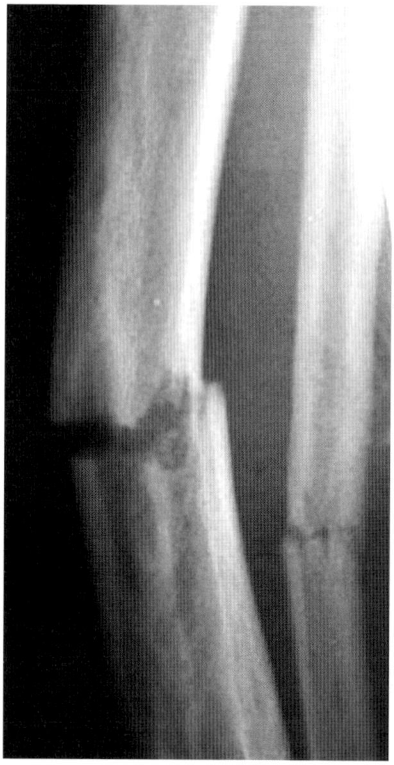

Fig. 7.45. Paget's of tibia and fibula with pathological transverse fractures.

Arthritis
Osteoarthritis

- Osteoarthritis (OA) is the commonest form of arthritis
- Occurs with advancing age, and repeated physical stress on joints
- Affects both large and small joints
- The hip and knee are most commonly affected
  The disease is characterized by:
- Articular cartilage loss followed by
- Bone repair, with osteophyte formation.

It can occur secondary to another underlying primary arthropathy, e.g. inflammatory arthropathies, avascular necrosis, trauma, neuropathic disorders.

Hip

- In both primary and secondary osteoarthritis, the hip is most commonly affected. The earliest radiographic change is apparent loss of joint space (thinning of the articular cartilage).
- Osteophytes develop and occasionally become large exostoses. The subarticular bone becomes

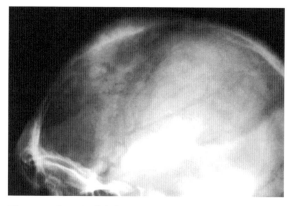

Fig. 7.46. Paget's of skull vault with mixed lucency and sclerosis, and vault thickening. The base of the skull is spared.

sclerotic (dense), with subarticular cysts developing (Fig. 7.48). In severe cases, these changes can lead to avascular necrosis.

Knee

- Apparent loss of joint space (cartilage loss), periarticular osteophytes, subchondral sclerosis and subarticular cysts

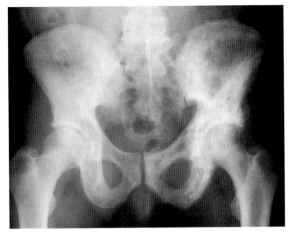

Fig. 7.47. Paget's disease of the left hemipelvis, with expanded bone and coarsened trabecular pattern.

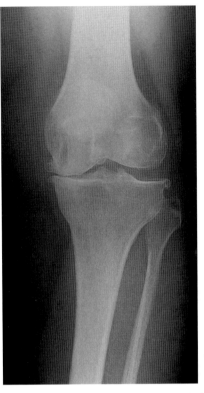

Fig. 7.49. Osteoarthritis of knee. AP weight-bearing view shows loss of joint space in medial compartment (with resulting varus deformity), periarticular osteophytes, and subarticular sclerosis.

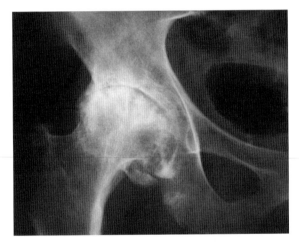

Fig. 7.48. Osteoarthritis of hip. Loss of joint space, especially in the superior weight-bearing aspect, with subarticular sclerosis and marginal osteophytes.

- Loss of articular cartilage is generally worse in the medial joint space (the more weight-bearing region), leading to a varus deformity. Weight-bearing (erect) views are helpful for displaying joint space (cartilage) loss (Fig. 7.49).
- Fragments of bone from the joint surface can form intra-articular loose bodies. These can accelerate the degenerative process.

Hands
- The thumb base (first carpometacarpal joint) and distal interphalangeal (DIP) joints are most affected (Fig. 7.50).

Gout
- A metabolic arthropathy which characteristically involves the first metatarsophalangeal joint of the foot, and occurs most often in middle-aged and elderly males.

Radiological Findings
Erosions
- Due to uric acid deposition
- Appear at joint margins, and "undercut" the articular cortex, and have a "punched out" appearance (Fig. 7.51).
- In severe gout, the bone can be completely resorbed.
- In the hand, gout tends to involve the distal interphalangeal joints, unlike rheumatoid arthritis, which affects the metacarpophalangeal and proximal interphalangeal joints.

Cartilage destruction
- A late finding (unlike rheumatoid), with bone destruction preceding cartilage loss

145

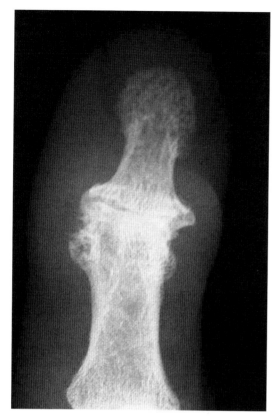

Fig. 7.50. Typical osteoarthritis changes at the distal interphalangeal joint (Heberden's nodes would be evident clinically).

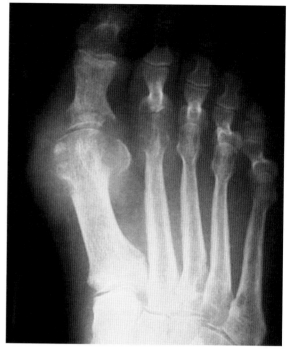

Fig. 7.51. Gout – erosions at margins of first and second metatarsophalangeal joints.

Osteoporosis
- Only if joint is immobilized (unlike rheumatoid)

Tophi
- Soft tissue swellings that can calcify (rheumatoid nodules do not calcify)

Rheumatoid arthritis (RA)
- Rheumatoid arthritis (RA) is an autoimmune disease characterized by a symmetrical inflammatory polyarthritis, particularly affecting small joints.

Hand and wrist (and equivalent joints in feet)
- Typically metacarpophalangeal joints
- Soft tissue swelling is the earliest finding, then periarticular osteoporosis
- Bony erosions develop at margins of the articular cartilage (Fig. 7.52)
- Progressively, cartilage and bone are destroyed, and marked resorption of the bones may occur
- Hand deformities include the "boutonnière" and "swan neck" deformities of the fingers, and ulnar

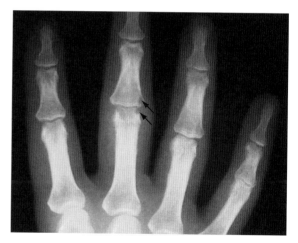

Fig. 7.52. Rheumatoid arthritis. Erosions at articular margins of the proximal interphalangeal joint of middle finger (arrows). Note soft tissue swelling and periarticular osteoporosis around the joint.

deviation/subluxation at the metacarpophalangeal joints (Fig. 7.53)
- Ulnar styloid resorption is typical
- Tendon sheath involvement may cause tendon rupture, e.g. extensor carpi ulnaris
- Ankylosis (joint fusion) can occur late

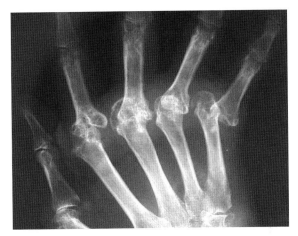

Fig. 7.53. Rheumatoid arthritis with ulnar deviation/subluxation at the metacarpophalangeal joints.

Elbow
- Common site
- Soft tissue abnormalities occur earliest, e.g. olecranon bursitis, joint effusion
- Later periarticular erosions and joint space loss occur leading to joint derangement

Shoulder
- Both glenohumeral and acromioclavicular joints can be involved
- Soft tissue involvement may cause rotator cuff rupture
- Cartilage loss leads to loss of joint space followed by erosions
- Bone erosions cause resorption of the distal clavicle.

Hip
- Cartilage loss with loss of joint space is the earliest finding
- Periarticular erosions occur later
- This process leads to medial displacement of the femoral head
- Osteoporosis and avascular necrosis can result from steroid therapy, and typically complicate severe disease

Knee
- Joint effusions are common, along with cartilage loss
- Erosions can develop at the periphery of the articular surfaces
- Baker's cysts due to the inflammatory process are relatively common. These can rupture, causing acute pain, mimicking deep vein thrombosis

Spine
- Atlanto-axial joint (a synovial joint) involvement is important. Soft tissue laxity causes subluxation, and there may be dens erosion leading to potential spinal cord compression.
- It is important to assess stability, as cervical manipulation or intubation may damage the cervical cord secondary to the spinal instability.

Seronegative arthritides
This is a group of conditions which include:
- Ankylosing spondylitis.
- Psoriatic arthritis.
- Reiter's syndrome.
- Inflammatory bowel disease.

Ankylosing spondylitis
- Occurs in late adolescent men (women less often) with onset of sacroiliitis.
- Symmetrical, with erosions of both ilium and sacrum, loss of joint space, and eventually ankylosis (Fig. 7.54(a)).
- These changes then ascend in the spine, with erosions of the vertebral margins, then bony healing and ankylosis, with the advanced deformity known as a "bamboo spine" (Fig. 7.54(b)).
- Trauma can cause pathological horizontal fractures through an ankylosed spine due to lack of flexibility of the spine.

Psoriatic arthritis
- Up to 20% of patients with skin manifestations of psoriasis develop arthritis.
- The hands and feet are most affected, with asymmetrical erosions particularly of the distal interphalangeal joints.
- Progressive destruction of the distal interphalangeal joints leads to a "cup and pencil" deformity.
- Large joint involvement is uncommon, but sacroiliitis is seen in up to 50%.

Reiter's syndrome
- Occurs in young males and is usually sexually transmitted.
- Arthritis conjunctivitis and urethritis are usual presenting symptoms.

147

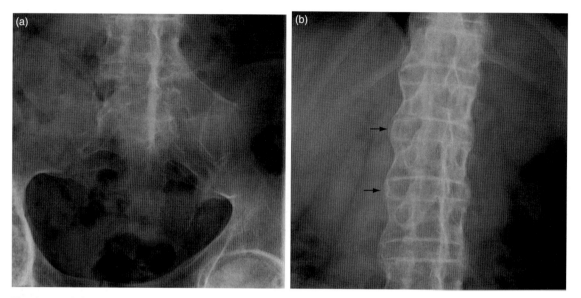

Fig. 7.54. Ankylosing spondylitis with (a) advanced sacroiliitis with bony ankylosis of both sacroiliac joints and (b) marginal bridging new bone formation (arrows) referred to as syndesmophytes (so-called "bamboo spine").

- Usually affects the feet, with erosions at the metatarsophalangeal joints and calcaneal spurs.
- Sacroiliitis can occur late.

Inflammatory bowel disease
- Up to 10% of patients with ulcerative colitis and Crohn's disease develop arthritis.
- Peripheral arthropathy and sacroiliitis are most common, with the arthritis activity related to the activity of the inflammatory bowel disease.
- Patients have high HLA-B27 antigen levels.

Osteomyelitis and septic arthritis
Etiology
- Organisms are most often staphylococcal, and sometimes streptococcal or *E. coli,* and infection can occur via three pathways:
  - Blood-borne
  - Adjacent infection (e.g. dental)
  - Penetrating injuries (including surgery).
- Predisposing factors – foreign bodies, diabetes.

Acute osteomyelitis
Early changes
- Typical age range – 5 to 20 years
- Blood borne organisms enter via diaphyseal nutrient artery, passing into and lodging in the metaphysis.

- Infection spreads along the bone, raising the periosteum, particularly in young children, in whom the periosteum is only loosely attached. This occurs after 7 days.
- In young children, the growth plate is avascular, barring the passage of organisms. After skeletal maturity, vascular continuity allows spread into the epiphysis.
- In neonates, early epiphyseal involvement is frequent, because the periosteum is loosely attached, and vascular channels pass through the growth plate. A joint effusion indicates septic arthritis.
- In older children and young adults, pyogenic infection spreads along the medullary cavity, causing patchy bone destruction and formation of cortical sinuses.

Early diagnosis
- Usually plain radiographs are normal until 7–10 days. Periosteal reaction is the earliest finding. There may be metaphyseal osteopenia due to hyperemia, and faint areas of lucent bone destruction (Fig. 7.55).
- Antibiotic treatment must be commenced before radiographic bone changes appear, preferably within 24 to 48 hours after onset of symptoms.
- Radioisotope scans help in early detection and localization.

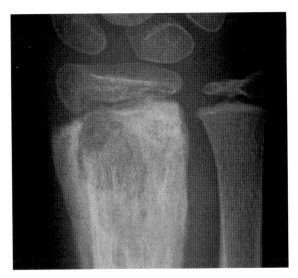

Fig. 7.55. Osteomyelitis of radius in a child (note unfused epiphyseal growth plates). Bone destruction in metaphysis with overlying periosteal reaction.

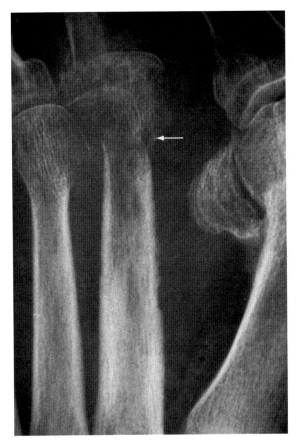

Fig. 7.57. Osteomyelitis of the second metatarsal (arrow) in a diabetic patient.

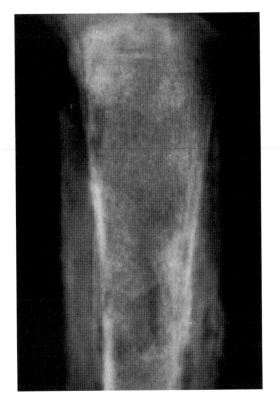

Fig. 7.56. Osteomyelitis of proximal tibia. Sequestrum of bone is developing surrounded by new bone formation.

Later changes

- New bone (the involucrum) forms beneath the elevated periosteum, and can envelop the whole shaft. It may be perforated in places with sinuses (cloacae), that discharge pus into the soft tissues and, ultimately, to the skin.
- As the periosteum is raised, necrosis occurs secondary to venous occlusion and interruption of nutrient artery blood flow. Segments of devascularized cortex form sequestra (Fig. 7.56).
- If acute osteomyelitis reaches this stage, spontaneous healing is rare.

Brodie's abscess

- A localized infection (usually due to *Staphylococcus aureus*), most often seen in the metaphysis before epiphyseal closure, and can be present for months or years. It often involves the tibia or femur.
- It has a circumscribed area of bone destruction (lucency) with a surrounding ill-defined area of bone reaction (sclerosis), ranging from a few millimeters to centimeters in size.

149

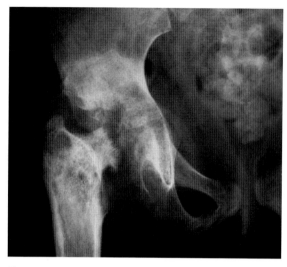

Fig. 7.58. Marked destruction of cartilage and adjacent bone resulting from untreated septic arthritis.

Diabetes and prostheses
- In diabetes, the foot is most commonly involved, secondary to superficial ulceration and infection (Fig. 7.57).
- Osteomyelitis is a serious complication around orthopedic prostheses.

Vertebral osteomyelitis
- Infection of the intervertebral disk (diskitis) is characterized by disk and vertebral end-plate destruction.

- It is most common in the lumbar spine.
- Isolation of the organism usually requires needle aspiration (under CT or fluoroscopic guidance).

Tuberculosis
- Occurs via hematogenous spread, usually from lungs.
- Bone changes progress insidiously, and are usually subacute or chronic. Often affects ends of long bones (e.g. proximal femur, proximal humerus) or spine.
- Unlike acute osteomyelitis, bone changes are present on initial X-rays.
- Sinuses from bone extend into adjacent soft tissue to form a "cold abscess."
- Calcified debris around a bone or joint is typical.

Septic arthritis
- It usually presents acutely, with normal initial bone density on radiographs.
- A joint effusion can widen the joint space, and is readily detected by ultrasound.
- If untreated, rapid cartilage destruction occurs, with loss of joint space, followed by bone destruction (Fig. 7.58) and ankylosis.
- Needle aspiration is usually required to identify the organism, and may be image-guided if necessary. Joint aspiration is urgent if there is clinical suspicion of septic arthritis.

Chapter 8

Gastrointestinal tract

Contents

Dysphagia
Barium swallow examination

- The barium swallow is the main radiological investigation for dysphagia, and is complementary to endoscopy. It provides morphological information as well as functional information about initiation of swallowing and peristalsis. Endoscopy provides more information about mucosal changes and allows biopsy when needed.
- The barium swallow is performed on a fluoroscopic table using barium sulphate suspension with the patient standing and/or lying. It is recorded as a series of static images, or as a "real time" recording (commonly referred to as videofluoroscopy).
- Videofluoroscopy has the advantages of allowing repeated review including in slow motion, which provides a more reliable assessment of motility disorders and can detect transient abnormalities more reliably than can static films alone.
- Videofluoroscopy is performed with a combination of dilute liquid barium and usually also a semi-solid bolus such as a piece of bread

soaked in barium to mimic normal foods. The semi-solid bolus is an important part of the study when assessing motility disorders and in detecting subtle stricturing.

Points to remember when requesting contrast studies of the esophagus
- Barium is used for all contrast studies except if there is a high likelihood of an esophageal tear into the mediastinum or peritoneum. In these circumstances a water-soluble contrast is used.
- If there is a high likelihood of tracheal aspiration, or a tracheo-esophageal fistula, some water-soluble contrast agents must be avoided as they can cause major life-threatening pulmonary edema if aspirated.
- Videofluoroscopy should be requested if the question relates to esophageal motility. It is superior to a static film study alone in most cases of dysphagia where the cause is unclear.

Causes of dysphagia
The many causes of dysphagia can be grouped into neuromuscular disorders and mechanical disorders, and mechanical causes can be subdivided into extra-mural, mural and luminal.

Neuromuscular disorders
- Oropharyngeal level
  - Stroke
  - Myopathies
- Esophagus
  - Cricopharyngeal dysfunction
  - Achalasia
  - Scleroderma
  - Diffuse esophageal spasm

Mechanical
- Intraluminal
  - Foreign bodies

- Mural
  - Benign strictures – reflux, corrosive
  - Mucosal folds – cricopharyngeal web, Schatzki's ring
  - Malignant – esophageal carcinoma
- Extramural
  - Goiter
  - Zenker's (pharyngeal) diverticulum
  - Mediastinal lymphadenopathy – e.g. metastatic lung carcinoma
  - Thoracic aortic aneurysm
  - Left atrial enlargement

Some of the more common or important causes are discussed below.

Cricopharyngeal dysfunction
- Cricopharyngeus normally relaxes as the food bolus reaches it. It can cause dysphagia (localized to the neck) by relaxing too late or relaxing incompletely.

Achalasia
- Achalasia leads to dysphagia by a combination of failure of relaxation of the lower esophageal sphincter and progressive loss of normal peristaltic activity (Fig. 8.1).
- It quite common for achalasia to be complicated by aspiration pneumonia.

Reflux esophagitis and stricture
- Chronic gastro-esophageal reflux leads to esophagitis that can lead to stricturing (Fig. 8.2), sometimes in the mid esophagus where the refluxed gastric contents tend to pool in the supine position.
- As a general rule all esophageal strictures should undergo endoscopy and biopsy to exclude malignancy. They may also require treatment by endoscopic dilatation.

Shatzski's ring
- A Shatzski's ring consists of a mucosal fold that occurs occasionally at the gastro-esophageal mucosal junction and is always associated with a sliding hiatus hernia (often small). These "rings" seldom cause obstruction but are considered potentially symptomatic if the lumen is reduced to 1 cm.

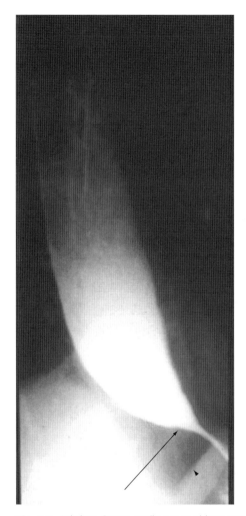

Fig. 8.1. Achalasia. Barium swallow in an oblique projection (patient upright and turned toward the left). The esophagus is mildly dilated and the barium is pooling above the lower esophageal sphincter (arrow) which has failed to relax normally (left hemidiaphragm – arrowhead).

Esophageal carcinoma
- Squamous cell carcinoma is more common than adenocarcinoma (Fig. 8.3). The majority of adenocarcinoma arises in the lower third of the esophagus in the setting of pre-existent Barrett's esophagus

Staging of esophageal carcinoma
Staging of esophageal carcinoma relies mainly on
- Local extension – endoscopic ultrasound (EUS) is the best modality for assessing early local extension through the esophageal wall. Lymph nodes can be assessed, particularly if the EUS allows US guided lymph node biopsy.

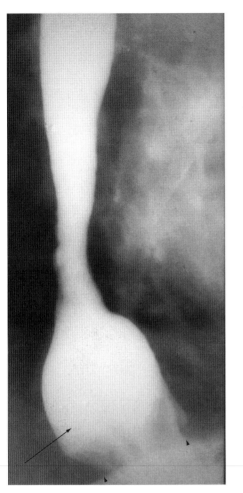

Fig. 8.2. Reflux esophagitis. Single contrast barium swallow showing sliding hiatus hernias (arrow) and mild degree of esophageal stricturing above it. Diaphragm is marked by arrowheads.

- Local and distant – CT of chest and upper abdomen, for assessment of extension into mediastinum, pleura, lungs, lymph nodes of mediastinum and upper abdomen, and the liver. PET/CT is more sensitive than CT alone for staging and is generally used if conventional CT shows no obvious metastases.

Goiter
- Thyroid enlargement may compress the upper esophagus and this is more likely if there is retrosternal extension of the goiter through the fixed dimensions of the thoracic inlet.

Zenker's (pharyngeal) diverticulum
- Zenker's diverticulum arises posteriorly at the junction of the hypopharynx and esophagus.

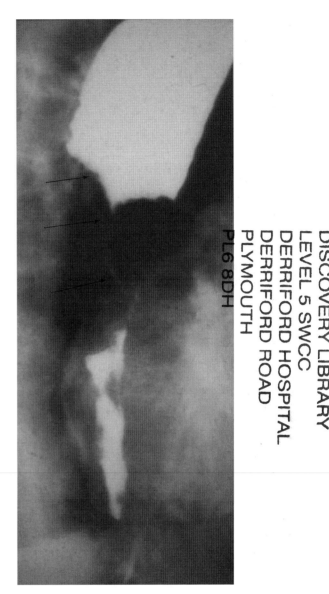

Fig. 8.3. Constricting carcinoma of mid esophagus (arrows) that is producing almost total occlusion.

It can act as a cause of dysphagia particularly if large, as it can retain swallowed food. It also is at risk of metaplasia and adenocarcinoma if there is chronic stasis of food within it.

Tracheal aspiration, gastro-esophageal reflux and hiatus hernias
- The barium swallow can also assess the following, which may exist with or without dysphagia
  - Laryngeal/tracheal aspiration of barium and therefore food and liquids

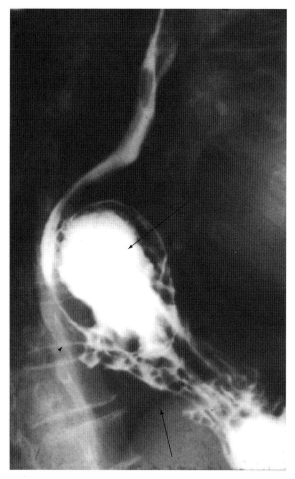

Fig. 8.4. Mixed sliding and para-esophageal hernia. The gastro-esophageal junction (arrowhead) lies above the level of the diaphragm (short arrow) which indicates a sliding component of hernia and there is also a para-esophageal component (long arrow).

- Gastro-esophageal reflux. Reflux is seen with the patient lying supine.
- The demonstration of reflux does not necessarily mean that it is symptomatic (this is usually a straightforward clinical assessment), and conversely the failure to demonstrate reflux on a barium study does not exclude symptomatic reflux.
- Reflux may exist with or without hiatus hernia, although it is much more common if a hiatus hernia is present.
- Hiatus hernias may be sliding (commonest), para-esophageal ("rolling") or a mix of the two (Fig. 8.4).

Acute abdominal pain
Causes
- Acute abdominal pain in the adult has a number of important causes including the following (some of these are discussed in other sections):
  - Perforated stomach or bowel
  - Biliary colic and acute cholecystitis
  - Appendicitis
  - Acute pancreatitis
  - Bowel obstruction
  - Bowel infarction
  - Ruptured abdominal aortic aneurysm
  - Ruptured ectopic pregnancy and complicated ovarian pathology
  - Diverticulitis
  - Renal colic

Plain films
- Chest radiograph
  - Look for free intraperitoneal gas (pneumoperitoneum) beneath one or both hemidiaphragms
- Plain abdominal X-ray. Look for
  - Free gas beneath diaphragm or elsewhere in abdomen
  - Evidence of bowel obstruction
  - Calcified gallstones
  - Urinary tract calculi
  - Pancreatic calcification
  - Calcified aortic aneurysm

Perforated gastrointestinal tract
- Common causes are perforated peptic ulcer, infarcted bowel, and diverticular disease
- The main radiographic sign is a pneumoperitoneum (Fig. 8.5)

Pitfalls in diagnosing bowel perforation
- Pneumoperitoneum is also seen for a few days post-laparotomy/laparoscopy.
- Normal bowel gas.
- Patient to ill for erect radiograph. If the patient is not well enough to sit upright for an erect film, then a left lateral decubitus film (patient lying on left side) can be used. Free intraperitoneal gas will tend to accumulate just medial to the right lateral abdominal wall.

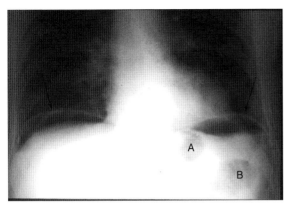

Fig. 8.5. Lower part of an erect chest radiograph showing free gas beneath both hemidiaphragms (arrows). Normal gas is seen in stomach (A) and splenic flexure of colon (B).

- False-negative plain films. Approximately 25% of patients with perforated stomach or bowel will not have detectable free intra-abdominal gas on plain radiographs. Free gas is often more easily recognized on the chest X-ray than on the abdominal film.
- Retroperitoneal perforation. Perforation of a retroperitoneal portion of bowel leads to retroperitoneal gas.

Additional imaging tests
- If confirmatory evidence of perforation is needed the following can be used
  - Radiographic contrast study using oral water-soluble contrast agent. If a perforation is present in the stomach or duodenum, this will usually be shown by the leakage of contrast. Barium is not used as it can produce severe fibrosing peritonitis if it spills into the peritoneum.
  - Abdominal CT. CT can demonstrate much smaller amounts of intraperitoneal gas compared with plain films as well as show a range of pathologies.

Biliary colic and acute cholecystitis
- Biliary colic and almost all cases of acute cholecystitis are due to gallstones. The main exception is acute acalculous cholecystitis, which is usually confined to patients who are very ill from other causes.
- Biliary colic is characterized by an episode or episodes of right upper quadrant or epigastric pain, which may radiate around the right upper abdomen/chest.

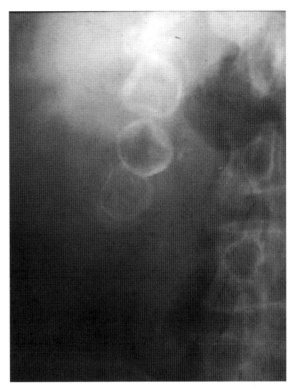

Fig. 8.6. Calcified peripheral layer in multiple faceted gallbladder stones.

- Acute cholecystitis pain is more sustained and is typically associated with right upper quadrant tenderness, fever and elevated white cell count.

Radiological diagnosis of gallstones
Plain abdominal radiographs
- Less than 10% of stones contain sufficient calcium to be detectable on a plain radiograph (Fig. 8.6).

Ultrasound
- The most valuable radiological test for diagnosis of gallbladder stones with a sensitivity and specificity >95%. On ultrasound gallstones appear as an echogenic focus (often mobile) within the gallbladder, producing an acoustic shadow (Fig. 8.7).
- Very small stones can be detected on ultrasound, although the small false-negative rate of <5% is usually caused by small stones, particularly in more obese patients.

CT
- Not indicated for suspected biliary colic, as only a minority of stones are calcified

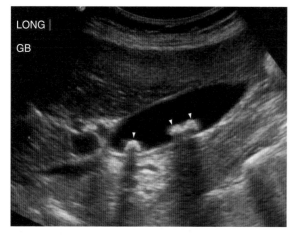

Fig. 8.7. Ultrasound shows three stones as echogenic foci (arrowheads) casting acoustic shadows.

Acute cholecystitis

- Ultrasound is the test of first choice for suspected cholecystitis (Fig. 8.8). The ultrasound signs are:
  - Gallbladder stones (except for the uncommon acalculous cholecystitis)
  - Gallbladder wall thickening resulting from edema (>3mm thickness)
  - Tenderness localized to the gallbladder (so-called sonographic Murphy's sign)
  - Fluid or abscess adjacent to the gallbladder
- HIDA scanning
  - Useful if cholecystitis not confirmed on ultrasound is still suspected clinically.
  - HIDA scanning is a nuclear medicine technique which uses an iminodiacetic acid (IDA) derivative labeled with ^{99m}Tc. This is injected intravenously and the agent is excreted into the bile. If there is no isotope activity in the gallbladder at 2–4 hours, but activity is seen in bile ducts, this is evidence of acute cholecystitis (see Chapter 5).
- Abdominal CT
  - CT scanning is not performed as a first line investigation for suspected acute cholecystitis but is often helpful in acute abdominal pain of unclear origin as it can show a wide range of pathologies.
  - The signs of acute cholecystitis on CT are (Fig. 8.9):
    - Gallbladder wall thickening
    - Abnormal gallbladder wall contrast enhancement

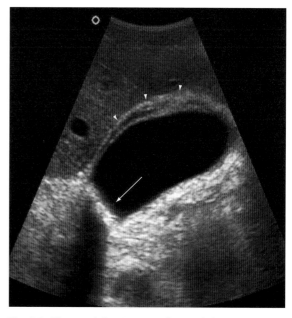

Fig. 8.8. Ultrasound showing signs of acute cholecystitis with a gallstones (arrow) impacted in the gallbladder neck and thickened gallbladder wall (arrowheads).

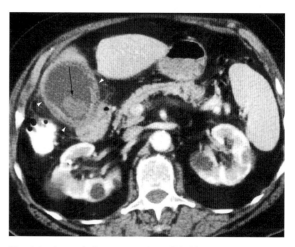

Fig. 8.9. Acute cholecystitis on CT. Gallbladder wall is thickened (arrowheads), there is edema in fat adjacent to gallbladder. A large gallstone is also seen in this case (arrow). Bilateral renal cysts are an incidental finding.

  - Fluid/edema adjacent to the gallbladder
  - Gallstones seen in minority

Appendicitis

- Imaging is helpful in cases which are clinically not diagnostically straightforward. This is more the case in females where the differential diagnosis includes gynecological causes of pain.

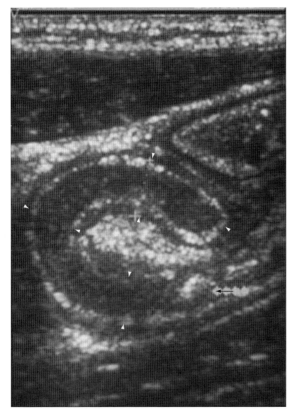

Fig. 8.10. Ultrasound showing an enlarged appendix (arrowheads) of 7mm diameter with an appendicolith within its lumen (arrow).

- The two most useful tests are ultrasound and CT, which have similar diagnostic accuracy for appendicitis, although ultrasound is more useful if a gynecological cause of pain needs exclusion.

Ultrasound
The signs of appendicitis on ultrasound are (Fig. 8.10):
- Thickened appendix – >5–6mm diameter
- Peritoneal fluid localized to the appendiceal region
- An appendicolith in the appendiceal lumen (this does not indicate appendicitis as an isolated finding)

CT
- Similar diagnostic accuracy to ultrasound for diagnosis of appendicitis.
- Can show alternative diagnoses in the region although is inferior to ultrasound for showing gynecological causes of abdominal pain.
- CT signs of appendicitis are (Fig. 8.11):

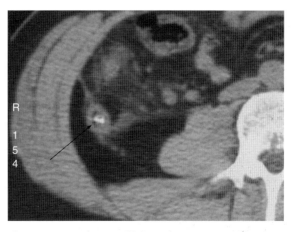

Fig. 8.11. Appendicitis on CT. Appendix in cross section appears round and contains an appendicolith (arrow) and is surrounded by areas of intermediate density representing inflammatory change in the adjacent fat.

- An enlarged fluid-filled appendix
- Surrounding inflammatory changes or abscess
- Appendicolith may be seen.

Acute pancreatitis (see section below)

Bowel ischemia/infarction (see section below also)
- Bowel infarction is most often seen in the setting of acute abdominal pain
  - In combination with bowel obstruction (e.g. strangulated hernia)
  - In acute hypotension, usually in the elderly
  - In patients with vascular disease or a source of systemic thromboembolism (e.g. cardiac source)
- In these settings it is frequently suggested by the presence of raised serum lactic acid.

Pancreatitis and pancreatic tumors
Acute pancreatitis
Diagnosis
- Most patients with acute pancreatitis have a straightforward diagnosis based on clinical features and serum amylase.
- Occasionally the diagnosis is not clear and CT of the abdomen may suggest the diagnosis because of characteristic peripancreatic inflammatory changes.

157

Aetiology

- The main causes of pancreatitis are alcohol and gallstones, with some being idiopathic or due to a variety of uncommon causes.
- Gallstone pancreatitis
  - At presentation, it is important to look for evidence of gallstone pancreatitis as its treatment differs, generally requiring cholecystectomy or early endoscopic biliary sphincterotomy.
  - Unless there is a clear history to support an alcohol etiology, it is important to perform ultrasound and consider cholangiography (MRCP, or CT-intravenous cholangiography) to establish a diagnosis of gallstone pancreatitis.

Radiology findings

- The role of radiology is to:
  - Identify those cases due to gallstones (gallstone pancreatitis)
  - Detect and monitor complications of pancreatitis
- Plain abdominal radiographs may show
  - Localized ileus in central/upper abdomen
  - Calcification of chronic pancreatitis
- Chest X-ray may show
  - Pleural effusions or areas of atelectasis and air space opacity in more severe cases, or these changes may develop later
- Ultrasound
  - Used at presentation to look for gallbladder calculi as a possible etiology
- CT
  - Performed at presentation particularly when the diagnosis is uncertain
  - Most common early finding is peripancreatic edema in the peripancreatic fat planes (Fig. 8.12).
  - Used later to detect and monitor complications

Local complications

- Pancreatic necrosis
- Pancreatic pseudocyst and abscess
- Hemorrhage
- Pancreatic ascites
- Fistulae – e.g. to pleural space, causing large pleural effusions with high amylase content

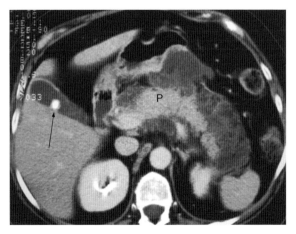

Fig. 8.12. Acute pancreatitis on CT (intravenous contrast enhanced). Intermediate density surrounds the pancreas (P) representing peripancreatic edema in the retroperitoneal fat. A high density gallbladder calculus is shown (arrow).

Pancreatic necrosis

- Contrast-enhanced CT can be used to provide a guide as to the presence and extent of pancreatic necrosis, as it has prognostic implications and may influence the decision to operate. Normally the pancreas enhances with intravenous contrast. Lack of enhancement in part or all of the pancreas is a marker of necrosis in those areas.

Pancreatic pseudocyst and abscess

- Pancreatic pseudocysts may develop in or around the pancreas. They commonly lie in the lesser sac but they can extend well away from the pancreas and may be multiple or multiloculated.
- Most pancreatic pseudocysts resolve without intervention. If persistent and large, or if a pancreatic abscess develops, surgical, endoscopic, or percutaneous drainage is required.

Hemorrhage

- Pancreatitis, with or without pseudocysts, can erode the wall of local arteries, and lead to false aneurysm formation and hemorrhage.
- If bleeding is suspected in the setting of pancreatitis (GI bleeding or intra-abdominal bleed), then angiography is indicated, with embolization of any bleeding site if possible.

Chronic pancreatitis

- The pancreas undergoes atrophy and fibrosis, the pancreatic ducts may dilate or develop strictures, and calculi develop in the pancreatic

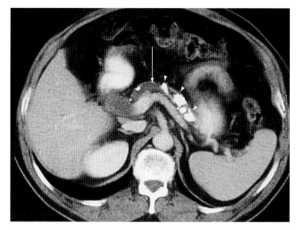

Fig. 8.13. Chronic pancreatitis on CT. The pancreatic duct is dilated (arrow), contains extensive calculi (arrowheads) and is surrounded by very thinned atrophic parenchymal glandular tissue.

ducts. Some or all of these changes are manifest on plain films, CT, ultrasound, ERCP, and MRCP (Fig. 8.13).

Pancreatic tumors

The most common tumors are:

- Adenocarcinoma (ductal origin)
- Cystic tumors
- Islet cell tumors (apudomas)

Pancreatic adenocarcinoma

Clinical presentation

- Pain – typically epigastric with radiation to back
- Jaundice – bile duct obstruction
- Gastric outlet obstruction

Imaging diagnosis depends on the mode of presentation. CT and ultrasound are the usual modes, as well as cholangiography in patients presenting with jaundice, either ERCP or MRCP (see Jaundice section below).

Staging carcinoma of pancreas

Pretreatment staging includes assessment of local extension, liver and lymph node metastases, local vascular involvement using a combination of CT and ultrasound, and in some patients endoscopic ultrasound, MRI, or laparoscopy.

Carcinoma of pancreas – treatment

- Only a small minority of patients have early disease, which allows complete resection.
- Palliative treatment includes biliary stenting in those patients with bile duct obstruction (see Jaundice section below)

Pancreatic endocrine tumors

A variety of tumors arise from the islet cells:

- Insulinoma
- Gastrinoma (these also may arise in or around wall of duodenum)
- Glucagonoma
- Others – somatostatinoma, VIPoma, non-functional tumors

The majority present with symptoms reflecting their endocrine function and are diagnosed on clinical features confirmed with laboratory tests.

The main role of imaging is to localize the tumor prior to surgery. Intra-operative localization (including intra-operative ultrasound) is frequently successful, but it is usual practice to attempt pre-operative localization with a combination of imaging tests including CT, ultrasound, endoscopic ultrasound, MRI, and occasionally angiographic techniques.

Pancreatic cystic tumors

- These uncommon tumors have a range of histological types, the majority being benign but with some being malignant, or having malignant potential.
- Differentiation from pancreatic pseudocysts is usually possible on clinical features (history of pancreatitis).
- Imaging characteristics sometimes suggest which group the tumor belongs to, but frequently it is unclear.

Bowel obstruction

- The clinical and radiological features depend on the site of obstruction, whether it is mechanical or functional, how long it has been present, and whether it is complete obstruction or not.
- The causes can be grouped into
  - Mechanical
  - Functional – also referred to as adynamic obstruction or ileus
- The causes can also be divided according to anatomical level
  - Gastric outlet
  - Small bowel
  - Large bowel

Gastric outlet obstruction

- Mechanical
  - Gastric carcinoma

- Carcinoma of pancreas (and other neoplasms)
- Gastric volvulus
- Peptic ulcer – now uncommon
- Adynamic
  - Motility disorders
  - Gastroparesis – e.g. diabetic

Radiological findings
- The majority of patients with suspected gastric outlet obstruction undergo endoscopy, at which time the cause will be apparent if it involves the mucosa.
- Some mechanical causes are well shown by contrast studies or CT (e.g. carcinoma of head of pancreas). If the obstruction is long-standing the stomach will usually be very distended.
- Gastric motility disorders can be evaluated on contrast studies or by nuclear medicine gastric emptying studies.
- Gastric volvulus may be difficult to diagnose at endoscopy and is best appreciated on a contrast study (barium meal). It is often associated with a hiatus hernia and can be complicated by gastric ischemia or infarction.

Small and large bowel obstruction
Causes
Mechanical obstruction
- Small bowel
  - Adhesions – commonest mechanical cause
  - Hernias – inguinal, femoral, internal
  - Inflammatory strictures – Crohn's disease
  - Inflammatory masses – e.g. appendicitis
  - Tumor – secondary more often than primary
  - Intussusception – intermittent obstruction
  - Gallstone "ileus"
- Large bowel
  - Carcinoma
  - Volvulus – sigmoid more common than cecal
  - Diverticular disease

Adynamic obstruction (ileus) – small or large bowel
- Peritonitis – localized or generalized
- Post-operative – lasts 2–3 days usually
- Ischemia
- Pseudo-obstruction – idiopathic or associated with another condition, e.g. scleroderma

Radiological features of bowel obstruction
The radiological changes reflect three processes:
- Bowel dilatation
  - Normally the small bowel measures up to 2.5–3 cm in diameter and the colon up to 6–8 cm.
- Fluid and gas accumulation
  - Gastrointestinal secretions and swallowed gas lead to air–fluid levels.
  - Normally there may be two to three fluid levels of 2–3 cm in length.
  - Abnormal fluid accumulation is best appreciated in erect films (or decubitus), seen as longer fluid levels (Fig. 8.14(a)).
  - Occasionally the fluid accumulation occurs with little gas accumulation and fluid levels may then be short.
- Emptying of bowel distal to obstruction

Differentiating small and large bowel obstruction
Differentiation between small and large bowel obstruction on plain films depends on recognizing:
- What bowel is dilated – bowel dilates down to the level of obstruction.
- What bowel is not dilated or is empty.
  Small bowel is recognizable by one or more of the following (Fig. 8.14):
- It is central within abdomen
- It is smaller caliber than large bowel
- It has valvulae conniventes
- The loops are more numerous than large bowel
  Large bowel, in contrast, has the following features (Fig. 8.15):
- Is larger caliber
- Has haustral folds – less numerous than valvulae conniventes and tend not to extend across whole diameter
- Lies around periphery of abdomen with exception of transverse colon and sigmoid colon which extend into central abdomen

Determining the cause of obstruction
- Differentiating between mechanical obstruction and adynamic obstruction (ileus) is most often a clinical differentiation with little radiological difference between the two. An ileus may affect small bowel, large bowel, or both.

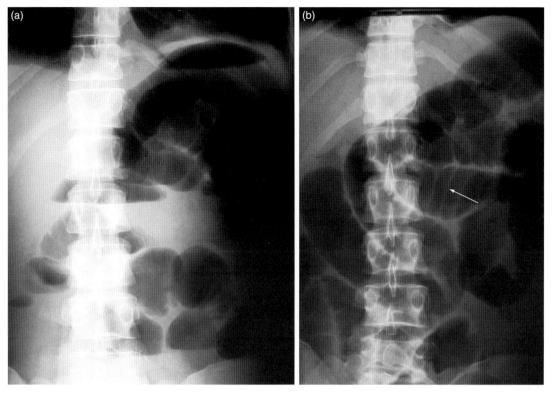

Fig. 8.14. Small bowel obstruction. (a) Erect film shows multiple long fluid levels in dilated small bowel centrally. (b) Supine film shows multiple loops of gas-containing small bowel loops centrally in abdomen. Valvulae conniventes appear as thin mucosal folds extending across the diameter of the bowel (arrow).

Plain films

- The cause of mechanical obstruction is not often apparent on plain radiographs. Some causes that can be identified on plain films are
  - Sigmoid volvulus (Fig. 8.16), cecal volvulus
  - Gallstone ileus – impacting gallstone visible in about 30% of cases
  - Hernias – may be shown as bowel loops extending inferiorly in inguinal region

CT

- CT is being used increasingly in evaluation of abdominal pain as well as suspected bowel obstruction and may define the cause.

Contrast enema

- A contrast enema can be useful:
  - If it is unclear as to whether there is a large bowel obstruction present
  - To determine the cause of a large bowel obstruction
- During an acute presentation a water-soluble enema is preferred. If the history is of intermittent

or incomplete large bowel obstruction then barium is generally preferred (the image quality is superior with barium) (Fig. 8.17).

Contrast meal and follow-through

- Water-soluble studies are useful in an acute presentation to help determine the level and nature of obstruction only if the obstruction is proximal (i.e. gastric outlet obstruction or very proximal small bowel obstruction). With more distal obstruction, the contrast becomes too dilute to provide any structural detail.
- Barium meal and small bowel "follow-through" studies are useful for intermittent small bowel obstruction to help confirm the diagnosis and define the cause (Fig. 8.18).

Bowel obstruction and ischemia
Strangulation

- Strangulation describes the combination of bowel obstruction and associated bowel ischemia/ infarction.
- It is potentially a complication of obstruction due to:

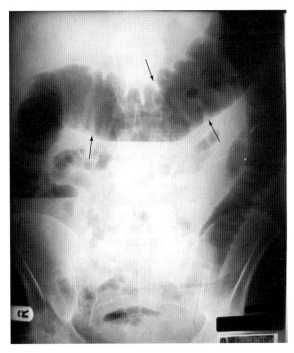

Fig. 8.15. Large bowel obstruction (distal). The dilated bowel is peripheral in the abdomen. Haustral folds (arrows) are seen most easily in the transverse colon in this patient.

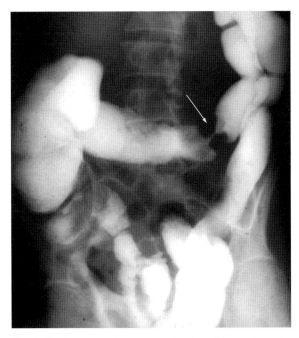

Fig. 8.17. Carcinoma of transverse colon (arrow) in a patient who had recent episodes of large bowel obstruction.

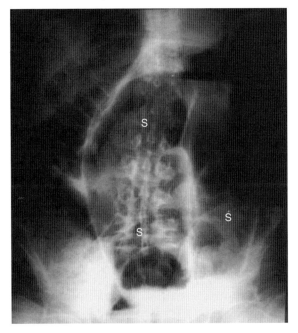

Fig. 8.16. Sigmoid volvulus. The sigmoid loop (S) is characteristically extending superiorly out of the pelvis. The bowel has perforated in this case, an ischemic complication of volvulus.

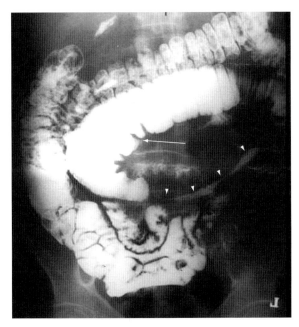

Fig. 8.18. Barium small bowel follow-through shows dilated small bowel (arrow) proximal to a long stricture (arrowheads), which was due to Crohn's disease.

- Hernias – including internal hernias
- Volvulus – e.g. sigmoid volvulus, cecal volvulus
- Closed loop obstruction associated with adhesions
- It arises by occlusion of venous outflow followed by compromise of arterial inflow

Cecal ischemia associated with large bowel obstruction

If large bowel obstruction is unrelieved, the proximal large bowel may undergo marked dilatation. In the cecum/proximal-ascending colon, where the diameter is normally larger, this can lead to sufficient tension in the colon wall to impede perfusion and cause ischemia, infarction and perforation, unless decompressed surgically. The chances of perforation are substantial if the diameter reaches 10 cm.

Inflammatory bowel disease

The most common forms of inflammatory bowel disease are Crohn's disease and ulcerative colitis.

The role of radiology is to:

- Assist in diagnosis and assessment of extent particularly in suspected Crohn's disease
- Detect and monitor complications, such as toxic megacolon, or in Crohn's disease, abscesses, strictures, and fistulae

Endoscopy and biopsy provides the diagnosis in most cases of colitis, terminal ileal Crohn's disease (ileoscopy), and Crohn's involving upper GI tract (esophagus, stomach or duodenum)

Plain abdominal X-rays

- Provide information about severity and extent of colitis.

Barium studies

- Not commonly used to diagnose inflammatory bowel disease involving upper GI tract or colon as endoscopy allows direct visualization and biopsy
- Useful in assessment of the small bowel, either as a barium follow-through or with administration of barium through a nasojejunal tube (small bowel enteroclysis).

Isotope white cell scans

- The patient's white cells are labeled with an isotope and reinjected prior to imaging.
- Can assist in establishing the diagnosis of inflammatory bowel disease, determining its extent and detecting abscesses.

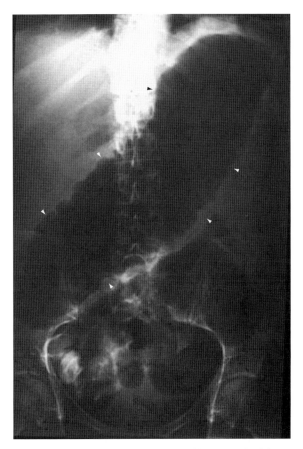

Fig. 8.19. Toxic megacolon with marked dilatation and mild mucosal thickening affecting of the transverse colon (arrowheads).

Colitis

Plain abdominal films (AXR)

In patients presenting with an acute episode of colitis a plain AXR is useful in assessing:

- Extent of colonic involvement
  - Areas that are acutely inflamed do not retain feces so appear empty.
  - Inflamed areas show mucosal swelling and wall thickening.
- Presence of toxic megacolon
  - Acute dilatation of the colon in acute colitis (Fig. 8.19).
  - Potentially dangerous because of the risk of perforation. Patients are systemically unwell.
  - The decision to operate (colectomy) is based on a combination of clinical features and the presence of progressive colonic dilatation. Daily abdominal films may be needed to aid assessment.

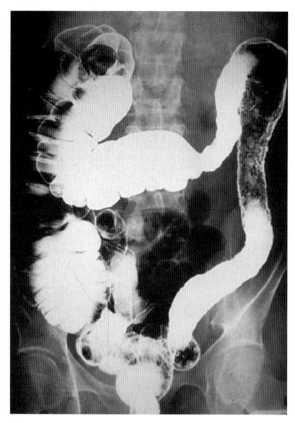

Fig. 8.20. Double contrast barium enema. Ulcerative colitis extending from rectum to distal transverse colon. Ulceration and "inflammatory" polyps produce an irregular surface.

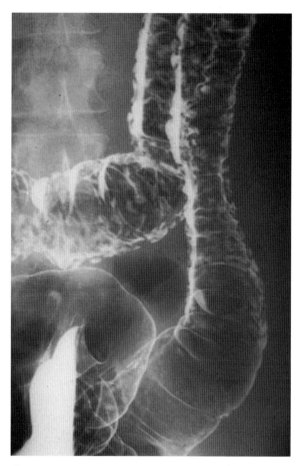

Fig. 8.21. Double contrast barium enema. Crohn's colitis with ulcers in splenic flexure.

Double contrast barium enema (DCBE) and colitis

Ulcerative colitis

- Colitis in ulcerative colitis (UC) virtually always involves the rectum and extends in continuity for a variable distance.
- Early change is that of granular mucosa. In more severe cases there is shallow ulceration. The mucosa becomes oedematous and produces areas mimicking polyps between the ulcers ("pseudopolyps" or "inflammatory polyps") (Fig. 8.20).
- The normal haustral folds are lost, and in chronic UC the colon becomes shortened and develops a "lead pipe" appearance.
- Small bowel is not involved except for about 10% who get "backwash ileitis."
- Carcinoma in ulcerative colitis.
  - The risk of carcinoma is influenced by a number of factors including severity of disease (especially at onset), and duration of disease.
  - Surveillance is by regular colonoscopy.

Crohn's colitis

- Crohn's colitis spares the rectum in about 50%, and frequently spares other areas so that the disease is not in continuity.
- The earliest changes are small aphthous ulcers. These then become larger and deeper (Fig. 8.21).
- Strictures may develop due to fibrosis.

Crohn's disease of small bowel

- Terminal ileum commonest site (Fig. 8.22)
- Segmental – more than one segment of small bowel may be affected

Chapter 8: Gastrointestinal tract

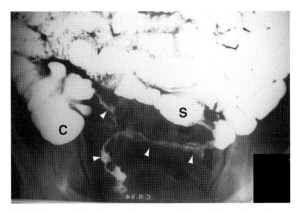

Fig. 8.22. Crohn's disease. Barium small bowel follow-through showing long segment of ulcerated strictured ileum (arrowheads). S – small bowel proximal to stricture, C – cecum.

- Strictures – may produce small bowel obstruction (Fig. 8.18)
- Fistulae – to adjacent small or large bowel, bladder, vagina/uterus, skin
- Abscess formation

CT and MRI
- Can show small bowel changes and detect complicating abscesses, which in some patients can be treated with percutaneous drainage.
- MRI in particular has the ability to assess extent, assess inflammatory activity and evaluate suspected abscesses and fistulae.
- Both CT and MRI can be combined with intraluminal contrast agents given orally or via a nasojejunal tube, so-called enterography or enteroclysis, respectively. These techniques can be used in a range of clinical settings to evaluate the small bowel.

Colorectal cancer
- Colorectal cancer is the second most common cause of cancer-related death worldwide.
- Almost all are adenocarcinoma.
- Most arise from adenomas, larger polyps carrying a higher risk of malignancy (increasing size of polyp corresponds to increasing risk of malignancy i.e. 6–9mm polyp has up to 1% risk of being malignant compared with up to 10% for a 10mm polyp).

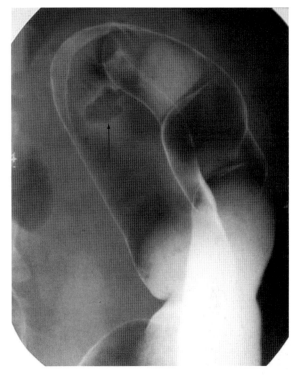

Fig. 8.23. Double contrast barium enema. Colonic pedunculated polyp, in this case malignant, at the splenic flexure (arrow).

- Genetic risk factors exist in addition to increased risk in some polyposis syndromes (highest in familial adenomatous polyposis) and in longstanding active ulcerative colitis.

Site
- Approximate distribution is:
  - Rectosigmoid 50%
  - Cecum/ascending colon 25%
  - Descending colon 15%
  - Transverse colon 10%

Morphologic types of colorectal cancer
- Polypoid mass (Fig. 8.23)
- Circumferential (annular or stenosing) – "apple-core" lesions (Fig. 8.17)
- Diffuse (infiltrating)

Role of radiology in diagnosis of colorectal cancer
Barium enema
- Prior to endoscopy, radiology was the main method of confirming a diagnosis of suspected colon cancer without resorting to an operation.

This was achieved by distending and opacifying the colon with barium contrast given via a rectal tube after the bowel had been cleansed with a suitable bowel preparation (single contrast barium enema – SCBE). This technique was sensitive to large masses and stenosing lesions but less sensitive to smaller masses and polyps.

- The SCBE was superseded by a technique using barium to coat the mucosal surface and the colon which is then distended with air ("double-contrast barium enema" – DCBE) (Fig. 8.23). This technique proved significantly more sensitive to the detection of both polyps and colon cancers. However, neither technique was able to provide a tissue diagnosis.

- The advent of colonoscopy has been associated with a progressive decline in the use of radiological tests in making a diagnosis of CRC. Colonoscopy is more sensitive in the detection of CRC and polyps in addition to providing the ability to obtain a tissue biopsy and even removal of some lesions, especially small polyps. Currently, if CRC is clinically suspected, most patients would undergo a colonoscopy unless there is a clinical reason to do otherwise.

- Currently, the main role of radiology in diagnosis of CRC is:
  - In patients where colonoscopy has been incomplete, that is, the cecum is not reached, or where colonoscopy for some reason cannot be performed.
  - When CRC is discovered as an incidental finding during a radiology test performed for another clinical reason. These tend to present at an earlier stage than those that present symptomatically.

Virtual colonoscopy/colonography

- In more recent years spiral multislice CT scan (or less commonly MRI), using special 3D software reconstructions, has enabled a view of the mucosal surface of the colon from the luminal perspective and hence is often referred to as "virtual colonoscopy" (Fig. 8.24)

- Current data suggests that it is at least as accurate for diagnosis of polyps and for carcinoma as DCBE.

- In the patient who has undergone incomplete colonoscopy it offers the advantage that patients

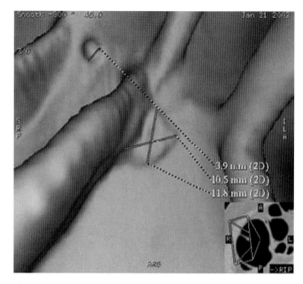

Fig. 8.24. Virtual colonoscopy (intraluminal view) shows two sessile polyps (shown by callipers).

can have a virtual colonoscopy on the same day as the failed colonoscopy and avoid the need for a repeat bowel preparation (DCBE is rarely possible after failed colonoscopy due to the presence of too much colonic air). This is particularly important because for most patients the worst aspect of colonoscopy, DCBE, or virtual colonoscopy is the discomfort and inconvenience of the bowel prep.

Radiology in diagnosis of complications of colorectal cancer

- Large bowel obstruction. Due to the associated risks and increased chance of an incomplete colonoscopy in this instance, and the likelihood that the patient will require surgery regardless of the cause, a single contrast (e.g. Gastrograffin) water soluble enema is usually performed. Water-soluble contrast agents are used rather than barium as they are safe if spilt into the peritoneal cavity during surgery, whereas there is a high risk of severe chronic peritonitis if barium spills into the peritoneal cavity.

- Perforation and associated local abscess formation is another complication of CRC and CT is valuable in its diagnosis.

- Suspected fistulae to adjacent organs can be assessed with contrast studies.

Role of radiology in staging of colorectal cancer

- Regardless of tumor staging, surgery usually is performed in patients with CRC for symptomatic reasons. Therefore, for most patients radiology only has a role in staging in the post-operative setting. The exception is in the patient with rectal carcinoma (see below).
- CT for determining local spread, lymph node involvement, and distant tumor spread is only used to stage CRC (often in the peri-operative period) if liver metastases are suspected or adjunctive therapy is considered (radiotherapy or chemotherapy).
- Knowledge of local extent of rectal carcinoma is important in pre-operative treatment planning and is best assessed with endorectal US or MRI.

Endorectal ultrasound

- Endorectal ultrasound (EUS) of the rectum is performed using a specifically designed US probe inserted into the rectal lumen. It is highly accurate in evaluating size of tumor and extent of invasion through the wall.

Rectal MRI

- Rectal MRI is accurate in assessing level of wall invasion and involvement of adjacent organs/structures. It offers the advantage over EUS of being able to determine whether a rectal tumor that has invaded into the peri-rectal fat has invaded beyond the fascial plane that separates the peri-rectal fat and the adjacent extraperitoneal fat, which can influence surgery.

Positron emission tomography (PET)

- PET scanning (preferably in combination with CT) (see Chapter 5) is used to detect suspected recurrent CRC, for example, on the basis of elevated CEA.
- It is sensitive for detection of small volumes of cancer and can differentiate it from scar tissue.

Role of radiology in screening for colorectal cancer

The justification for screening is that CRC is common and if detected early is potentially curable or preventable by removal of premalignant adenomas.

Colon polyps and cancers are detectable with colonoscopy, sigmoidoscopy, DCBE, and virtual colonoscopy with high accuracy. Sigmoidoscopy is confined to assessment of the rectum and sigmoid colon, while DCBE and virtual colonoscopy are insensitive to small polyps and both require subsequent colonoscopy (or surgery) for biopsy or removal of detected polyps.

In CRC screening, the list of possible diagnostic tests includes:

- Fecal occult blood test (FOBT) performed on stool samples. This may be combined with sigmoidoscopy
- Sigmoidoscopy – most CRC occur within the rectum or sigmoid colon
- Colonoscopy
- DCBE
- Virtual colonoscopy

Each has advantages and disadvantages. There is currently worldwide interest in virtual colonoscopy as a screening test as initial studies suggest it approximates the accuracy of colonoscopy without the risks, cost, and invasiveness, and is better tolerated by patients. Further studies are required to determine which CRC screening test(s) are most appropriate for population screening.

Patients at high risk for CRC (family history, genetic factors, polyposis syndromes, long term ulcerative colitis) all undergo regular screening colonoscopy.

Colonic diverticular disease

Clinical presentations

- Incidental finding on imaging or colonoscopy
- Pain
- Altered bowel habit
- Bleeding – sometimes life-threatening
- Abscess formation
- Fistula
- Perforation
- Portal pyemia – liver abscess

Radiological features

- Most often seen on contrast enemas or CT
- Sigmoid colon is the most commonly affected site

Barium enema

- The bowel wall becomes thickened which reduces caliber and produces a "saw-tooth" or concertina-like appearance.
- The diverticula project as out-pouchings, which tend to fill with barium (Fig. 8.25).

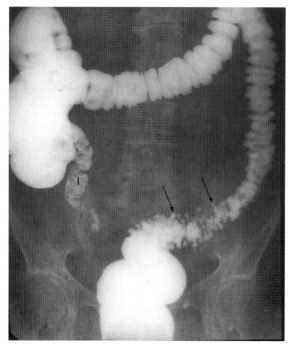

Fig. 8.25. Diverticular disease affecting the sigmoid colon (arrows) on single contrast barium enema. Barium has refluxed into the terminal ileum (I).

CT
- Diverticular disease is seen very commonly as an incidental finding on CT.
- The value of CT lies in its ability to demonstrate pericolic inflammatory changes and abscesses complicating diverticular disease.

Complications
- Stricturing secondary to local muscularis hypertrophy
- Abscesses (Fig. 8.26)
- Perforation – retroperitoneal or intraperitoneal
- Fistulae – to bladder, vagina, small bowel most commonly
- Bleeding – can be major

Radiology in gastrointestinal bleeding
The cause of gastrointestinal bleeding is most often diagnosed at endoscopy (upper or lower). In patients with negative or non-diagnostic endoscopy, radiology may show the site and possibly the cause of bleeding, and may be therapeutic.

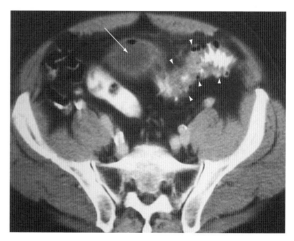

Fig. 8.26. Diverticular disease of sigmoid colon, which is thick-walled (arrowheads), complicated by a pericolic abscess (arrow).

Guides to source of bleeding
- Hematemesis – proximal to the duodenojejunal junction.
- Melaena – upper GI tract down to the level of proximal small bowel
- Bright red PR bleeding – left colon or rectum, unless blood loss is very rapid from upper GI tract.
- Dark red PR bleeding – proximal colon or small bowel.

Active bleeding
If endoscopy is non-diagnostic three imaging modalities may be used, namely angiography, isotope blood loss study and CT.

Angiography
- Arteries examined are celiac artery, superior mesenteric artery (SMA), inferior mesenteric artery.
- Bleeding localized by identifying
  - Contrast extravasation – requires rapid bleeding to be occurring at the time of angiography or
  - Abnormal circulation – e.g. angiodysplasia, tumor circulation

Therapeutic angiography
- Embolization of a bleeding site is possible in some patients. In the small bowel (distal to duodenum) and in the large bowel there is a risk of local bowel ischemia or infarction.
- Vasoconstrictor infusion – this may help arrest bleeding at least temporarily.

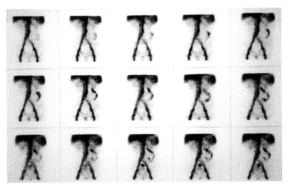

Fig. 8.27. ^{99m}Tc-labeled red blood cell scan. Serial images up to 60 minutes show isotope accumulating in bowel suggesting bleeding in region of splenic flexure.

- Gastro-esophageal variceal bleeding – may be treated by transjugular intrahepatic portosystemic shunt (TIPS) and variceal embolization.

Isotope blood loss study
- Uses labeled colloid or labeled red blood cells.
- Requires active bleeding during the study but detects smaller rates of bleeding than does angiography and is probably more sensitive than CT (Fig. 8.27).
- Can help localize bleeding and direct subsequent angiography or guide surgery.

CT
- Spiral CT with rapid scanning and arterial phase contrast enhancement is an alternative to isotope blood loss studies in rapid bleeding.
- The precise bleeding site is identifiable if there is sufficient contrast extravasation at the time of scanning and this can accurately guide therapeutic angiography or surgery (Fig. 8.28).

Intermittent bleeding or occult bleeding
Upper and lower endoscopy are routine and capsule endoscopy may be used. Diagnostic imaging tests are:
- Angiography, isotope blood loss scan or CT – performed during an episode of active bleeding.
- Angiography and CT – when performed between episodes of active bleeding rely on demonstrating pathology rather than bleeding.
- Small bowel barium study has a low yield but if upper and lower endoscopy are negative may demonstrate a bleeding source (e.g. small bowel tumor).

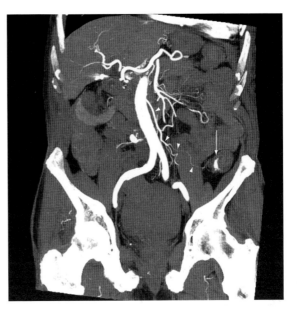

Fig. 8.28. Coronal CT during arterial phase showing contrast extravasating (arrow) into the descending colon from a branch of the inferior mesenteric artery (arrowheads). In this case the cause was diverticular disease.

- Meckel's diverticulum isotope scan – uses ^{99m}technetium pertechnetate which localizes in gastric mucosal cells, present in almost all cases that bleed. The gastric mucosa is responsible for local peptic ulceration.
- Barium enema or CT colonography – if colonoscopy not possible.

Mesenteric ischemia
Mesenteric ischemia presents in a range of clinical patterns, ranging from acute dramatic presentations with high morbidity and mortality, to presentations with less dramatic symptoms and signs, but which may be disabling for patients and difficult to diagnose.

Causes of intestinal ischemia
- Arterial occlusion
  - Large artery – thrombosis and embolus
  - Small artery – arteritis and radiation
- Venous occlusion
  - Clotting tendency
  - Carcinoma, e.g. pancreas
  - Sepsis
- Associated with bowel obstruction
  - Volvulus

- Hernia
- Large bowel obstruction with marked cecal distension
- Non-occlusive hypoperfusion
  - Associated with acute hypotension

Patterns of clinical presentation

- Acute bowel ischemia/infarction
- Ischemic colitis
- Mesenteric angina

Which of these clinical pictures develops, is determined by site and extent of arterial occlusion, rapidity of onset, adequacy of existing collateral arterial pathways, and general cardiovascular function. More rapid and more extensive occlusion leads to acute presentation with risk of infarction. The effect of collaterals is important and natural collateral pathways exist between the three main arteries supplying the gastrointestinal tract, namely the celiac artery, superior mesenteric artery (SMA), and inferior mesenteric artery (IMA). If occlusion of the celiac artery, for example, is preceded by long-term stenosis at its origin, the effects are less dramatic since collateral arcades from the SMA will more likely compensate.

Acute mesenteric ischemia and infarction

- Common causes and approximate incidence
  - 50% SMA embolism/thrombosis
  - 25% non-occlusive – secondary to hypotension
  - 25% other – IMA occlusion, mesenteric venous thrombosis, arteritis
- This excludes the other major group which occurs in association with bowel obstruction, i.e. bowel strangulation.
- Patients generally present with abdominal pain, signs of peritonitis, raised white cell count. One of the key markers is elevated serum lactate level. Mortality is up to 50%–70% and is higher with delayed diagnosis.

Plain abdominal and chest films

The findings include:

- Ileus – bowel dilatation and fluid accumulation (air–fluid levels) (Fig. 8.29)
- Pneumoperitoneum – indicates infarction and bowel perforation
- Bowel mucosal thickening – results from edema ± hemorrhage
- Intramural bowel gas

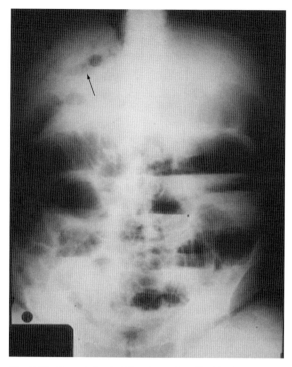

Fig. 8.29. Erect abdominal film shows ileus (fluid levels in dilated bowel, mainly small bowel) and gas in the portal vein branches within liver (arrow).

- Gas in portal veins – this is a sign of bowel infarction and loss of bowel mucosal integrity. It is associated with a high mortality rate (Fig. 8.29).

CT

- Abdominal CT is more sensitive than plain abdominal films in detection of ischemia.
- Signs are
  - Mucosal thickening
  - Intramural bowel gas
  - Pneumoperitoneum
  - Portal vein gas
  - Peritoneal fluid
  - Abnormal bowel wall contrast enhancement, which may be either increased or absent
  - May show major vessel occlusion (arterial or venous)

Doppler ultrasound and angiography

- Have little role in acute mesenteric ischemia

Ischemic colitis

- Most often the diagnosis is suspected on the basis of colonoscopy and biopsy.

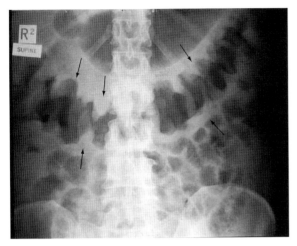

Fig. 8.30. Ischemic colitis. Marked mucosal thickening in transverse colon (arrows). The haustral folds are broader than normal and the overall colon wall thickness is increased. This same pattern can be seen in inflammatory bowel disease.

- Distribution is variable but the most at risk site is the region of the splenic flexure because it is a "watershed" zone between SMA and IMA supply.

Plain films
- Mucosal thickening may be evident in part or all of colon (Fig. 8.30)

Doppler ultrasound and angiography/CT angiography
- May be helpful in detecting the underlying cause of ischemic colitis

Mesenteric angina
- Clinical features of mesenteric angina are post-prandial pain, often associated with weight loss, and classically a history of "being afraid to eat."
- Since the collateral pathways between celiac, SMA and IMA can be very efficient, and because coincidental vascular disease is common, the commonly accepted requirement for a diagnosis of ischemia as the cause of pain is for at least two of the three arteries to be occluded or severely stenosed.

Doppler ultrasound and angiography/CT angiography
- Doppler ultrasound is used as a "screening" test
  - The celiac and SMA are usually easily seen and so can be assessed. The IMA is often difficult to assess.

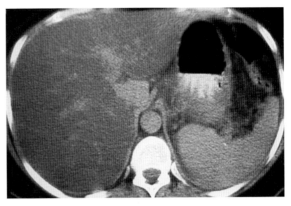

Fig. 8.31. Fatty liver (non-contrast CT). The fatty change lowers the density of the liver and results in the intrahepatic blood vessels and the spleen appearing higher density than liver.

- If both celiac and SMA are normal or near normal the diagnosis of mesenteric angina is effectively excluded. If one is severely stenosed or occluded, the diagnosis remains possible and angiography or CT angiography is considered.
- Celiac or SMA angioplasty can be performed in selected cases

Chronic liver disease
Common causes
- Non-alcoholic fatty liver disease (NAFLD)
- Alcohol-related liver disease
- Hepatitis related – especially B and C
- Hemochromatosis
  In these patients the major roles of radiology are to:
- Suggest or confirm the presence of cirrhosis or NAFLD
- Guide liver biopsy
- Provide surveillance for and targeted biopsy of possible hepatocellular carcinoma (HCC)

Hepatic steatosis (fatty change)
- Ultrasound
  - Detects fatty change readily as it produces increased echogenicity and sound attenuation
  - Can monitor substantial changes in its severity
- CT
  - Fatty change seen as decreased density of the liver (Fig. 8.31)
- Because fatty change can be patchy, and also focal areas can be spared from fatty change, this

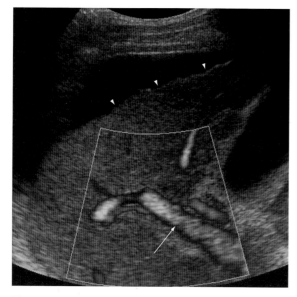

Fig. 8.32. Ultrasound shows ascites surrounding cirrhotic liver which has a nodular surface (arrowheads). The portal vein is patent as shown by Doppler (arrow).

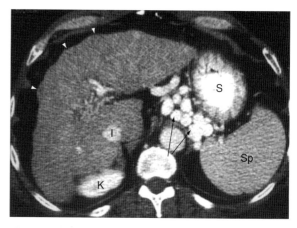

Fig. 8.33. Liver cirrhosis on contrast enhanced CT. The liver is slightly small and the surface is irregular (arrowheads). Prominent portosystemic collateral veins (arrows) have resulted from portal hypertension. Oral contrast lies in the stomach (S); Sp – spleen, I – inferior vena cava, K – top of right kidney.

condition sometimes creates "pseudotumors" on imaging, that is, a focal area that might be misdiagnosed as a tumor. Occasionally additional scans (including MR) and rarely biopsy, are required to resolve the nature of the focal change.

Cirrhosis

- No imaging modality is sensitive for the diagnosis of the early stages of cirrhosis.
- More advanced cirrhosis is usually recognizable on US and CT.

Ultrasound

The main ultrasound changes in cirrhosis are:

- Heterogeneous echo pattern
- Surface nodularity (Fig. 8.32)
- Small liver with advanced cirrhosis
- Small right lobe and relatively larger caudate and left lobes
- Regenerative nodules are sometimes visible – these may mimic HCC
- Changes of portal hypertension if present

These changes are detected in only about two-thirds of patients with cirrhosis, so a negative ultrasound does not exclude cirrhosis.

CT

As with ultrasound, CT is not sensitive for diagnosis of early cirrhosis but advanced cirrhosis has the following appearances on CT (Fig. 8.33):

- Surface nodularity
- Small liver with very advanced disease
- Small right lobe and larger caudate and left lobe

Ultrasound guided liver biopsy

- Liver biopsy in chronic liver disease is performed to:
  - Establish the nature and severity of the liver disease – "non-targeted" biopsy.
  - Determine the nature of any focal lesion, usually to exclude or confirm HCC – "targeted" biopsy.
- US is the generally preferred modality for guidance.
- Prior to biopsy any coagulation disorder must be reversed.
- Larger core biopsy needles (e.g. 14 gauge) are used for non-targeted biopsies.
- Targeted biopsy for suspected HCC is usually with a core biopsy needle (e.g. 18 gauge) for histopathology. Cytology is often misleading.

Transjugular liver biopsy

- Sometimes used for liver biopsies in patients who have irreversible coagulopathy.
- A needle biopsy system is guided from an internal jugular vein puncture down the superior vena

cava, and into the inferior vena cava. Then a hepatic vein is catheterized, and a biopsy is obtained centrally from within the liver. If the biopsy site bleeds, the blood tracks back into the vascular system, avoiding hematoma and blood loss.

Hepatocellular carcinoma (HCC) surveillance
- Patients with cirrhosis as well as those with chronic hepatitis B (with or without cirrhosis) are at increased risk of developing HCC. More than 80% of patients with HCC have cirrhosis.
- Symptomatic HCC carries a poor prognosis (<20% 1-year survival) so there is a potential gain from detecting HCC when small (<3–5 cm) prior to symptomatic presentation.
- Small HCC are more amenable to treatment, whether by surgical resection (about 20% of patients are suitable) or by other treatments, most often direct ablation (e.g. using percutaneous alcohol injection or radiofrequency ablation).
- Surveillance usually comprises a combination of periodic serum alpha-fetoprotein level and ultrasound performed typically 12-monthly in patients at risk. Arterial phase contrast-enhanced CT helps confirm and assess extent of suspected HCC found at US prior to biopsy and treatment.

Portal hypertension
- The most common cause of portal hypertension is cirrhosis
- Results in substantial morbidity mainly as a result of gastro-esophageal variceal bleeding

Diagnosis
- Diagnosed most often by endoscopic demonstration of gastro-esophageal varices
- Pressure measurements – invasive and not commonly measured in clinical practice
- Imaging signs of portal hypertension (usually on US or CT)
  - Portosystemic collateral veins including a patent paraumbilical vein
  - Reversal of flow in the portal vein (Doppler ultrasound)
  - Portal vein enlargement
  - Ascites – not invariable and not specific
  - Splenomegaly – present in only about 50%–60% of cases and not specific.

Causes
- Classified as pre-hepatic (e.g. portal vein thrombosis), hepatic (e.g. cirrhosis) and post-hepatic (Budd–Chiari syndrome)
- Imaging with ultrasound and/or CT can usually assign patients into one of these categories.

Therapy
- The main interventions for portal hypertension are:
  - Endoscopic therapy for bleeding gastro-esophageal varices – sclerotherapy or banding.
  - Portosystemic therapeutic shunts. These may be surgical or radiological transjugular intrahepatic portosystemic shunts (TIPS). TIPS can be combined with embolization of bleeding varices. Surgical and TIPS shunt scan be monitored by Doppler ultrasound.

Jaundice
- The main value of radiology is in evaluating patients with cholestatic/obstructive jaundice as suggested by:
  - Dark urine
  - Pale stools
  - Pruritus
  - Increased alkaline phosphatase and gamma-glutamyl transferase, out of proportion to rise in the transaminase enzymes.
- Cholestatic/obstructive jaundice can occur at a number of blocks in the excretory pathway of bilirubin. The main aim of radiology is to detect major bile duct obstruction which is:
  - Obstruction to both right and left hepatic ducts, or
  - Obstruction to common hepatic or common bile duct (referred to collectively as common duct).
- Radiology detects duct obstruction most often by detecting duct dilatation above the level of obstruction. Duct dilatation:
  - Occurs in >95% of cases of duct obstruction (exceptions can be stones or benign strictures).
  - Is recognized most easily by ultrasound. The common duct measures up to 6–8 mm in normal patients (this increases in the elderly and in patients who have had a previous cholecystectomy).

- Once duct obstruction is suspected the questions are:
  - Anatomical level
    - High (hilar) – close to confluence of right and left hepatic ducts
    - Low – around the level of the pancreatic head
  - Cause of obstruction.

Causes of bile duct obstruction (* common causes)

- Benign
  - Stones*, post-operative strictures, primary sclerosing cholangitis
- Malignant
  - Carcinomas of pancreas*, ampulla, bile duct (cholangiocarcinoma), gallbladder
  - Metastases*

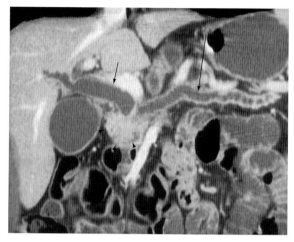

Fig. 8.34. CT coronal reformat shows dilated bile duct (short arrow) which is obstructed by a carcinoma in the head of pancreas (arrowheads). The tumor also obstructs the pancreatic duct which is dilated (long arrow).

Imaging modalities

- After an initial ultrasound other imaging tests are commonly used:
  - Computed tomography (CT)
  - Cholangiography – endoscopic retrograde cholangiography (ERCP), or magnetic resonance imaging and magnetic resonance cholangiopancreatography (MRCP)

Computed tomography (CT)

CT is used to attempt to answer the questions about "level" and "cause" of obstruction if these have not been answered by ultrasound (Fig. 8.34).

Cholangiography

- If the ultrasound and CT scans have not provided the answer to the questions about "level" and "cause," some type of cholangiography is then usually required
- Cholangiography simply means creating an image of the lumen of the bile ducts. The methods available in jaundiced patients are:
  - Endoscopic retrograde cholangiography (ERCP) – increasingly used only as part of intervention
  - Magnetic resonance cholangiopancreatography (MRCP) – now commonplace
  - Percutaneous transhepatic cholangiography (PTC) – performed in fluoroscopy with a fine needle. Now usually performed only as part

of a percutaneous transhepatic interventional procedure

Choledocholithiasis

- Choledocholithiasis (stones in common duct) is a relatively common cause of obstructive jaundice which is benign and treatable but if unrecognized can lead to cholangitis and septicemia with significant morbidity and mortality.
- The classic presentation is a combination of pain, jaundice, and fever (Charcot's triad). Not all three of these clinical elements are always present, and patients may not be jaundiced.

Ultrasound

- Sensitivity in jaundiced patients up to 60% (very high positive predictive value).
- Sensitivity in non-jaundiced patients substantially lower

CT–intravenous cholangiography

- Plain CT detects only about 50% of bile duct stones. The majority do not contain sufficient calcium to make them apparent on CT.
- CT combined with intravenous cholangiography (CT–IVC), however, is highly accurate in diagnosing choledocholithiasis, provided that the patient is not jaundiced. The contrast agent is excreted like bilirubin, and if serum bilirubin is elevated more than twice normal the contrast is not excreted. Duct stones show up as low density filling defects in the opacified bile.

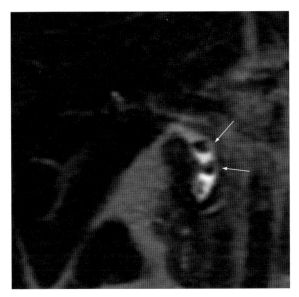

Fig. 8.35. MRCP shows stones in the common bile duct (arrows).

MRCP

- MRCP is used increasingly for suspected choledocholithiasis (Fig. 8.35).
- It may be less accurate than CT–IVC for very small stones but has the similar accuracy for larger stones and has the advantage that it can be used in the presence of jaundice since it does not rely on hepatic excretory function.

ERCP

- If the investigations suggest choledocholithiasis, ERCP can be performed at which time endoscopic sphincterotomy and stone removal is usually possible (Fig. 8.36).

Endoscopic ultrasound (EUS)

- EUS uses high frequency ultrasound on the end of an endoscope (a different endoscope to that used for ERCP).
- It is relatively expensive and invasive, and requires operator experience to achieve high accuracy.

What imaging test to request if choledocholithiasis is suspected?

- Ultrasound – first test; lower sensitivity but high positive predictive value
- CT – not usually helpful
- CT–IVC – accurate if serum bilirubin near normal (less than twice normal)
- ERCP – invasive but therapeutic

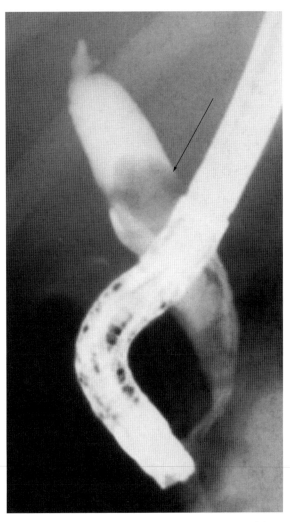

Fig. 8.36. ERCP showing relatively large stone in common bile duct (arrow) prior to removal with endoscopic sphincterotomy and stone basketing.

- MRCP – accurate except for very small stones and can be used in presence of jaundice
- Endoscopic ultrasound – very accurate; more invasive and more technically demanding

What imaging test to request if bile duct obstruction is suspected?

- Ultrasound
- CT
- ± Cholangiography (usually MRCP; ERCP if endoscopic intervention planned)

Biliary stenting

- In patients with malignant biliary obstruction the majority of tumors are not resectable. Biliary stents (plastic or metal mesh) are placed thorough the level of obstruction to allow bile to pass from the liver into the bowel.

- Stenting is performed, if possible, from an endoscopic approach, rather than a percutaneous transhepatic approach, as it is usually safer and more comfortable for the patient and requires less time in hospital. Sometimes, however, a percutaneous approach is necessary.

Liver tumors and other focal pathologies
Clinical presentation
- Incidental finding:
  - Many liver masses are found incidentally on CT or ultrasound.
  - Common lesions include cysts, hemangiomas and, less commonly, focal nodular hyperplasia (FNH).
  - Important because of the risk of benign pathologies being mistaken for malignant disease.
- Upper abdominal pain
- Bile duct obstruction
- Bleeding:
  - Uncommon but potentially life-threatening.
  - Mostly seen with hepatocellular carcinoma and, occasionally, adenoma.
- Tumor staging
- Surveillance for hepatocellular carcinoma:
  - In patients with risk factors (e.g. cirrhosis, hepatitis B).
- Palpable mass on physical examination.

Radiological appearances of specific pathologies

Cysts
- Common incidental finding on ultrasound (Fig. 8.37) or CT (Fig. 8.38)
- Can be characterized accurately by ultrasound
- Multiple cysts seen in approximately 30% of patients with adult polycystic kidney disease

Hemangioma
- Common incidental pathology
- Major clinical issue is establishing confident benign diagnosis

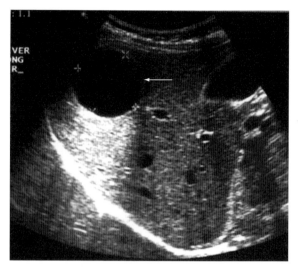

Fig. 8.37. Ultrasound – typical appearance of simple cyst (arrow) with no internal echoes and no perceptible wall, with posterior acoustic enhancement.

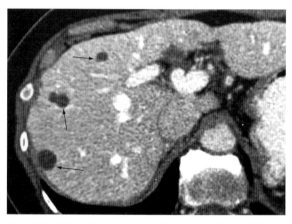

Fig. 8.38. CT – typical appearance of several small simple liver cysts (arrows) with low density and no perceptible wall.

- Should not be biopsied (can cause life-threatening bleeding)
- Typically echogenic on ultrasound
- Vast majority can be diagnosed with a combination of ultrasound and CT (Fig. 8.39). Contrast-enhanced ultrasound can be helpful where available.

Focal nodular hyperplasia (FNH)
- Benign condition which is usually incidental.
- Very vascular and often have a central "scar" and a spoke-wheel pattern of arterial branching, the

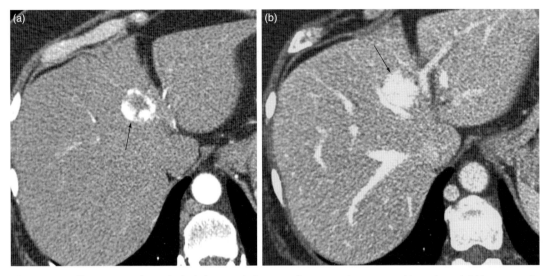

Fig. 8.39. CT of hemangioma (arrows) which shows typical pattern of contrast enhancement with patchy and vivid contrast enhancement in the early phase (a), and complete enhancement on later phase scan (b).

latter often evident on ultrasound. Contrast enhanced ultrasound can be helpful.
- Biopsy can usually, and should, be avoided as it carries a significant risk of hemorrhage.

Adenoma
- Benign tumor, seen almost exclusively in females
- Often an incidental lesion, but of importance because they have some malignant potential, cannot be confidently diagnosed on imaging without core biopsy and may spontaneously bleed

Metastases
- Liver is a common site for metastases from a wide range of primary tumors.
- Liver metastases are most often detected on CT (Fig. 8.40) or ultrasound, with MRI and PET/CT useful in some settings.

Hepatocellular carcinoma (HCC)
- Occurs mostly but not exclusively in patients with cirrhosis.
- Larger when presenting with symptoms, and small when detected in surveillance programs in patients at risk.
- Contrast-enhanced CT including an early ("arterial") phase (Fig. 8.41) is more sensitive for detection of HCC than ultrasound but is more expensive. Most surveillance programs therefore combine ultrasound and serum alpha-fetoprotein

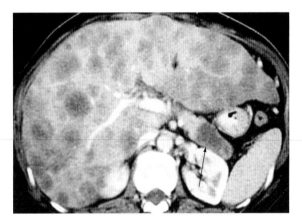

Fig. 8.40. CT scan (post-intravenous contrast) shows multiple liver metastases. Most contain low density central areas corresponding to areas of degeneration. The primary tumor is in tail of pancreas (arrow).

levels, with CT used to clarify any equivocal results.
- Percutaneous core biopsy (ultrasound or CT guided) is generally performed to confirm the imaging suspicion of HCC. Histopathology is more reliable than cytopathology alone.

Abscess (Fig. 8.42)
- Most are pyogenic and caused by bacteria normally found in the gut
- Pyogenic abscesses arise via two main routes:

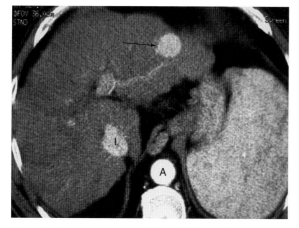

Fig. 8.41. Contrast – enhanced CT in early ("arterial") phase of scan. This shows a small enhancing nodule in left lobe (arrow) representing an HCC. Since the hepatic arteries provide most of the blood supply to HCC tissue and only about 30% of supply to the remainder of the liver, the arterial phase of the scan is much more sensitive in detecting HCC than is the later ("portal") phase. I – inferior vena cava, A – aorta.

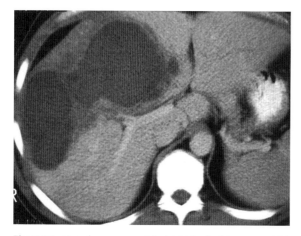

Fig. 8.42. Liver abscesses – mainly right lobe (in this case amebic).

- Biliary – e.g. with bile duct stones or malignant biliary obstruction
- Hematogenous – most often via the portal circulation from bowel pathology
- Amebic abscesses are seen in endemic areas and in travellers to those areas.

Hydatid cysts
- Usually present as an incidental finding or when complicated, for example, by bacterial infection
- Usually diagnosable by combination of serology and imaging findings, which typically includes

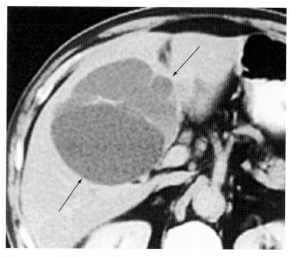

Fig. 8.43. CT (contrast enhanced) showing multiloculated hydatid (arrows).

multiple cystic elements, frequently with calcification of the wall (Fig. 8.43)

Image-guided biopsy and needling
- Liver cysts, hemangiomas, and focal nodular hyperplasia are generally diagnosable on a combination of ultrasound and CT, with MRI required sometimes.
- Most other lesions that are suspicious for tumors require biopsy. This is usually possible as a percutaneous procedure with ultrasound or CT guidance.
- Fine caliber needles (e.g. 22G) are safer and are adequate for cytology, whilst larger needles (e.g. 18G) are needed for histology which may be required, for example, in suspected HCC.
- Needle aspiration is also used for suspected abscess, and can be followed by insertion of a catheter for abscess drainage.

Radiological techniques for treating liver tumors
Interventional radiological techniques can be used to treat liver tumors in a variety of ways.

Angiographic techniques
- Selective catheterization of the hepatic artery supply to liver tumors can be used
  - To embolize the tumor and deprive it of its blood supply. Used to control bleeding, e.g. from HCC.

- To deliver cytotoxic agents. This can be combined with embolization, so-called transarterial chemoembolization (TACE).

Physical tumor ablation

- Percutaneous ethanol injection (PEI). Pure ethanol is injected under imaging guidance. Used for HCC up to about 3 cm in diameter.

- Percutaneous radiofrequency ablation (RFA). A needle is introduced into the tumor and a radiofrequency electrical current applied to produce local heating and necrosis. Most suitable for HCC but also used in selected patients with metastatic disease. Used to treat tumors up to about 5 cm in diameter.
- Percutaneous ablation of HCC is used widely, since about 80% of patients with HCC are not suitable for resection, usually because of cirrhosis.

Contents

Renal failure and renal artery stenosis

Renal failure

- The causes of renal failure can be divided into:
  - Pre-renal, e.g. hypotension, renal artery stenosis/occlusion
  - Renal parenchymal, e.g. glomerulonephritis
  - Post-renal – urinary obstruction
- The role of medical imaging is to:
  - Identify features that suggest
    - Urinary tract obstruction
    - Renal parenchymal disease
    - Renal artery stenosis
  - Provide a guide for safe renal biopsy
- If urinary tract obstruction is suspected then interventional radiological techniques can be used to provide treatment.

Ultrasound

- The usual first imaging test in assessment of renal failure.
- Can quickly assess renal size (Fig. 9.1) and is a screening test for hydronephrosis (Fig. 9.2).
- Normal size range is 10–13 cm and is related to patient size, and decreases in the elderly.
- Small kidneys imply chronic renal parenchymal disease and indicate that at least a component of the renal impairment will be irreversible.
- Conditions such as polycystic renal disease will be detected.

- Dilatation of the urinary tract does not always indicate the presence of current obstruction. It may result from previous obstruction or from chronic vesicoureteric reflux. Antegrade pyelography or nuclear medicine scans can confirm significant obstruction.

Computed tomography (CT)

- CT is often used to further evaluate urinary obstruction when suspected on ultrasound, or in the context of renal colic.
- CT may demonstrate calculous obstruction or tumor obstruction.
- It is usually performed without i.v. contrast because of the risk of further renal impairment due to the contrast medium.

Nuclear medicine (see Chapter 5)

- Small amounts of radioactive materials, which undergo glomerular filtration (e.g. DTPA) or tubular excretion (e.g. MAG_3) are injected intravenously and the kidneys are imaged over a period of time with a gamma camera (Fig. 9.3).
- Semi-quantitative renal function can be determined, with the ability to determine relative function between the two kidneys. An assessment of urinary drainage can be made.

Intravenous urogram

- IVU is of limited value in assessing renal failure because renal excretion is poor.
- Furthermore, the intravenous contrast may further compromise renal function. Intravenous contrast should be avoided in patients with renal impairment whenever possible.

Interventional techniques for urinary tract obstruction

- If there is any suggestion of urinary tract obstruction (i.e. obstruction to the outflow of urine) as the cause of renal impairment then

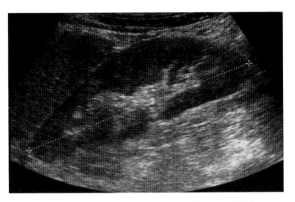

Fig. 9.1. Ultrasound (longitudinal section) of a normal kidney showing renal parenchyma surrounding the echoes of the renal sinus, including the non-dilated pelvicalyceal. The callipers measure the renal length.

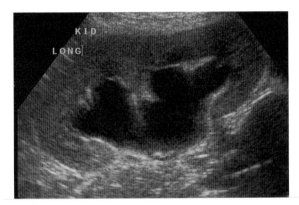

Fig. 9.2. Ultrasound shows hydronephrosis with distension of the pelvicalyceal system which appears black (anechoic). The renal parenchymal thickness is normal which means that the obstruction is not longstanding.

direct pyelography, either retrograde or antegrade should be considered.

- Temporary or permanent decompression of an obstructed urinary system can be performed percutaneously (percutaneous nephrostomy) or by retrograde ureteric catheterization (which requires cystoscopy) in the following situations:
  - Bilateral ureteric obstruction (e.g. due to pelvic tumor)
  - Unilateral ureteric obstruction of a previously solitary functioning kidney
  - Unilateral obstruction complicated by infection of that kidney.
- The combination of infection and obstruction leads to rapid renal damage and demands urgent relief of obstruction (as well as treatment of the infection). This group of patients may have normal serum creatinine as the opposite kidney may be functioning normally.

- If obstruction is bilateral, usually only one side needs decompression to reverse renal failure and the side with better preservation of renal parenchyma on ultrasound or CT is chosen.
- If the obstruction is at the level of bladder outlet (e.g. chronic retention from prostatomegaly), a simple urinary bladder catheter may at least partially reverse renal impairment, prior to more definitive treatment.

Renal impairment due to chronic disease

- With most causes of chronic renal disease leading to renal failure, ultrasound will show small kidneys with reduced renal parenchymal thickness.
- Adult polycystic renal disease
  - Autosomal dominant polycystic kidney disease (ADPKD or PKD) may present with renal impairment.
  - Involves the liver in approximately 30% of patients.
  - Other common clinical features are hypertension and abdominal masses.

Renal artery stenosis (RAS)

- Renal artery stenosis (RAS) can cause hypertension and/or renal impairment.
- A number of investigations can be used to diagnose renal artery stenosis:
  - Nuclear medicine scan – captopril renography
  - Doppler ultrasound
  - CT angiography (CTA)
  - MR angiography (MRA)
  - Conventional angiography
- In patients with renal impairment the tests which use radiographic contrast or gadolinium (CTA, conventional angiography, MRA) are avoided, as they have the potential to exacerbate renal impairment. Conventional angiography is restricted, if possible, to those patients where another modality has suggested RAS and renal artery angioplasty is considered worthwhile.
- Doppler ultrasound and nuclear medicine scans have been the two main "screening" tests for RAS, with imperfect but acceptable diagnostic accuracy.

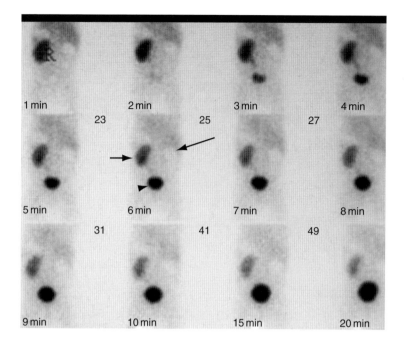

1 min 2 min 3 min 4 min
23 25 27
5 min 6 min 7 min 8 min
31 41 49
9 min 10 min 15 min 20 min

Fig. 9.3. MAG$_3$ nuclear medicine scan shows markedly impaired function in the right kidney. Posterior view with sequential images taken over 20 minutes. Activity is seen in left kidney (arrow) and bladder (arrowhead) with drainage from kidney to bladder over time. The right kidney is seen as lacking activity (long arrow). In this case the renal impairment was caused by long-term obstruction of the right ureter.

MRA

- Has high accuracy for RAS diagnosis and is non-invasive but is less available and more expensive.
- If there is significant renal impairment MR contrast agents should be avoided because they can cause, rarely, nephrogenic systemic fibrosis as a severe adverse reaction.

CTA

- Has a high accuracy but is contraindicated if significant renal function impairment exists.

Captopril renography (see Chapter 5)

- In renal artery stenosis there is elevation of renin secretion and increased conversion of angiotensin 1 to angiotensin 2. This results in increased tone in the post-glomerular arterioles maintaining glomerular filtration in spite of reduced renal artery perfusion pressure.
- The captopril renal scan uses this principle of reversible renal function as a way of diagnosing renal artery stenosis. The scan is performed with an intravenously injected tracer such as technetium-DTPA, which undergoes glomerular filtration. On a separate occasion the study is performed following pre-treatment with captopril which blocks conversion of angiotensin 1 to angiotensin 2 so that, in the presence of renal artery stenosis, glomerular filtration is diminished, including the filtration of technetium-DTPA.

Conventional angiography and angioplasty

- Angiography is usually used to confirm RAS detected on another modality with a view to proceeding to renal artery angioplasty if the stenosis is pronounced (at least 50%) (Fig. 9.4).

Urinary tract calculi

The main roles of radiology are to:

- Confirm diagnosis of urinary calculus.
- Determine size and location of urinary calculi.
- Detect presence of obstruction to outflow of urine from renal pelvis or ureter and, if present and associated with renal impairment or infection, to establish drainage by percutaneous nephrostomy tube placement into the pelvicalyceal system.
- Monitor the function of the affected kidney.
  The main clinical presentations of stones are:
- Renal or ureteric colic
- Hematuria
- Urinary tract infection
- Renal function impairment (secondary to ureteric obstruction)

Abdominal X-ray (AXR)

- Visibility of urinary calculi on AXR depends on composition, size and location.

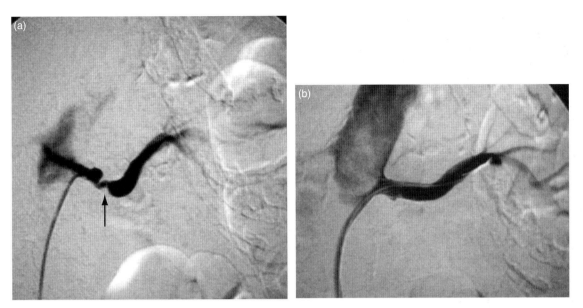

Fig. 9.4. Left renal artery stenosis (arrow) shown on selective angiogram before (a) and after (b) angioplasty and stenting.

- 80%–90% of calculi are visible, these mostly being calcium phosphate or oxalate, and struvite stones.
- Cystine stones (in cystinuria) are faintly opaque, and urate and xanthine stones are non-opaque.
- Small opaque stones may be obscured by overlying structures.
- Vascular calcification (e.g. phleboliths in pelvis) can be confused with stones.

Intravenous urography (IVU) (see Chapter 4)
An IVU is of value because:
- Opacities can be confirmed to lie in ureter
- The degree of obstruction can be assessed
- Underlying structural abnormalities of the urinary tract can be shown

In the setting of acute renal colic a limited number of films are taken. When a calculus is obstructing urinary drainage the renal excretion of the contrast is delayed. An IVU can demonstrate obstruction even in the absence of hydronephrosis (Fig. 9.5).

Role of computed tomography (CT)
- CT is the most sensitive imaging test for diagnosis of urinary calculi as all calculi appear dense, and overlying structures are not a problem as they can be with AXR (Fig. 9.6).

- CT can also show hydroureter and hydronephrosis as signs of obstruction. It may also suggest alternative diagnoses to renal colic.
- CT–IVU is tending to replace conventional IVU (Fig. 9.6(b)).
- A disadvantage of CT is a higher radiation exposure when compared to an AXR or limited IVU. A plain CT just for detection of calculi is lower dose than a more detailed study of the abdomen. The approximate relative radiation doses are:
  - AXR 0.4 mSv
  - Plain CT abdomen and pelvis 3 mSV
  - Detailed CT abdomen 15 mSv
  - Limited IVU (3 films) 1.2 mSv
  - Annual background 2.0 mSv

The role of ultrasound (US)
Ultrasound and urinary tract calculi
- Insensitive for detecting small renal calculi but can detect larger renal calculi (Fig. 9.7)
- Detects bladder calculi
- May detect stones in the very proximal or very distal ureter but misses the remainder of the ureter
- Can assess renal size and hydronephrosis. In acute urinary tract obstruction, however,

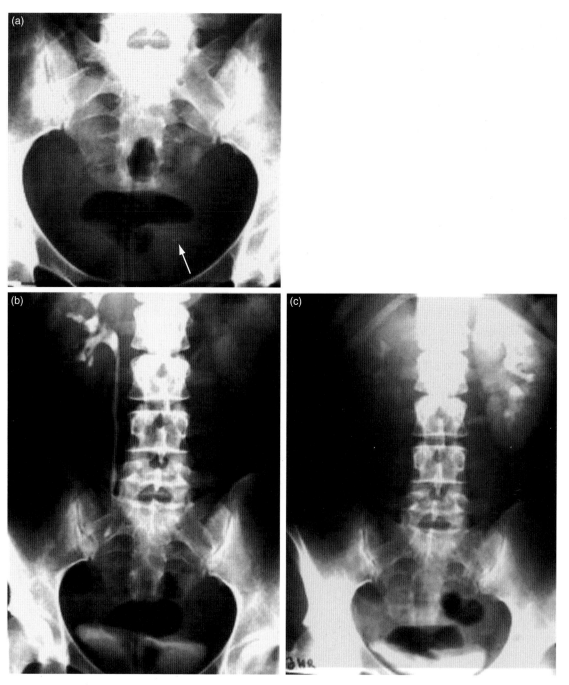

Fig. 9.5. (a) AXR shows two small calculi in lower end of left ureter (arrow). These can be difficult to differentiate from a phlebolith (calcification in small vein thrombus) without subsequently seeing the exact position of the ureter or demonstrating ureteric obstruction. (b) IVU 5 minutes after contrast agent injection shows drainage from right kidney and ureter, but poor function on left side. (c) IVU 3 hours after contrast injection shows delayed excretion from left kidney because of poor function secondary to ureteric calculus obstruction.

hydronephrosis may be minimal so US may not detect acute obstruction

- Detection of calculi is not dependent on stone composition

Interventions and urinary calculi
Antegrade pyelogram
- Through a fine caliber needle, contrast is directly injected into the renal collecting system usually to

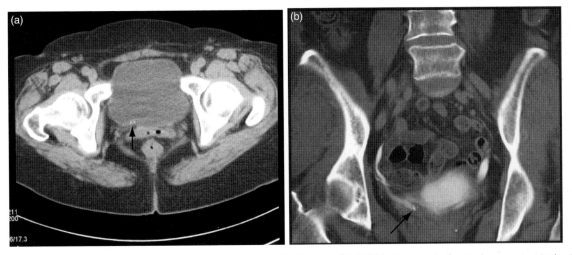

Fig. 9.6. (a) Plain CT shows small calculus (arrow) at lower end of right ureter. (b) CT–IVU with coronal reformat shows contrast in the right ureter down to the stone (arrow).

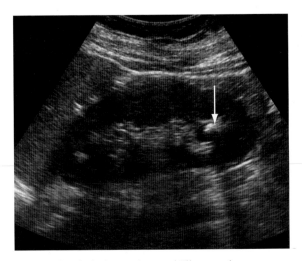

Fig. 9.7. Renal calculus on ultrasound. The stone shows as echogenic focus (arrow) casting an acoustic shadow. This is not a sensitive test for renal calculi.

assess ureteric obstruction or as the initial step in performing a nephrostomy.

Retrograded pyelogram
- Via cystoscopy the ureters are cannulated and retrogradely injected with contrast to assess the ureters and pelvicalyceal systems.

Nephrostomy
- A small self-retaining tube is inserted percutaneously into the kidney to achieve temporary external drainage, to overcome obstruction to the ureter.

- This track subsequently may be used to remove calculi or place a ureteric stent.

Ureteric stent
- A small caliber tube is inserted through the obstructed ureter to establish flow of urine, with one end placed in the renal pelvis and the other in the bladder. This can be done either antegrade or retrograde.

Nuclear medicine (see Chapter 5)
- A nuclear medicine renogram provides a means of assessing relative function between right and left kidneys which can influence how renal stones are treated.

Urinary tract infection (UTI)
Role of imaging
- UTIs in a male and recurrent UTIs in a female warrant investigation for underlying causes such as
  - Urinary calculi
  - Congenital anomaly of urinary tract – especially in childhood
  - Reflux of urine from bladder into ureters (vesico-ureteric reflux) – especially in childhood
  - Urinary tract obstruction
- Imaging may reveal consequences of infection such as renal scarring.

IVU
- IVU is useful in assessment of congenital or acquired problems that interfere with urinary drainage and will show calculi.

185

Ultrasound

- Useful for assessment of hydronephrosis, renal scarring, and residual post-micturition bladder volume.

UTI and urinary tract obstruction

- In patients acutely unwell with a UTI, especially if upper urinary tract infection is suspected (e.g. loin pain) it is important to exclude urinary tract obstruction (e.g. due to calculus) as obstruction must be relieved urgently, usually by nephrostomy.
- US can be used to detect obstruction, although if calculi are thought likely, then either CT or IVU is preferred.

UTI and abscesses

- It is important in septic patients to exclude renal or perirenal abscesses, and CT is more reliable than is US.
- Abscesses usually can be aspirated diagnostically or therapeutically under imaging guidance with a needle and catheter.

Hematuria and renal masses
Causes of hematuria

- Renal parenchyma – renal tumor, renal infarct, glomerulonephritis
- Renal collecting system – renal calculus, urothelial tumor, infection
- Ureter – calculus, urothelial tumor
- Bladder (prostate) – infection, urothelial tumor, trauma, prostate disease
- Urethra – infection, trauma

  The role of imaging is mainly in assessing causes that are "post-glomerular," i.e. not due to glomerulonephritis.

Imaging tests for hematuria

- Abdominal X-ray
  - Opaque urinary calculi
- Intravenous urography (IVU)
  - Assess pelvicalyceal systems, ureters and bladder
- Ultrasound
  - Assess renal size for evidence of chronic parenchymal disease
  - Screening test for renal mass lesions (clearly differentiates cysts from solid masses)
  - Can detect polypoid bladder tumors (not sensitive for "flat" or very small tumors)
- CT
  - Best test for renal tumors – performed before and with IV contrast. Good for staging.
  - Performed without contrast it is accurate in showing urinary tract calculi (including those not opaque on plain AXR)
  - Excellent for renal trauma
- Interventional radiology
  - Often used for treatment of an intrarenal false aneurysm secondary to trauma, including trauma caused by percutaneous intervention or renal biopsy.

Renal masses

The more common renal masses are:

- Cyst
- Renal cell carcinoma
- Abscess

  Other, less common, causes include metastases, lymphoma, and a range of benign tumors.

Renal cysts

- Renal cysts are very common and uncommonly produce symptoms.
- If large, they may produce discomfort.
- Some renal cysts can be difficult to differentiate from atypical renal tumors but usually the combination of CT and US allows this differentiation (Fig. 9.8).
- In the vast majority of patients ultrasound is sufficient for a confident diagnosis of a benign cyst.
- Cysts in polycystic kidney disease appear the same as single cysts but become very numerous (Fig. 9.9).

Renal carcinoma

- Renal masses tend to be found on CT, US, or IVU, either coincidentally or as a consequence of investigation for hematuria or pain (Figs. 9.10, 9.11).
- Surgery for renal carcinoma is often curative if diagnosed early, so detection of small tumors is important.
- Contrast-enhanced CT is the most reliable way of assessing renal tumors and their local spread.

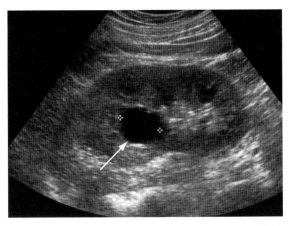

Fig. 9.8. Simple renal cyst. Longitudinal ultrasound section of right kidney showing cyst in central kidney (arrow). Note the thin walls and absence of internal echoes.

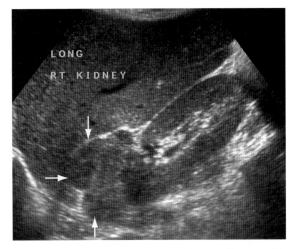

Fig. 9.10. Renal carcinoma. Longitudinal ultrasound section of the right kidney, which shows a solid mass projecting from the upper pole (arrows).

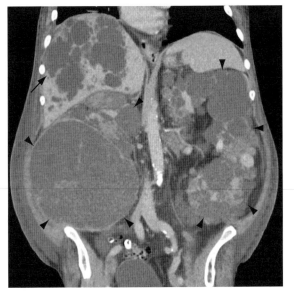

Fig. 9.9. Adult polycystic kidney disease. Coronal contrast enhanced CT shows very numerous cysts in both kidneys (arrowheads), resulting in overall marked enlargement. Benign cysts appear as low density (water density) round masses with no detectable wall and with no contrast enhancement. Multiple cysts also involve the liver (arrow).

- The tendency of renal carcinoma to extend into the renal vein is characteristic and can be evaluated with CT, US, or MRI.

Urothelial tumors
- Urothelial tumors, usually transitional cell carcinoma (TCC), of the pelvicalyceal system or ureters are usually detected by IVU or CT–IVU, or retrograde (or occasionally antegrade) pyelography.

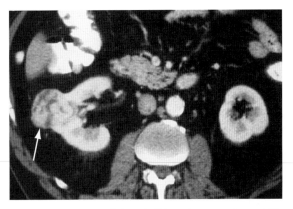

Fig. 9.11. Carcinoma of the right kidney. Contrast-enhanced CT shows a small solid mass projecting laterally from the right kidney (arrow) and showing patchy contrast enhancement.

- Urothelial tumors of the bladder are accurately diagnosed by cystoscopy (which also provides the opportunity for biopsy and treatment) but may be detected first by IVU, ultrasound or CT (Figs. 9.12, 9.13).

Prostate
Benign prostatic hyperplasia
- Extremely common and incidence increases with age.
- Leads to voiding difficulties with advancing age in males and tends to present as frequency and/or nocturia, and is frequently termed "bladder neck obstruction" (BNO).

187

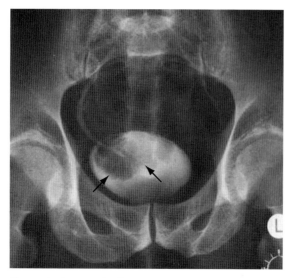

Fig. 9.12. Transitional cell carcinoma (TCC) of the bladder. View of bladder during an IVP showing the TCC as a filling defect on the right side (arrows).

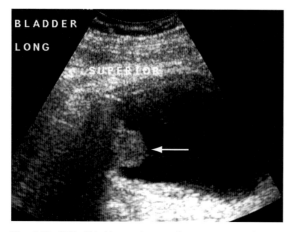

Fig. 9.13. TCC of bladder on ultrasound appearing as a echogenic polypoid nodule (arrow) projecting from the bladder wall.

- The bladder tends to empty incompletely and it may become quite distended. The bladder wall muscle hypertrophies and bladder diverticulae may develop.
- UTIs are quite a common complication.
- Occasionally BNO leads to renal impairment in which case there is evidence of hydronephrosis, e.g. on ultrasound.
- Enlargement of the prostate does not correlate closely with the degree of bladder neck obstruction (i.e. marked obstruction can occur with relatively minor degrees of prostatomegaly and vice versa).

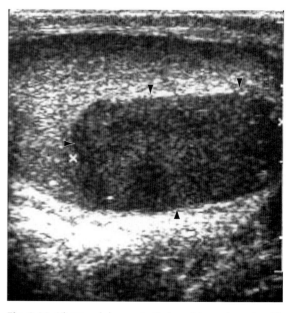

Fig. 9.14. Ultrasound shows a testicular solid mass (arrowheads) which in this case is a seminoma.

- Ultrasound can provide the following information:
  - Assessment of residual bladder volume post-micturition
  - Assessment of "back-pressure" effects on the kidneys
    - Hydronephrosis
    - Renal parenchymal thinning
  - Assessment of degree of prostatomegaly
    - Transabdominal assessment is very approximate only.
    - Transrectal ultrasound (TRUS) is more accurate but not routinely indicated.
- IVU can provide similar relevant information to ultrasound, although ultrasound provides adequate information in most patients with otherwise uncomplicated BNO.

Prostate cancer
- Initial assessment of "at-risk" males is digital rectal examination (DRE) and a blood assay of prostate specific antigen (PSA).
- The role of imaging is to:
  - Perform targeted prostate biopsy using transrectal ultrasound (TRUS) for guidance
  - Stage prostate cancer – including assessment of local, nodal, bone, or lung spread.

Transrectal ultrasound guided prostate biopsy (TRUS)

- TRUS guided prostate biopsy is indicated if there is suspicion of prostate malignancy on DRE or PSA grounds.
- Biopsies are taken of any suspicious areas as well as random samples from a number of areas of the gland as many cancers are not apparent on ultrasound.

Scrotal masses and pain

Scrotal pain

- Ultrasound (US) is the main imaging modality used for evaluation of scrotal pain, masses and trauma.
- Epididymitis, orchitis, and epididymo-orchitis show on ultrasound as swelling and usually increased blood flow of the affected parts, often with a hydrocoele. US also can demonstrate complicating testicular abscesses.

- Testicular torsion is mainly a clinical diagnosis but US can help confirm or exclude the diagnosis by assessment of blood flow by Doppler, or by demonstrating epididymo-orchitis as an alternative diagnosis.
- In trauma US helps detect testicular rupture which requires surgery, and shows hematocoeles.

Scrotal mass

- Usually it is clear as to whether the mass is scrotal or inguinal in origin.
- The key question in assessment of a scrotal mass is whether it is testicular in origin or not.
- Most extratesticular scrotal masses are not tumors whereas most intratesticular masses are tumors.
- US is sensitive for detection of testicular tumors (Fig. 9.14) and can also show extratesticular masses such as cysts of the epididymis.

Contents

Acute headache

The main differential diagnoses are:
- Subarachnoid hemorrhage (SAH)
- Meningitis
- Migraine

Influence of presenting clinical features on differential diagnosis
- Sudden onset suggests SAH or migraine
- Mild fever suggests meningitis (caveat – patients with SAH can have mild fever; meningitis sufferers are occasionally afebrile)
- Nuchal rigidity or photophobia suggest SAH or meningitis

Eye signs in acute headache
Subarachnoid hemorrhage
- Subhyaloid hemorrhages pathognomonic
- Cup shaped when patient examined sitting because of blood fluid behind hyaloid membrane

Meningitis
- Papilledema in chronic
- Normal in acute

Migraine
- Normal

Tests in acute headache
Lumbar puncture
Must be performed if meningitis thought possible, and if the CT is negative.

CT brain
- If performed within 24 hours, 90% of patients will have detectable blood in subarachnoid space. At 1 week, only 70% are positive.
- Advantages of CT
  - Detects subarachnoid hemorrhage with high sensitivity in first few days (Fig. 10.1).
  - Determines probable site of bleed in many cases.
  - Detects complications of SAH (see below).
  - Excludes high pressure due to meningitis complications (hydrocephalus, abscess), ensuring lumbar puncture can safely be performed.

Subarachnoid hemorrhage (SAH)
Causes
- Berry aneurysms – the most common cause of non-traumatic SAH
- Arteriovenous malformation
- Trauma
- Secondary to intracerebral hemorrhage
- Bleeding diathesis/anticoagulation
- Idiopathic – no cause found in 20%

"Berry" aneurysms
- Berry-shaped "blow-outs" in cerebral arteries at bifurcations or branching.
- Cerebral arteries have only one layer of elastica in media that is deficient at bifurcations.
- Association with polycystic kidneys, aortic coarctation, fibromuscular dysplasia of arteries.
- Incidence in "normal" population is 2%.
- Multiple in 25% of cases.

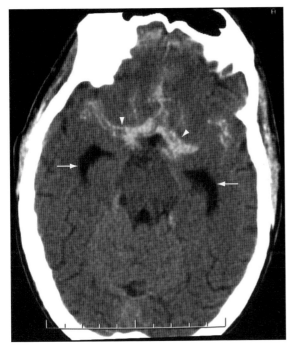

Fig. 10.1. CT shows subarachnoid blood in the basal cisterns (arrowheads) as well as enlargement of the temporal horns of the lateral ventricles (arrows) indicating complicating hydrocephalus.

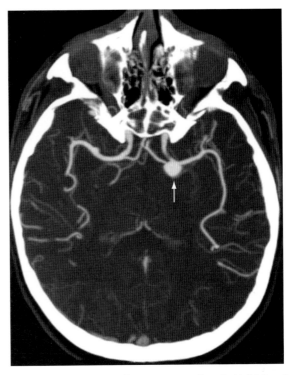

Fig. 10.2. CT angiogram shows aneurysm of terminal left internal carotid artery (arrow).

- The main sites are:
  - 30% – anterior communicating artery
  - 30% – posterior communicating artery
  - 30% – middle cerebral artery
  - 10% – posterior (vertebrobasilar) circulation

Complications of subarachnoid hemorrhage
- Vasospasm after 3 days, potentially producing infarction.
- Intracerebral hemorrhage – implies previous hemorrhage with adhesions in subarachnoid space.
- Hydrocephalus – can be treated by insertion of intraventricular shunt.
- Rebleed, if untreated, with 50% mortality.

Management
- Confirm diagnosis – CT or lumbar puncture.
- Determine cause
  - Cerebral angiography or CT angiography (CTA) (Fig. 10.2).
  - If CTA is negative, cerebral angiography is performed with both carotid and vertebral artery territories selectively studied. It is performed as soon as possible, because vasospasm develops after 3 days. With the

bleeding source treated, vigorous conservative treatment of spasm is possible.
  - If CTA is positive for an aneurysm, a decision can usually be made to treat aneurysms either surgically or by endovascular coils.
- Treatment of cause
  - Most common treatment is surgical clipping or endovascular coiling of aneurysms via selective cerebral angiographic placement.

Stroke and transient ischemic attacks
Definitions
- Stroke
  - Sudden onset of a neurological deficit of vascular origin lasting more than 24 hours.
- Transient ischemic attack (TIA) ("warning stroke")
  - Sudden onset of a neurological deficit of vascular origin lasting less than 24 hours.

Stroke types
- Ischemia leading to infarction 80%
- Hemorrhage 20%
  - Subarachnoid hemorrhage 50%
  - Intracerebral hemorrhage 50%

Cerebral infarcts
Causes
- Emboli from:
  - Carotid bifurcation atheroma, or
  - Heart – thrombus on cardiac infarct surface, or from left atrium in atrial fibrillation.
- Thrombosis
  - Superimposed on underlying atheromatous disease in intracranial arteries.
- Hemodynamic
  - Hypoperfusion due to severe stenosis of major vessels and/or prolonged hypotension.
- Venous infarct
  - Less common than other causes
  - Commonly secondary to venous sinus thrombosis with retrograde propagation into cerebral veins.
  - Are characteristically hemorrhagic

Pathology
The first 6 hours
Whatever the cause, the following processes occur if circulation/oxygenation is not restored. Knowledge of these pathological processes helps in understanding the radiology of cerebral infarcts.
- Loss of function – may occur within 5–6 seconds, e.g. Stokes–Adams attack
- Prolonged decreased cerebral blood flow leads to loss of function of sodium pump
- Sodium, water, and some calcium pass into the intracellular space producing cellular swelling or cytotoxic edema
- Edema particularly involves the metabolically active neurones in the gray matter (cortex).

After the first 6 hours
- Endothelial cells malfunction with loss of normal tight junctions. The blood–brain barrier is disrupted, and water leaks into the extravascular space, producing vasogenic edema.
- Cerebral swelling within 24 to 48 hours – the usual cause of death in large infarcts.
- After 5–7 days, new capillaries grow into the infarcted areas and phagocytes ingest and remove necrotic cells.
- After 3–4 weeks, the infarcted brain has shrunk and consists largely of glial cells (gliosis).

CT of ischemic stroke
- The initial modality of choice is CT, because it is fast, available, and quickly differentiates infarct from hemorrhage.
- The appearance of an infarct depends upon when the patient is scanned.

The first 6 hours
- CT is normal in up to 50% of cases. Abnormal CT signs include:
  - Swelling, e.g. cortical sulcal obliteration.
  - Decreased density due to cytotoxic edema, e.g. loss of the normal gray–white differentiation (Fig. 10.3(a)).
  - Occasionally the actual thrombo-embolus is seen as a curvilinear density in the course of the affected artery.

After 6 hours
- The infarcted area becomes lower density and more readily recognized (Fig. 10.3(b)).
- Swelling can increase dramatically in the first 3 days.
- Hydrocephalus may result from the swelling in cerebellar infarcts.
- A small proportion of infarcts undergo hemorrhagic transformation, particularly if thrombolytic or anticoagulant drugs are used.
- After about 4 weeks, the infarcted area is atrophic, with sharply defined margins. This appearance is permanent.

MRI of ischemic stroke
The first 6 hours
- The most sensitive MRI technique in the early phase is diffusion-weighted imaging (DWI).
- Ultrafast DWI sequences measure the rate of water diffusion at the microscopic level.
- Soon after an infarct, cytotoxic (intracellular) edema is predominant, so diffusion is restricted and appears as a high signal.
- Restricted diffusion is present in almost 100% of acute infarcts in vivo.
- DWI can differentiate between a TIA and a completed infarct.

Radiology of TIAs
- If the patient presents within the first few hours after a neurological deficit, it is not clinically possible to differentiate a stroke from a TIA, hence the value of DWI and MRI.

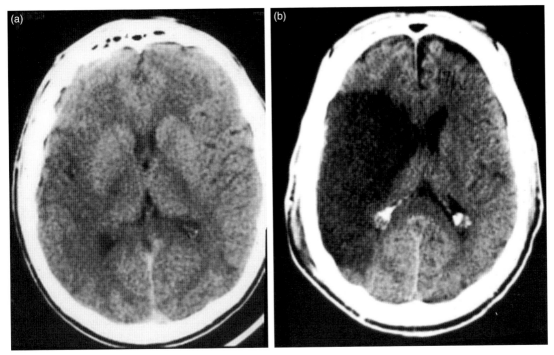

Fig. 10.3. Cerebral infarct. (a) At 5 hours: loss of gray–white differentiation in right frontal and temporal lobes. The abnormal cortex has decreased in density. (b) At 3 days: swelling and more sharply demarcated decreased density in right middle cerebral artery territory.

Investigation of TIAs

- Either a CT or MRI should be performed to exclude other conditions that can simulate ischemia, e.g. subacute subdural hematomas, tumors.
- Digital subtraction angiography (DSA) of the carotid circulation is the "gold standard" for vessel assessment, but is invasive, with a risk of 0.5% to 1% of stroke.
- Non-invasive investigation is best performed by magnetic resonance angiography (MRA), which can demonstrate the intracranial and cervical circulation.
- Alternatively, duplex Doppler ultrasound evaluates the cervical carotid bifurcation, with greater than 90% accuracy in experienced hands.
- Also, echocardiography, especially trans-esophageal echocardiography, is used to exclude a possible cardiac source of emboli.
- Whilst MRI, including DWI + MRA is the most desirable method for investigation of TIAs, CT and duplex Doppler ultrasound are more widely available and constitute a satisfactory alternative approach.

Primary intracerebral hemorrhage

- Almost always associated with hypertension
- 90% occur in four deep sites, namely the putamen, brainstem, cerebellum and thalamus

Radiology of intracerebral hemorrhage

- Clinical differentiation between hemorrhage and infarct is notoriously inaccurate, so a diagnostic test is necessary.
- CT is almost 100% sensitive and is very fast (can be performed on uncooperative patients) (Fig. 10.4)
  - Acute hemorrhage seen as an area of increased density (white) in, for example, the basal ganglia, often with mass effect
  - May also show hydrocephalus.

Secondary intracerebral hemorrhage

Hemorrhages occur secondary to:

- Arteriovenous malformations (AVMs) (children and young adults)
- Aneurysms (adults)
- Amyloid angiopathy (elderly)

193

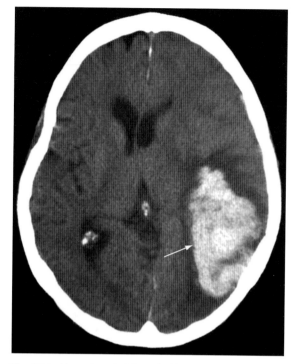

Fig. 10.4. Hemorrhage in left cerebral hemisphere (arrow) with some surrounding edema, and causing midline shift to the right (subfalcine herniation).

- Tumors, such as gliomas or metastases (particularly melanoma)
- Traumatic contusions
- Venous infarcts
- Bleeding diathesis

Consider an underlying cause whenever a bleed occurs in an unusual location, or in a younger patient without hypertension.

Arteriovenous malformations (AVMs)
- Consist of multiple abnormal arteriovenous communications without intervening capillaries
- Best assessed by MRI and DSA

Aneurysms
- The first rupture of an aneurysm usually results in a subarachnoid hemorrhage.
- If the aneurysm is not treated, adhesions may direct a subsequent bleed into the adjacent brain. These hemorrhages usually occur adjacent to the common aneurysm sites:
  - Medial frontal lobe for anterior communicating aneurysms.

- Temporal and inferolateral frontal for middle cerebral aneurysms.
- Medial temporal for posterior communicating aneurysms.
- Subarachnoid hemorrhage is usually also present.

Amyloid angiopathy
- Abnormal amyloid in blood vessel walls.
- Peripheral (lobar) hemorrhages, often multiple, in hypertensive patients over 65.

Tumors
- Tumors prone to hemorrhage are often aggressive:
  - Primary – glioblastoma multiforme
  - Secondary – melanoma (third commonest metastasis to brain after lung and breast).

Trauma
- Hematomas and confluent contusions can simulate other causes of hemorrhage (see section on head trauma in Chapter 7).

Venous infarcts
- Especially post-partum women, women on older types of contraceptive pill, and clotting factor abnormalities, e.g. lupus anticoagulant.
- Venous sinuses first affected, producing raised intracranial pressure type headaches.
- Retrograde propagation into cerebral veins results in hemorrhagic infarcts.
- CT and MRI show peripheral hemorrhages and clot in the involved sinuses.

Summary of investigation pathways
Stroke

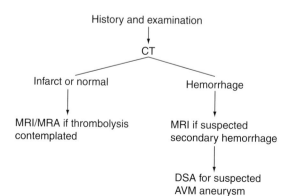

Transient ischemic attacks (TIAs)

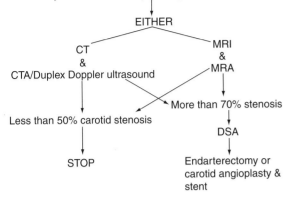

Intracranial tumors

- Classification is based on assumed cell of origin. Fundamental groups are:
  - Glial and non-glial tumors
  - Intra-axial and extra-axial, i.e. of brain or external to brain
- Pediatric
  - Intracranial tumors are more common than in adults
  - More common in posterior fossa (up to 70%)

General working classification
Primary (70%–75%)
- Intra-axial
  - Glioma (40%–50%)
    - Astrocytoma – 70% of gliomas
    - Oligodendroglioma
    - Ependymoma
  - Lymphoma
- Extra-axial
  - Meningioma
  - Chordoma
  - Osteosarcoma/chondrosarcoma
  - Neurofibroma and schwannoma
  - Pituitary adenoma
  - Pineocytoma/pineoblastoma

Secondary (25%–30%)
- Intra-axial
  - Carcinoma
  - Melanoma

- Extra-axial
  - Carcinoma
  - Melanoma
  - Lymphoma

Clinical presentation
Focal neurological deficit
- Often gradual onset, deficit depends on tumor location.
- False localizing signs can occur due to raised intracranial pressure (ICP).
- Sensori-neural hearing loss occurs with eighth cranial nerve neuromas, or occasionally in brainstem lesions.

Seizures
- The second most common mode of presentation.

Raised intracranial pressure
- Headache – with tumors, headache is commonly more severe on waking, and decreases during the day after rising.
- Nausea and vomiting can be misinterpreted as a gastrointestinal disorder.
- Visual symptoms may result from papilloedema or from tumor involving the visual pathway.
- Decreased conscious state occurs with severe elevation of ICP.
- If raised ICP is suspected, further clinical assessment (e.g. neurologist or neurosurgeon) and imaging are indicated.
- Acute presentations may follow bleeding into the tumor or acute hydrocephalus.

Role of radiology
Detection
- CT
  - CT is widely available, and is commonly still the first investigation performed. It is very sensitive for calcification, hemorrhage, and bony destruction.
  - If CT is unequivocally normal in non-specific presentations of headache or seizure, it is usually the only investigation performed.
- MRI
  - If there are more site-specific questions (e.g. hearing or visual loss), or a strong degree of clinical suspicion, then MRI is necessary to exclude pathology.

- Superior for almost all aspects of neuroimaging, and if it were more widely available would be the first line of investigation.
- Intravenous contrast
  - Should be administered when tumor is suspected (with either CT or MRI), or vasogenic edema identified. It makes most lesions more conspicuous because of contrast uptake across a disrupted blood–brain barrier.
- Cerebral edema
  - Most intra-axial pathology causes edema, which can be classified into vasogenic or cytotoxic.
  - Vasogenic edema does not respect boundaries of a single vascular territory, predominantly involves white matter, and has finger-like projections at its margins.
  - Cytotoxic edema has sharp margins, involves both white and gray matter, and often appears wedge-shaped (see Stroke section).
  - Vasogenic edema is associated with a disrupted blood–brain barrier, and may indicate inflammatory or neoplastic pathology (Fig. 10.5); cytotoxic edema is typically the result of infarction.

Characterization

- Deciding whether the lesion is intra-axial or extra-axial is the first step in narrowing the differential diagnosis.
- Extra-axial lesions often have a broad meningeal base, a dural tail of enhancement, or cause changes in the overlying cranial vault (hyperostosis or destruction).
- The presence or absence of calcification and hemorrhage are also important.

Guide for biopsy

- Stereotactic biopsy or resection uses imaging data to allow real time representation of the image superimposed with the surgical instrument, to target the lesion, minimizing the normal tissue affected.

Delivery of therapy

- Radiotherapy and chemotherapy can be delivered to specific sites directed by imaging.

Surveillance

- The phakomatoses, especially tuberous sclerosis and neurofibromatosis, have increased incidences of tumor.

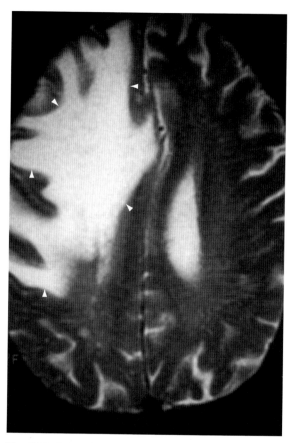

Fig. 10.5. T2-weighted MR scan shows vasogenic edema (arrowheads) associated with an underlying metastatic carcinoma (actual metastasis is not visible on this sequence).

Radiological appearances
Glioma
Astrocytoma (Grade 1 in 3-tier WHO classification)

- 25% of astrocytomas
- The least malignant astrocytoma, macroscopically often indistinguishable from normal brain, merging imperceptibly with surrounding brain without easily defined margins. Occurs in young age group, and can "de-differentiate" into higher grades of tumor.
- On CT may only see subtle mass effect on adjacent normal structures, or an area of low density with little or no enhancement. Calcification occurs in 15%.
- MRI shows a poorly defined mass with abnormal signal and minimal enhancement. Vasogenic edema surrounding the tumor is absent or minimal.

Anaplastic astrocytoma (Grade 2 in 3-tier classification)

- Found in older age group, usually without necrosis or hemorrhage.
- Generally larger and more heterogeneous.
- Greater mass effect and more likely to enhance (Fig. 10.6).

Glioblastoma multiforme (Grade 3 in 3-tier classification)

- The commonest and most malignant astrocytoma; found in the older age group. Pathologically characterized by increased features of malignancy, necrosis and hemorrhage.
- CT and MRI show a heterogeneous infiltrative lesion, with areas of necrosis and hemorrhage. In general, enhancement is widespread and intense.
- Vasogenic edema is common and often extensive.
- Usually solitary, but can spread along fiber pathways, e.g. across the corpus callosum ("butterfly glioma"), or along the internal capsule into the brainstem. Less commonly can be multifocal.
- On histology, tumor cells are identified beyond the margins of the MRI abnormality.

Metastatic tumor

- Most common primary sites are lung, breast, colon, and melanoma. Parenchymal intra-axial lesions are more common than meningeal spread. Usually multiple, lying at the gray/white matter junction.
- Non-contrast CT may reveal masses, vasogenic edema, or be entirely normal. Whenever tumor is suspected, IV contrast should be administered, as most metastases enhance.
- MRI is more sensitive than CT.
- Hemorrhagic metastases are commonly from melanoma, renal cell carcinoma, lung and choriocarcinoma.

Meningioma (Fig. 10.7)

- Common, especially in elderly females. Suspect underlying neurofibromatosis when found in younger patients or if multiple.
- Benign, often large at presentation as they are slow growing. Common sites include the convexity, the falx, and around the sella turcica and sphenoid bone.
- The key to diagnosis is to recognize the site of origin as extra-axial.

- CT shows a hyperdense or isodense lesion, calcified (20%), associated with hyperostosis of adjacent bone, with homogeneous vivid contrast enhancement. Vasogenic edema within adjacent brain is common.
- MRI is better able to confirm an extra-axial site (Fig. 10.7), and can also show enhancement of adjacent dura ("dural tail of enhancement"), which is relatively specific for meningioma.

Primary CNS lymphoma

- Increasingly common.
- Usually separated into primary CNS lymphoma, and those associated with HIV infection or immunosuppression.
- Solitary or multiple, typically in contact with the ventricles, hyperdense on CT, with prominent enhancement.
- The enhancement and mass effect can decrease significantly after administration of IV corticosteroid.

Pituitary adenoma

- Tumors of the anterior pituitary that can be hormonally active or inactive. Active lesions tend to present earlier, at a smaller size. Hypersecretion of prolactin, TSH, ACTH, GH cause well-defined clinical presentations, that prompt laboratory assessment of hormone levels, and pituitary MRI. CT is inferior to MRI for pituitary imaging.
- Direct sampling of blood from the inferior petrosal sinus can localize a tumor causing Cushing's disease, which may be too small to see.
- Differential diagnoses must be considered, as surgery is usually trans-sphenoidal, with limited access beyond the sella. Other conditions that cause masses in or near the sella include cavernous carotid artery aneurysm, craniopharyngioma, Rathke's cleft cyst, meningioma, and hypothalamic/chiasmatic glioma.
- Microadenomas (<10mm) may displace the infundibulum to the opposite side, bulge the surface of the gland superiorly, or erode the floor of the sella turcica. Dynamic scans immediately after IV contrast administration increases detection.
- Macroadenomas (>10mm) can compress or invade the optic chiasm, third ventricle, cavernous, and sphenoid sinuses (Fig. 10.8).

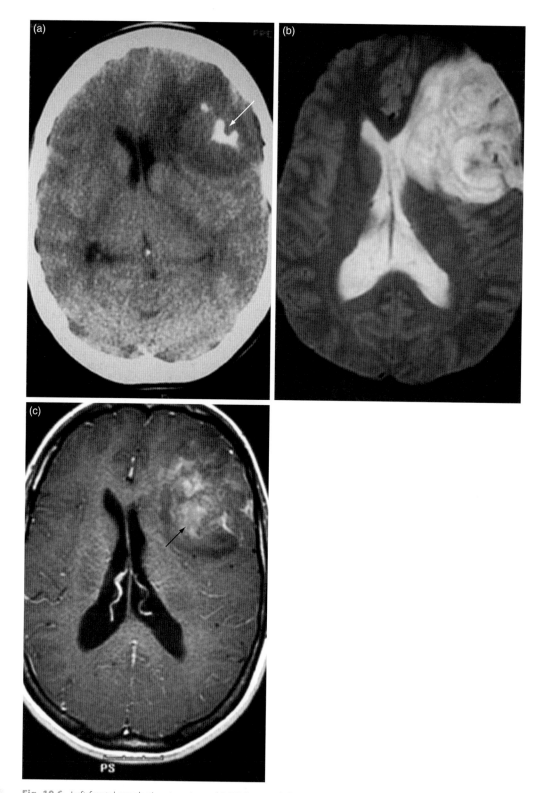

Fig. 10.6. Left frontal anaplastic astrocytoma. (a) CT shows calcification (arrow), (b) T2-weighted MRI shows the lesion as hyperintense with minimal vasogenic edema, and (c) some scattered areas of enhancement on T1 post-intravenous contrast MRI (arrow).

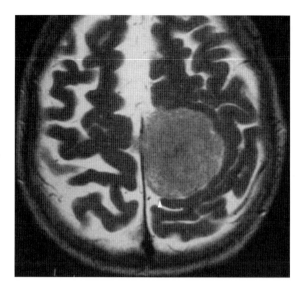

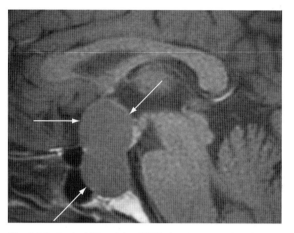

Fig. 10.8. Sagittal T1-weighted MRI of a pituitary macroadenoma, projecting into the suprasellar cistern (arrows).

Fig. 10.7. T2-weighted MRI image shows a tumor. Although it appears to lie within the top of the left cerebral hemisphere, closer inspection shows a CSF cleft (arrowhead) between the mass and displaced normal brain. All features indicate an "extra-axial" site of origin, typical of a meningioma.

Schwannoma
- Can involve any cranial nerve. The most common is an acoustic schwannoma causing sensori-neural hearing loss.
- MRI is the most sensitive test.
- Tumors may arise de novo, but if bilateral indicate neurofibromatosis type 2.

Multiple sclerosis
Key concepts
- Multiple sclerosis is common and causes significant disability in relatively young patients. Clinical features include a relapsing and remitting course, eventually with less complete remissions, and accumulating disability.
- Diagnosis can be difficult, and has been improved with MRI, which can allow an earlier diagnosis. In addition MRI can help exclude other diseases and give some prognostic information. CT has a low sensitivity.
- Can occur at any age, although rare in childhood and old age.
- "Plaques" of demyelination may be acute or chronic.
- Diagnosis requires that other possibilities are excluded, and that lesions are disseminated in time and space.

Clinical patterns
- Approximately 50% present with weakness or numbness in one or more limbs.
- 25% present with optic neuritis (pain and decreased vision).
- The remainder present with unsteady gait, brainstem symptoms (diplopia, vertigo, vomiting, trigeminal neuralgia), and abnormalities of bowel or bladder function.
- Nystagmus and ataxia are common.

Diagnosis
- MS can be diagnosed on a "typical" MRI, but often the appearances are only suggestive of the diagnosis.
- MRI can provide evidence of dissemination in time (by demonstrating plaques of different age, or an enhancing plaque at a site other than that causing the presentation) and dissemination in space.

Prognosis and monitoring treatment
- In general, imaging findings do not correlate with prognosis, although severity of appearance at first presentation does correlate with degree of disability.
- MRI can monitor the effect of therapeutic agents.

Radiological appearances
- Small hyperintense regions on T2-weighted images, typically in peri-ventricular and sub-cortical white matter, posterior fossa, and corpus callosum.

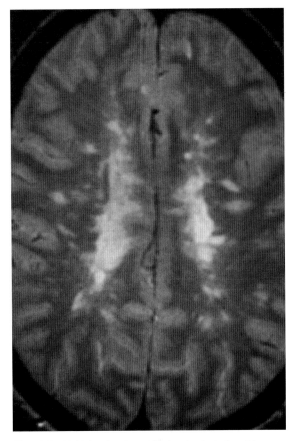

Fig. 10.9. Multiple sclerosis on MR showing typical ovoid peri-ventricular high signal lesions.

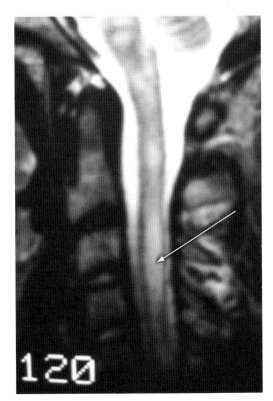

Fig. 10.10. Spinal cord involvement by multiple sclerosis with high signal on T2 images (arrow). Intracranial involvement is necessary for specific diagnosis of multiple sclerosis, otherwise all other causes of intramedullary lesions would have to be considered in this case.

- An ovoid appearance, perpendicular to the ventricular margins, with a horizontal orientation (so-called "Dawson's fingers" of peri-ventricular demyelination) is typical (Fig. 10.9).
- Targeted scans may show optic nerve signal abnormality in optic neuritis.
- Spinal cord involvement is common and may be the first presentation. With current MRI scanners, it is often possible to show the symptomatic cord lesion, but whether or not a cord lesion is shown, intracranial imaging should still be performed.
- Intramedullary lesions of the cord are often relatively non-specific and can appear identical to cord tumor, infarction, and transverse myelitis. If typical intracranial MS lesions are shown, a more confident diagnosis of cord MS can be made.
- Natural history of lesions on imaging:
  - All lesions are initially hyper-intense on T2-weighted images due to edema (Fig. 10.10); then, approximately half resolve, while half

remain hyper-intense. Some of these become "black holes" on T1-weighted images.
- Contrast enhancement:
  - Enhancement reflects a breakdown in the blood–brain barrier, indicates active disease, and usually persists for a few weeks to a few months.

MRI differential diagnosis
- Age-related white matter changes
- Hypertension and other vascular risk factors
- Vasculitis
- Neurosarcoidosis
- Acute disseminated encephalomyelitis (ADEM)
- Migraine

Seizures
Definition of seizures
- Seizures are transient electrical events that disturb normal brain function.

- They may be thought of as an electroclinical event, but in fact consist of transient complex alterations in blood flow, metabolism, biochemistry, and neurotransmitters as well as electrical events.

Who gets seizures?

- They occur in normal or abnormal brains.
- In a normal brain, sleep deprivation, hypoglycemia, hypoxia, and drugs can precipitate seizures.
- May also occur spontaneously in a structurally normal brain where there is an underlying biochemical or genetic predisposition to seizures
- Seizures presenting late in life are often associated with a structural abnormality.
- When a focal structural abnormality is found as the cause of seizures, surgery may be performed to remove the abnormality. Surgery has been particularly successful in mesial temporal sclerosis.

Classification of seizures

- Seizures are classified according to mode of onset.
- If they are bilaterally symmetrical and without local onset at the beginning, they are known as generalized seizures, e.g. tonic clonic seizures, where the patient loses consciousness and has uncontrolled movements of the limbs.
- If the onset is focal, e.g. involving one limb, then they are called partial seizures. These are further subdivided into simple partial where there is no loss of consciousness and complex partial where the patient temporarily loses consciousness.

Epilepsy

- Epilepsy is a chronic disorder in which seizures are the major symptom and occur periodically.
- Prevalence is 5–8 cases per 1000.
- Incidence is 30–50 new cases per 100 000 of population per year.
- Associated disorders – many syndromes are associated, e.g. tuberous sclerosis and Sturge–Weber.

How is the diagnosis of epilepsy made?

- A combination of patient and eyewitness history, EEG, video monitoring and neuro-imaging.

- Video monitoring combined with EEG is useful to distinguish real seizures from pseudo-seizures (often psychogenic).

Role of imaging

- To find a focal abnormality that may be the seizure source. Clinical information and EEG often point to a particular brain region.
- Useful imaging modalities are
  - CT
  - MRI
  - SPECT – best performed at the time of the seizure, to localize abnormal blood flow
  - PET – to localize regions of decreased metabolism

Structural abnormalities that can cause seizures

- Tumors
  - First presentation may be seizures.
  - High grade primary and secondary tumors, and low grade primary tumors can present this way.
  - CT and MR are both used routinely.
- Migrational abnormalities
  - These are abnormalities of brain formation.
  - The normal migration of neurons to cortical gyri is interrupted. Although present at birth, patients may not become symptomatic until later in life.
- Vascular malformations
  - Abnormal collections of blood vessels.
  - Some are seen with angiography. These are usually arteriovenous malformations. They have a tendency to bleed and are usually removed surgically.
  - Other malformations are angiographically occult. These rarely cause clinical bleeds, but may cause seizures, and can be surgically removed.
- Mesial temporal sclerosis
  - Mesial temporal sclerosis is the most common cause of temporal lobe epilepsy. The patient presents with complex partial seizures.
  - Pathologically, there is neuronal loss and gliosis in the hippocampus (in the medial aspect of the temporal lobe) on the affected side.
  - The changes in the hippocampus are not seen on CT but well shown with MRI.
- Infections

201

Dementia

Definition

- A deterioration of intellectual and cognitive function, with little or no disturbance of consciousness or perception.
- A clinical syndrome of failing memory and loss of other intellectual functions due to chronic cerebral degenerative disease.
- Affects 1%–6% of the population over 65 years and 10%–20% aged over 80.

How is it diagnosed?

- Establishing deteriorating memory or mental function may require many assessments.
- Blood tests to check appropriate medication levels and exclude underlying metabolic, endocrine and nutritional causes.
- Lumbar puncture to exclude chronic infection.
- Many patients with depression present with failing memory. This is often difficult to distinguish from dementia.
- Mini Mental State Examination (MMSE) and the Hamilton Depression Rating Scale are useful tests in assessment of dementia and/or depression.
- CT or MR scan to exclude chronic subdural hematoma or tumors.
- Every effort should be made to exclude all treatable causes of dementia.

Causes of dementia

Reversible

- Intracranial masses: subdural hematoma, tumors
- Medication: chronic drug intoxication
- Metabolic: hypothyroidism, Cushing's syndrome
- Nutritional: vitamin deficiency, alcohol abuse
- Chronic infections: cryptococcus, syphilis
- Normal pressure hydrocephalus (NPH)
- Depression

Progressive

- Multi-infarct dementia
- Alzheimer's disease
- Frontal/temporal dementia
- Creutzfeldt–Jakob disease (CJD)
- Lewy body disease
- Neurodegenerative diseases: Parkinson's, Shy–Drager, Progressive Supranuclear Palsy, Huntington's disease, HIV

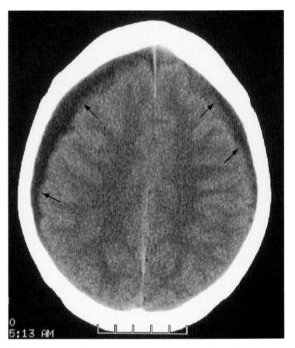

Fig. 10.11. CT demonstrates the presence of bilateral chronic subdural hematomas (arrows) in a 65-year-old patient with memory loss which improved following drainage of the collections.

Chronic subdural hematomas

- Chronic subdural hematomas are an important reversible cause of dementia (Fig. 10.11).

Normal pressure hydrocephalus

- Presents with ataxia, urinary incontinence, and memory impairment.
- CT and/or MR may suggest the diagnosis.
- Intracranial monitoring of CSF pressures may help in diagnosis.
- Response to neurosurgical shunting of the ventricles may be definitive.

Multi-infarct dementia

- Stepwise deterioration due to cerebro-vascular disease.
- Often a history of hypertension, cardiac disease, transient ischemic attacks (TIA), and stroke.
- MRI shows ischemic changes or infarcts.

Alzheimer's disease (AD)

- The commonest degenerative cerebral disease and the commonest cause of dementia.
- Affects all cerebral regions in the late stages but starts in the medial temporal lobe (especially the hippocampus). MRI shows atrophy of the

hippocampus and parahippocampal gyrus out of keeping with the atrophic changes in the remainder of the brain.

- Assessment of atrophy in patients is difficult because of the wide range in ventricular and sulcal sizes present in the cognitively normal aging population. Care must always be taken to match imaging findings with the clinical pattern.
- SPECT imaging or MR perfusion may show decreased flow in the temporal and parietal lobes.

Myeloradiculopathies

- It is essential to determine clinically whether the patient has an upper motor neurone or a lower motor neurone disorder.
- Myelopathy is defined as a disorder of the spinal cord. Patients generally have upper motor neurone signs:
  - Hypertonia (spasticity)
  - Hyperreflexia
  - Weakness
  - ± Sensory signs
- Radiculopathy is a disorder of the nerve roots. Patients generally have lower motor neurone signs:
  - Hypotonia
  - Hyporeflexia
  - Weakness
  - Sensory signs

Myelopathies

Etiology by anatomical group
- Intrinsic disease within the spinal cord – intramedullary
- Cord compression by a lesion external to the cord but within the subarachnoid space – intradural extramedullary
- Cord compression by a lesion outside the cord and meninges – extradural

Commonest causes
- Cervical spondylosis ± congenital spinal stenosis
- Cervical/thoracic disk herniations
- Trauma
- Tumors

Other important causes
- Congenital – spinal dysraphism
- Multiple sclerosis

- Transverse myelitis
- Ischemia
- Vascular malformations

Radiological investigations of myelopathies
- Modalities that may be useful are plain X-rays, MRI, myelography, CT, CT myelography
- MRI and plain X-rays are the most important and often the only modalities required. MRI can demonstrate intrinsic and extrinsic cord disease.
- Myelography and CT are reserved for those patients who cannot undergo MRI, e.g. patients with cardiac pacemakers or aneurysm clips.

Cervical spondylosis
- Very common degenerative disease of the cervical spine.
- Cord compression results from:
  - Degeneration of intervertebral disks and osteophyte formation impinging upon the anterior aspect of the spinal cord.
  - Osteoarthritis in uncovertebral and facet joints, with osteophytes that impinge upon lateral and dorsolateral aspects of the cord.
  - Thickening of the ligamentum flavum, impinging upon the cord dorsally.
- Congenital spinal stenosis may exacerbate the compressive effect of even mild degenerative changes (Fig. 10.12).
- MRI can demonstrate:
  - Narrowed vertebral canal
  - Osteophytes or disk herniations
  - Degree of cord compression
  - Edema or myelomalacia in the cord
- A significant proportion of elderly people have spondylosis and cord compression without symptoms or signs, so the clinical picture is important
- Hyper-intense signal within the cord on T2-weighted scans, due to either edema or myelomalacia, indicates that the cord compression is very likely to be significant.

Disk herniation
- A generic term that encompasses both annulus fibrosis bulge and herniation of the nucleus pulposis through the annulus. MRI often cannot differentiate between them, but treatment is unaffected.

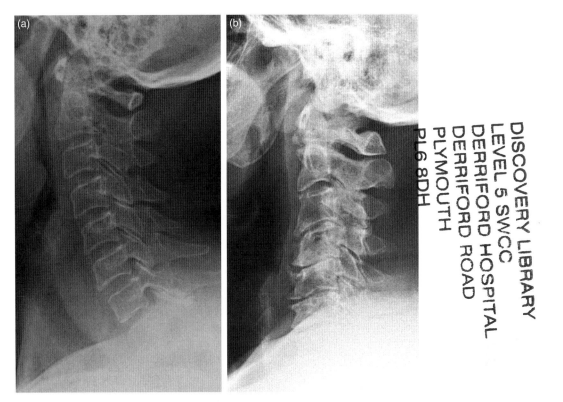

Fig. 10.12. Lateral cervical spine X-rays showing (a) normal sagittal diameter and, (b) stenosis associated with spondylosis. Normal diameter of the bony canal is ≥14 mm.

- Herniation is sometimes divided into four categories:
  - Diffuse disk bulge
  - Focal protrusion – can be focal annulus or nucleus pulposis bulge
  - Extrusion – large focal protrusion
  - Sequestration – complete separation of nucleus pulposis fragment. A sequestrated fragment can migrate as far as one whole vertebral body width from the "parent" disk.

Clinical sequelae
- Cervical – the posterior longitudinal ligament is thin and the cord occupies much of the cervical spinal canal, so disk herniation is likely to be directly posterior and impinge on the cord.
- Thoracic – the thoracic spinal canal is relatively small, so even small herniations present early with cord compression. Symptomatic herniations are, however, relatively rare because disk degeneration and herniation occur mostly where movement is free, i.e. cervical and lumbar spine, rather than thoracic spine.

- Lumbosacral – the conus medullaris usually terminates at the T12/L1 disk level, below which stretches the cauda equina. Most herniations are from L5–S1, L4–5 or L3–4 disks, so even large herniations present with lower motor neurone features.

MRI of cervical and thoracic disk herniations
- Rounded posterior extensions of disks (Fig. 10.13).
- Varying cord distortion/compression
- May see intrinsic cord hyper-intensity on T2-weighted images, as with spondylosis.

Acute cord trauma
MRI is increasingly important in the management of spinal trauma, for both prognosis and initiation of early decompressive surgery.
   Findings include:
- Extrinsic compression by bone fragments, extradural/subdural hematoma or, acutely, disk prolapse.

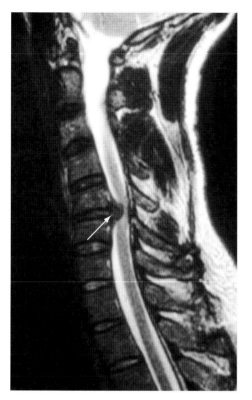

Fig. 10.13. T2 weighted sagittal scan shows a large focal disk protrusion at C5–6 impinging upon the cord (arrow).

- The following have increasingly worse prognosis (from above down):
  - Cord edema
  - Cord contusion
  - Cord hemorrhage
  - Cord avulsion

Chronic cord trauma

(1) The most important sequel to severe cord trauma is the development of cystic myelomalacia, which can then extend either superiorly or inferiorly as traumatic syringomyelia.

(2) Extension of a cyst superiorly can remove vital remaining cord function. Therefore, if any deterioration in function occurs (often painful), early MRI, followed by direct surgical drainage of the syrinx is vital.

Spinal tumors

Intrinsic (intramedullary) tumors of the spinal cord, or extrinsic compression from intradural or extra-dural extramedullary tumors can present with myelopathy.

Tumor location
The location of the tumor is best shown by MRI.
- Intramedullary tumors
  - Cord outline expanded
  - Subarachnoid space symmetrically narrowed
  - Dural outline undisturbed
- Intradural extramedullary tumors
  - Cord displaced
  - Subarachnoid space narrowed on one side, expanded on the other
  - Dural outline undisturbed
- Extradural tumors
  - Cord, subarachnoid space and dura displaced

Tumor type
- Intramedullary
  - Ependymoma – especially adults
  - Astrocytoma – especially children
- Intradural extramedullary
  - Meningioma
  - Neurofibroma
- Extradural
  - Metastatic deposits
  - Lymphoma

Radiological diagnosis of spinal tumors
Intramedullary tumors
- Astrocytomas and ependymomas are the common tumors
- These can be indistinguishable on MRI. The following features are more common in ependymomas
  - Hemorrhage, cyst formation (tumor syrinx), focal well-defined enhancing nodule, secondary deposits in subarachnoid space

Intradural extramedullary tumors.
- Meningiomas and neurofibromas are the common tumors.
- Meningiomas are commonly at the craniocervical junction and in the thoracic region, particularly in women.
- Neurofibromas commonly extend through intervertebral foramina to be both intradural and extradural and are often multiple in neurofibromatosis type 1.

Extradural tumors
- Metastases and lymphoma are the common tumors

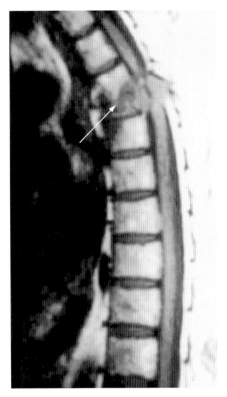

Fig. 10.14. Metastatic tumor from thoracic vertebra extends posteriorly to distort the cord (arrow).

- Metastases are initially blood borne to vertebrae from primary cancers, e.g. prostate, breast, lung or melanoma.
- Tumor tissue invades epidural fat to compress cord or cauda equina (Fig. 10.14).

Lymphoma

- More common in young adults.
- Largely indistinguishable from metastases on MRI.

Radiculopathies
Clinical features of radiculopathies
- Pain is much more common than with myelopathies.
- Lower motor neurone signs.
- Sensory symptoms in dermatomal distributions.
- Muscle atrophy more pronounced.
- More common in cervical and lumbar regions, and uncommon in thoracic region.
- *Note:* The first cervical root exits the spinal canal between the occiput and C1. There are eight

cervical nerve roots. Therefore, the first seven cervical nerve roots exit the canal through the intervertebral foramina above the similarly numbered vertebral body. C8 nerve root exits through the C7/T1 intervertebral foramen, and all the thoracic and lumbar nerve roots exit though the foramen below the like-numbered vertebra.

Causes of cervical radiculopathies
- Cervical spondylosis (can present with mixed clinical picture – a "radiculomyelopathy")
- Disk prolapse
- Trauma
- Thoracic outlet syndrome
- Tumor
  - Mostly extradural – metastases or lymphoma
  - Less commonly intradural/extramedullary

Cervical spondylosis
Plain X-ray
- Shows disk degeneration, with decrease in vertical height of the disk spaces and osteophyte formation (Fig. 10.15).
- Osteophyte encroachment upon intervertebral foramina is best seen on oblique views.
- *Note:* Cervical spondylosis is seen with almost equal prevalence in the asymptomatic population, so plain X-ray changes are not necessarily clinically significant.

MRI
- Shows osteophytes and disk protrusions encroaching upon nerve root sheaths and the spinal cord.
- The ligamentum flavum is often thickened, further contributing to nerve root and cord impingement.
- *Note:* Approximately 30% of all disk prolapses are asymptomatic. Therefore, radiological changes must be interpreted in conjunction with the clinical features.

Non-contrast CT
- Limited role because it cannot clearly show the subarachnoid space and its contents.
- It can differentiate between disk and osteophyte, which MRI cannot always do.

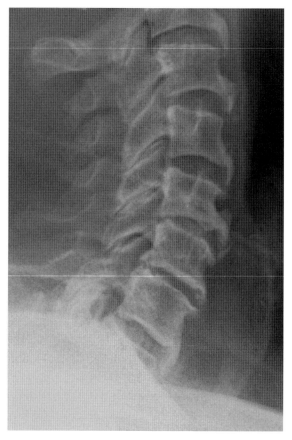

Fig. 10.15. Lateral view of cervical spine showing disk degeneration and osteophyte formation.

CT-myelography (myelography followed by CT)
- Intra-thecal contrast is injected to outline nerve roots and the cord as filling defects.
- Disk protrusions and osteophytes indent the contrast-filled nerve root sheaths and may deform the cord.
- CT-myelography is the procedure of choice when MRI is contraindicated.

Cervical disk prolapse
- More common than spondylosis in young adults.
- Often presents with acute onset of severe pain radiating down the arm.
- MRI is the best investigation.
- Plain X-rays have limited value as there may be no disk height loss in acute prolapses and, conversely, disk height reduction may be present without any disk prolapse.
- CT can show disk protrusions, but imaging of the lower cervical spine is problematic.

- CT-myelography performed if MRI contra-indicated.

Trauma (See also Chapter 7)
Nerve roots may be impinged on by fractures of
- Articular facets
- Pedicles
- Vertebral bodies

Because of the proximity of the transverse foramina (containing the vertebral arteries), there is a significant incidence of associated vascular injury, usually traumatic dissection.

Radiological modalities for investigation of spinal trauma
- Plain X-rays of cervical spine
- CT
- MRI if there is a neurological deficit
- Vertebral angiography if vertebral artery damage suspected (or CTA).

Thoracic outlet syndrome
The C8 and T1 nerve roots ascend slightly before exiting the thorax above the first rib and between the scalenus anterior muscle anteriorly, and scalenus medius posteriorly. The subclavian artery also passes between the scalene muscles. One or both roots can be impinged upon here by any of the following:
- Fibrous band from scalenus anterior to the first rib (commonest)
- First rib deformity secondary to fracture
- Primary bone tumor of first rib

Clinical presentation
- Pain in arm and/or hand, with paresthesia/anesthesia in C8 and T1 dermatomes (little finger, medial aspect of hand and forearm)
- Weakness and wasting of the intrinsic muscles of the hand, or
- Claudication in arm and reduced radial pulse.
- *Note:* It is rare for neurological and vascular symptoms signs to co-exist.

Radiological diagnosis of thoracic outlet syndrome
- Unlike the investigation of all the other cervical radiculopathies, MRI and CT have little to offer, as they cannot demonstrate the fibrous band.
- Plain X-rays – there is a strong association between a fibrous band and a cervical rib (Fig. 10.16), or even more strongly with a long pointed seventh cervical transverse process.

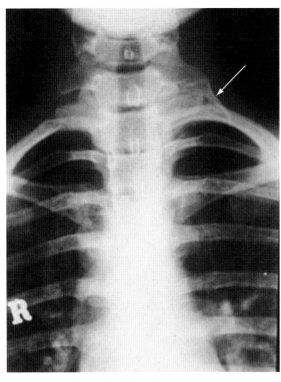

Fig. 10.16. Left cervical rib (arrow).

Extradural tumors
- See Myelopathies section
- Plain X-rays
  - Metastases often involve the neural arch structures and vertebral bodies, but not disks.
- MRI
  - The best modality because it shows tumor extent, and impingement on nerve roots and cord.

Intradural extramedullary tumors
- See Myelopathies section
- Over 90% of tumors are neurogenic (schwannomas, neurofibromas), or meningiomas.

Lumbar radiculopathies

Clinical presentation of lumbar radiculopathies
- Back pain and sciatica are the commonest symptoms.
- Because the spinal cord's lowermost tip, the conus medullaris, normally ends opposite the T12–L1 disk space, lower motor neurone signs are found.

Causes of lumbar radiculopathies
- Disk herniation
- Central and/or lateral spinal stenosis
- Tumor
- Epidural abscess

Lumbar disk herniation
- Can be sub-categorized:
  - Diffuse disk bulge – uniform bulging of annulus fibrosis
  - Focal protrusion – localized mass effect due to fissure in annulus
  - Extrusion – large localized mass effect due to extensive extrusion of nucleus pulposis through annular fissure
  - Sequestration – nucleus material migrates distant from original annulus defect
- Natural history
  - Most disk herniations become organized and regress both anatomically and symptomatically, given time.
  - Investigation of back pain and sciatica can therefore be delayed for 4 weeks to allow a trial of conservative therapy.
  - Only if conservative therapy is ineffective or neurological deficit is profound should radiological investigation be performed.

Radiology in lumbar disk herniation
- Plain X-rays
  - No role – very poor sensitivity and specificity, and unnecessary radiation dose.
- CT
  - Over 90% accurate for disk herniations, but will miss the occasional intrathecal tumor.
- CT-myelography
  - Not as accurate as CT for lateral disk herniations, but will detect intrathecal tumors.
  - Disadvantages: Radiation and toxicity of the contrast medium (seizures, chemical encephalitis).
- MRI
  - The best modality – the most accurate and no ionizing radiation (Fig. 10.17).

Lumbar spinal stenosis
- Can be divided into central and lateral spinal stenosis, although they frequently co-exist.

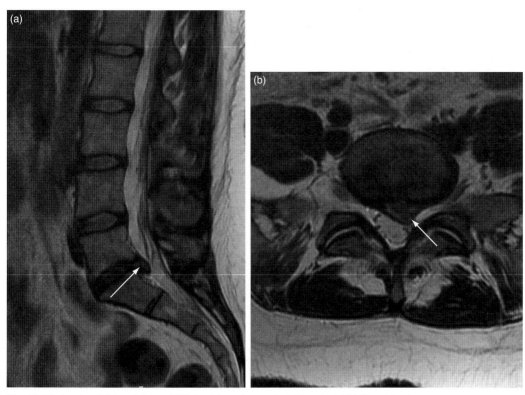

Fig. 10.17. Lumbar disk herniation at L5/S1 level (arrow) on sagittal (a) and axial (b) T2-weighted scans.

- Central spinal stenosis implies circumferential spinal canal narrowing, commonly due to a combination of a congenitally narrow canal, bulging degenerated disks and hypertrophied osteophytes from osteoarthritic facet joints.
- Lateral spinal stenosis refers to localized narrowing of the intervertebral foramina through which the nerve root passes as it exits the theca and the lumbar canal.

Clinical features
- Central stenosis produces the classic symptom complex of claudication of the cauda equina (back pain and sciatica particularly with exercise).
- The pain is relieved by rest and sitting (flexing) and simulates Leriche syndrome (claudicant pain due to occlusion of the distal aorta or common iliac arteries). Examination of the pulses is mandatory for patients with pain exacerbated by exercise.
- Lateral stenosis is more likely to produce unilateral pain, precipitated or exacerbated by exercise.

Radiology of lumbar spinal stenosis
- Both CT and MRI demonstrate encroachment upon individual nerve roots by bone, disk, and osteophyte, and thickened ligamentum flavum.
- MRI best demonstrates nerve root distortion.

Lumbar spine tumors
- See cervical radiculopathy/myelopathy sections
- Meningiomas are extremely rare in this region.
- Rarely, an ependymoma of the filum terminale or conus medullaris may present with radicular symptoms.

Epidural abscess
- Although uncommon, this diagnosis must not be missed, because an abscess is curable. Conversely, non-recognition can lead to paraplegia and even death.

Clinical features
- Pain and local tenderness are the principal clinical findings. Fever is not always present. Progressive paraplegia (or quadriplegia) is a later presentation.

Radiology of epidural abscess

- Plain X-rays are normal in the early stages. Because the disease generally begins as a diskitis, the diagnostic signs are erosion of the vertebral end plates and loss of disk height.
- Radionuclide scans show excessive uptake before plain X-ray signs appear, but have only limited specificity due to "hot spots" from degenerative disease.
- MRI is the modality of choice. The signs are:
  - Increased signal on T2-weighted scans in the affected disk and adjacent vertebral end plates.
  - Destruction of the vertebral end-plates
  - Decrease in disk height
  - Abnormal soft tissue or fluid in epidural space
- *Note:* Disk destruction is typical in vertebral osteomyelitis and only occurs very late with tumor infiltration.

Head and neck – other

An approach to masses in the neck

- Ultrasound, CT, and MRI are all used in the evaluation of a neck mass.
- CT is considered the primary imaging modality, and MRI tends to be utilized as a problem-solving tool or for detailed pre-operative assessment.
- Ultrasound may also be used as a problem-solving tool, and is the favored modality for image-guided biopsy or aspiration of a neck mass. An orthopantomogram (OPG) is frequently used to assess mandibular bony involvement by an oral cancer.

Common neck masses

- Tumor
  - Nodal metastases
    - Squamous cell carcinoma (SCC) of oropharynx, larynx, nasopharynx
    - SCC esophagus
  - Salivary gland tumors
  - Lymphoma
  - Neurogenic tumors
    - Schwannoma
    - Paraganglioma
  - Lipoma
  - Dermoid
- Infection
  - Dental sepsis with abscess

- Inflammatory nodal mass (e.g. tuberculosis)
- Parotid abscess
- Retropharyngeal abscess
- Congenital lesions
  - Thyroglossal duct cyst
  - Branchial cleft cyst
  - Ranula

Squamous cell carcinoma of the oral cavity and airways

- CT is used to evaluate the anatomical extent of a primary tumor involving the nasopharynx, oro/hypopharynx, or larynx.
- Small or superficial primary cancers, detected clinically by oral examination or laryngoscopy, are typically invisible on CT. The purpose of CT in these patients is to identify metastatic lymph nodes and adjacent bony involvement.
- MRI is the most accurate for suspected involvement of the base of skull, paranasal sinuses, intracranial extent, or infiltration along nerves.
- MRI of the hypopharynx and larynx is somewhat limited by motion artifact (due to involuntary swallowing).

Nasopharyngeal carcinoma (NPC)

- NPC may be difficult to detect clinically. Imaging is therefore important to establish local extent as well as nodal status (Fig. 10.18).
- Most tumors will have spread to lymph nodes at presentation.
- NPC has an increased incidence in Chinese.

Laryngeal carcinoma

- Virtually all are squamous cell carcinomas.
- They are divided into supraglottic, glottic, and subglottic tumors, according to location. Most tumors are glottic and relatively small at diagnosis, with a good prognosis.
- Evidence of cartilage invasion, contralateral lymph node involvement or spread beyond the capsule of a lymph node can be detected by CT.

Inflammatory conditions of salivary glands

- Sialolithiasis or intraductal calculi can result in duct obstruction, inflammation of the gland ± abscess. The parotid and submandibular glands

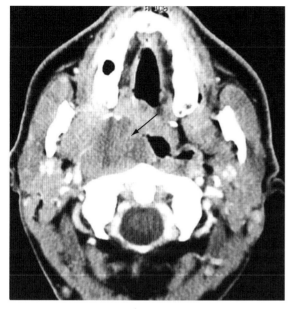

Fig. 10.18. Nasopharyngeal carcinoma. A large soft tissue mass is present within the right side of nasopharynx (arrow). The patient presented with a serous otitis media and trismus.

are chiefly involved. Duct strictures result in recurrent symptoms.

- Calculi are usually radio-opaque, detected on plain film or non-contrast CT.
- Sialography can be performed to assess for duct strictures, which can sometimes be treated using vascular angioplasty techniques.

Tumors of the salivary glands

- Both benign and malignant parotid tumors occur. Clinically, facial nerve pain or palsy indicates malignancy.
- The most common tumor of the parotid is a benign pleomorphic adenoma, but carcinomas also occur.
- Multiple tumors occasionally occur in one or both parotids.

Inflammatory conditions of the paranasal sinuses

- The paranasal sinuses may be initially assessed by plain films, looking for opacification and/or air–fluid levels.
- Coronal CT more accurately assesses the sinuses if indicated. It can distinguish a benign from an aggressive process, by demonstrating bony remodeling (benign) versus bony

destruction (aggressive infections or malignant tumors).
- Chronic or acute sinusitis is the most common abnormality detected on CT. Changes seen include:
  - Mucosal thickening
  - Air–fluid levels
  - Sinus opacification
  - Pseudo-polyps
  - Bony hyperostosis in the setting of long-standing inflammation
- Complications include mucous retention cyst, mucocoele, osteomyelitis
- Intracranial extension of infection.
  - Rarely, aggressive sino-nasal infections (aspergillosis and mucormycosis) are seen in diabetic or immunocompromised patients. These cause bony destruction and rapidly intracranial invasion with fatal results.

Tumors of the paranasal sinuses

- Benign and malignant tumors occur. The most common benign tumor is a papilloma.
- Juvenile angiofibroma is an unusual tumor with a classic presentation and imaging characteristics.
  - Highly vascular tumor within the nasal cavity, nasopharynx, and often pterygopalatine fossa, and typically presents with severe or recurrent epistaxis in a young male.
  - CT demonstrates a vascular soft tissue mass. Angiography is diagnostic and embolization may be used to pre-operatively devascularize the tumor. Biopsy typically results in hemorrhage, hence the need to make the diagnosis non-invasively.

Imaging of the temporal bone

- Thin section axial and coronal CT using a "bone window" algorithm is used. Usually both the normal and abnormal sides are imaged for comparison.
- MRI is used as an adjunct.

Temporal bone fractures

- These usually result from significant head trauma. Clinically, the patient may present with blood in the external auditory canal, CSF leak, tinnitus, vertigo, hearing loss, or facial nerve palsy.
- The most common type of fracture passes longitudinally through the bone (80%).

The ossicles are frequently disrupted resulting in conductive hearing loss. The tympanic membrane is typically involved. Up to 20% have facial nerve palsy.

- Transverse fractures are less common (20%). These typically involve the labyrinth and result in vertigo and sensorineural hearing loss. Up to 50% have facial nerve paralysis.

Cholesteatoma

- An acquired cholesteatoma is a small mass of keratin debris with a lining of squamous epithelium and produces local bone destruction.
- It results from epithelial cell migration into the middle ear following tympanic membrane rupture, in the setting of chronic middle ear infection and eustachian tube dysfunction.

Imaging of the temporomandibular joint (TMJ)

- The TMJ can be imaged using plain film, CT or MRI. Both normal and abnormal sides are routinely shown for comparison, with the joints in the open and closed mouth position.

Glomus tumors (paragangliomas)

- Arise from chemoreceptor cells, and present as a lump in the neck, or with symptoms referable to skull base involvement.
- Two typical sites within the skull base are glomus tympanicum at the cochlear promontory, and glomus jugulare at the jugular bulb.

- More inferiorly in the neck, glomus vagale is associated with the vagus nerve, and the carotid body tumor arises at the carotid bifurcation.
- These are well-circumscribed, highly vascular tumors.
- MRI, CT and angiography usually provide a definitive diagnosis.
- Pre-operative devascularization using micro-particle angiographic embolization is usually performed.

Congenital lesions

Thyroglossal duct cyst

- The thyroglossal duct extends from foramen cecum at the base of tongue to the thyroid. Cysts of the thyroglossal duct are the most common congenital neck lesion and occur in the midline, usually inferior to the hyoid bone.

Branchial cleft cyst

- Cysts derived from embryological remnants of the branchial pouches, usually first or second. They typically present as a neck lump when they become infected. They can be seen in the region of external auditory canal, within parotid, or near the angle of mandible.

Ranula

- This is a post-inflammatory retention cyst, which causes a painless sublingual swelling, that may extend into the submandibular space. The diagnosis is usually confirmed by CT.

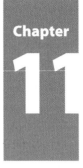

11 Vascular system

Contents

Lower limb arterial disease

Clinical features and etiology

- The main clinical features of lower limb arterial insufficiency are
  - Intermittent claudication
  - Skin ulceration
  - Rest pain
  - Gangrene
- The main causes are
  - Atherosclerosis – vast majority of cases
  - Embolism – may present as acute ischemia
  - Vasculitis – uncommon
  - Trauma

Imaging and non-invasive tests

The role of imaging and related non-invasive tests is to:

- To confirm the diagnosis of peripheral vascular disease.
- To determine the anatomical level of obstruction, its cause, and its severity.
- In selected patients to treat an arterial stenosis or occlusion using angiographic techniques via the lumen – angioplasty, stenting, and related techniques, often referred to as endovascular techniques.
- Monitor outcome of treatments.

Ankle brachial index (ABI)

A pneumatic blood pressure cuff is placed on the leg. The flow is then monitored in the dorsalis pedis or posterior tibial artery by using a simple Doppler probe. The cuff is inflated and released to determine the pressure required to abolish flow, and this is compared with the arm (brachial) systolic pressure. This yields a ratio of ankle to brachial pressure (ABI) and can be used to differentiate ischemic pain from other causes of pain and to grade severity of arterial disease.

The typical ABI values and the clinical correlation are:

> 0.9 normal

0.7–0.9 claudication range

0.5–0.7 ulceration range

< 0.5 rest pain range

Normal values can occur at rest in the presence of significant arterial stenosis or occlusion, and the ABI may only be low after exercise. For this reason, a normal ABI is usually followed by a post-exercise ABI (e.g. on a treadmill).

If an ABI is abnormal, it is often valuable to proceed to duplex ultrasound to determine the location of the disease and differentiate, for example, between a stenosis and an occlusion of the superficial femoral artery.

Ultrasound (US) imaging and Doppler

A combination of gray scale US imaging, spectral Doppler (Fig. 11.1) and color flow Doppler is used to detect and grade stenoses or occlusion in the arteries of the leg. Stenoses result in localized velocity increases. Velocity can be depicted as a color map or as a spectral waveform.

Ultrasound often allows decisions to be made about the best approach to treatment, for example, angioplasty versus surgical bypass grafting. Worksheets are typically used to record the findings of an ultrasound study.

Diagnostic angiography

This involves inserting a needle into the lumen of the artery, commonly in the femoral artery. A guidewire is inserted through the needle and this then serves as a means of introducing catheters into the arterial tree.

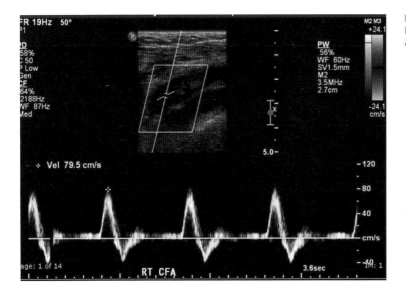

Fig. 11.1. Duplex US showing normal Doppler waveform in the common femoral artery.

With skill and a range of shaped wires and catheters most arteries of the body can be cannulated. Iodinated contrast is then injected to display the arteries and distal perfusion.

Interventional angiography

During lower limb angiography a range of treatments are possible:

- Angioplasty
  - Uses a small inflatable balloon to stretch an area of stenosis or occlusion.
  - In peripheral vessels the most common angioplasties are in iliac, superficial femoral (Fig. 11.2) and popliteal arteries.
- Stenting – uses a metal mesh cylinder to maintain lumen patency after angioplasty in some situations.
- Thrombolysis – using clot-dissolving materials such as urokinase to dissolve thrombus or embolus in vessels.

CT and MR angiography

CT angiography (CTA) is useful in selected patients and its applications are widening. Spiral CT with intravascular contrast allows images of arteries to be generated in an axial plane and reformats then can be created.

MR angiography (MRA) is proving useful in selected settings and is non-invasive but is less widely available.

Acute limb ischemia

Acute limb ischemia presents with the sudden onset of a painful, cold and pulseless limb.

The most common causes are thrombosis, usually superimposed on atheroma, and embolism. Less common causes are arterial injury or spontaneous intimal dissection.

Urgent diagnosis and treatment are important, as the limb can reversibly tolerate only about 6 hours of major ischemia.

Diagnostic angiography is generally the definitive test. It will show exactly the site of occlusion and the status of any collateral flow. Often the underlying pathology can be determined from the appearance, e.g. embolus or dissection. Acute thrombus or embolus can sometimes be removed and/or dissolved (thrombolysis) via an angiographic approach, although some patients require surgical thrombectomy or embolectomy.

Diabetic foot

Patients with long-standing diabetes often have problems due to lower limb ischemia often in combination with peripheral neuropathy and they are more prone to osteomyelitis. Toenail and skin infections are common, as is trophic skin ulceration. The combination of changes is commonly referred to as the "diabetic foot." The changes are a combination of the following.

Arterial insufficiency

In addition to large vessel arterial disease diabetics tend to have small vessel disease, which means that treatment of more proximal arterial stenotic/occlusive disease tends to yield less benefit compared with non-diabetic arterial disease.

Arterial calcification is common including in the small arteries in the feet, something that is virtually only seen in diabetics or in chronic renal failure (Fig. 11.3).

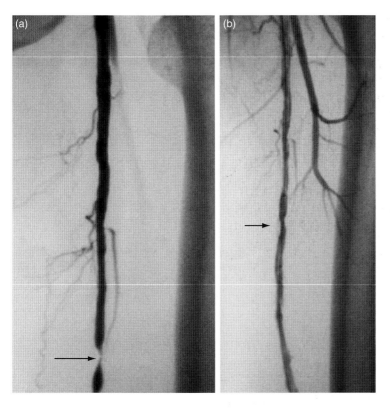

Osteomyelitis

The combination of deep skin ulceration and arterial insufficiency predisposes to osteomyelitis.

The early stages of osteomyelitis may be difficult to diagnose, and antibiotics are given if there is clinical possibility of osteomyelitis even if radiographic bone changes have not manifested. X-ray changes of bone loss may occur after 1–2 weeks (Fig. 11.4). MRI and nuclear medicine bone scanning will show changes at an earlier stage.

Neuropathic bone and joint changes

Neuropathic changes in the foot frequently affect the tarsometatarsal joints (mid foot) with joint sclerosis and bony fragmentation. The neuropathy and deformity of the foot increase the likelihood of skin ulceration.

Abdominal aortic aneurysm

- An abdominal aortic aneurysm (AAA) is a localized dilatation of 3 cm or more. The normal abdominal aorta is typically 1.5–2.5 cm diameter being larger above the renal arteries and in the older population.

- Prevalence is approximately 2%–3% of the population, most common in elderly males.
- Most abdominal aortic aneurysms are atherosclerotic in origin, although connective tissue disorders such as Marfan's syndrome occasionally may be responsible.
- Dissecting aneurysms occur where there has been a breech in the intima with blood flowing in the dissected plane within the vessel wall (see Chapter 6).
- False aneurysms occur where there has been a breech in the wall that is confined by the adjacent soft tissues.

Clinical presentation
- Pulsatile abdominal mass as a coincidental finding. Note that a normal aorta also may be palpable in thin people or be displaced by an adjacent mass, e.g. lymphadenopathy.
- Pain.
- Rupture – pain and collapse.
- Uncommonly, distal emboli, fistula to duodenum or inferior vena cava, infection.

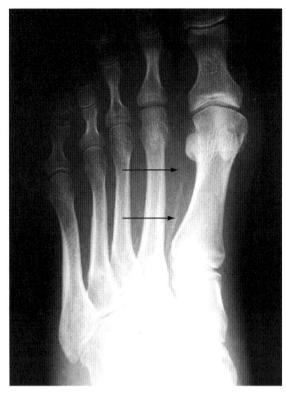

Fig. 11.3. Small artery calcification in the foot (arrows) in a diabetic.

Role of imaging

- Diagnosis
  - Usually with ultrasound (Fig. 11.5) or CT (Fig. 11.6).
  - Suspected rupture warrants urgent US or preferably CT (Fig. 11.7).
- Follow-up
  - AAA typically enlarge at 2–4 mm per annum.
  - Risk of rupture is much more likely if diameter >5 cm.
- Guide insertion of a covered stent within the aorta to treat and exclude the aneurysm.

Deep venous thrombosis and chronic venous insufficiency

Causes of a swollen limb include:

- Deep vein thrombosis (DVT)
- Chronic venous insufficiency (CVI)
- Infection, e.g. cellulitis
- Soft tissue mass
- Lymphatic obstruction

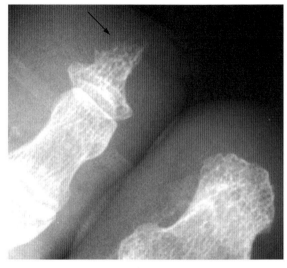

Fig. 11.4. Osteomyelitis in a diabetic – destruction of the terminal tuft of the second toe (arrow) due to osteomyelitis.

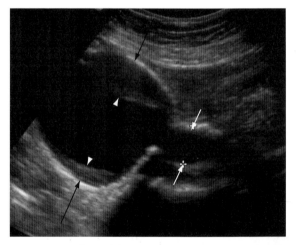

Fig. 11.5. Ultrasound examination in the saggital plane showing an aneurysm of the lower abdominal aorta (long arrows) which does not extend into the common iliac artery shown (short arrows). Mural thrombus within the aneurysm is partially echogenic (arrowheads).

- Injury including hematoma
- Pelvic mass compressing iliac veins
- Generalized causes of edema, e.g. cardiac or renal failure

  Imaging investigations commonly used:
- Venous imaging (DVT or CVI) – ultrasound or, less often, venography
- Cellulitis – ultrasound usually to exclude other cause and assess possible infected collections
- Imaging the soft tissues – commonly ultrasound, ± CT or, more usefully, MRI

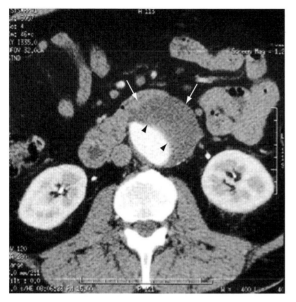

Fig. 11.6. Contrast-enhanced CT showing an infrarenal AAA (arrows), about 5 cm in diameter. Note the thrombus within it (arrowheads).

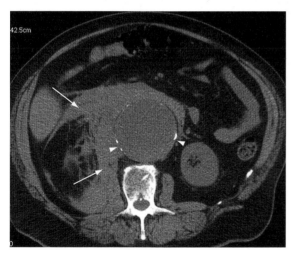

Fig. 11.7. Ruptured AAA (non-contrast CT). Note the hematoma extending around the aneurysm and into the right retroperitoneal space (arrows). The aneurysm wall is partially calcified (arrowheads).

- Lymphatic obstruction (rare)
  - Nuclear medicine imaging with subcutaneous injection of radio-labeled colloids
  - Lymphangiography – lymphatic in foot is cannulated and oil-based radiographic contrast injected
- Injury – ultrasound to evaluate muscle injuries and US or CT to evaluate hematoma; X-rays as appropriate for associated injuries.

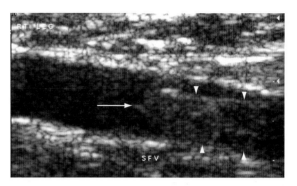

Fig. 11.8. Longitudinal US of superficial femoral vein showing echogenic thrombus (arrowheads) in the vein. The superior extent of the thrombus is seen (arrow). US can be used to follow known thrombus to assess central propagation or resolution.

Deep vein thrombosis
Ultrasound

- Suspected leg DVT is now first evaluated with ultrasound, preferably including color Doppler.
- This has high accuracy for femoropopliteal thrombosis, and acceptably high accuracy for calf vein thrombosis.
- US is less accurate for detection of isolated iliac vein thrombosis, and for assessing the extent of central propagation of DVT beyond the external iliac veins.
- Inferior vena cava (IVC) thrombosis – US is accurate for detection of thrombus in upper IVC (above renal vein level) but is much less accurate in lower IVC.

The ultrasound features of DVT are:

- Direct demonstration of thrombus in vein (Fig. 11.8)
- Non-compressible vein
- Absence of flow in vein

Venography

- Venography of the lower limb involves cannulation of a vein, usually on the dorsum of the foot, and injection of radiographic contrast agents of the same type as used in arteriography and CT. A tourniquet is applied to the ankle so that the contrast preferentially is directed into the deep veins of the calf and thigh.
- Thrombosis appears as filling defects within the opacified vein(s). This is an accurate technique, being more consistently accurate for calf vein

thrombosis, but of similar accuracy to US for femoropopliteal thrombosis.

- It has been largely replaced by US as it has the following drawbacks compared with ultrasound:
  - Patient discomfort
  - Contrast agent adverse effects (as for other radiographic contrast studies)
  - Ionizing radiation

Inferior vena caval (IVC) filters

- IVC filters are suitable for patients with lower limb DVT who have proven pulmonary embolism which continues despite adequate anticoagulation, or in whom anticoagulation is contraindicated.
- The filters are generally a metallic device inserted via a femoral or jugular vein which trap any embolus of significant size.
- They are placed inferior to the renal veins so that, if a large embolus is trapped and occludes IVC flow, there is no risk of renal vein thrombosis.

Venous thrombolysis

- Venous thrombolysis can be used where there is extensive occlusive thrombus in the iliofemoral vein(s) as it can reduce long-term chronic venous insufficiency.

Chronic venous insufficiency and varicose veins

- Chronic venous insufficiency manifests as varicose veins or changes of chronic venous stasis, with leg swelling, induration and ulceration.
- In both situations it is useful in planning surgical intervention to assess
  - Patency of deep and superficial venous systems.
  - Competence of valves in deep and superficial systems. Common sites of valvular incompetence are at the long saphenous–femoral junction in the upper medial thigh, and at the short saphenous–popliteal junction posterior to the knee.
  - Presence and location of incompetent perforating veins.
- Whilst some of this information can be assessed clinically, more detailed assessment is obtained using ultrasound.
- Valvular incompetence can lead to chronic venous stasis and/or varicose veins.

Contents

Lymphoma

Lymphomas comprise a variety of cancers of the lymphatic system. These solid tumors, arising in peripheral lymphoid tissues, are divided into two main groups:

- Hodgkin's disease (HD) – characterized by Reed–Sternberg cells
- Non-Hodgkin's lymphomas (NHL)

Hodgkin's disease (HD)

Incidence and epidemiology

- It occurs at any age, with two peaks of incidence, around adolescence, and in late middle and older age.
- The mean age at presentation is 32 years

Clinical presentation

- Often presents with palpable lymph nodes without other symptoms.
- If it begins in deep nodes, considerable spread may occur before presentation with symptoms referable to complications. These include:
  - Lymph node enlargement causing mediastinal compression (Fig. 12.1) or lymphedema
  - Hematological symptoms – anemia, neutrophilia, lymphopenia
  - Immunological symptoms – susceptibility to infection

- Other presenting symptoms include fatigue, weight loss, fever, night sweats, and pruritus
- Nodal involvement usually follows an anatomical progression, beginning in a single lymph node, then spreading to adjacent nodes, and then to the other organs

Staging

- The amount of spread at first presentation influences prognosis and therapy planning, so accurate staging is very important. The Ann Arbor staging classification is used.
- Staging is usually performed by CT scans of neck, chest, abdomen, and pelvis, after biopsy has confirmed lymphoma.
- ^{67}Gallium citrate scintigraphy and more recently, positron emission tomography (PET) using ^{18}F-flurodeoxy-glucose (^{18}F–FDG) can aid in more accurate staging and re-staging of both HD and NHL.

Radiology of Hodgkin's disease

Chest involvement

- Occurs in two-thirds of patients
  Common features:
- Hilar and/or mediastinal enlargement – present in the vast majority (Fig. 12.2). Nodes can calcify following treatment
- Pleural effusion – in 20%–50%
  Less common features:
- Coarse reticulonodular pattern due to direct extension into pulmonary lymphatics from the hila
- Pulmonary nodules
- Rarely, endo-bronchial involvement, with bronchial obstruction and distal collapse/consolidation
- Diffuse infiltration/consolidation

219

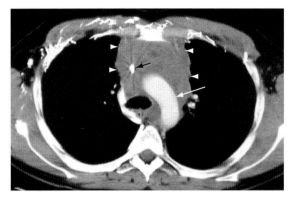

Fig. 12.1. CT scan shows homogeneous mass in the anterior and superior mediastinum (arrowheads). This encases the aortic arch (long arrow), and SVC (short arrow), with SVC compression. Note the enhancing chest wall venous collaterals.

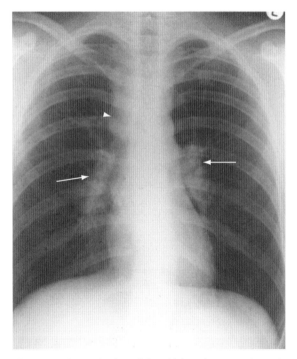

Fig. 12.2. Chest X-ray shows bilateral hilar enlargement (arrows), and right paratracheal enlargement (arrowhead). The most important differential diagnosis is sarcoidosis, which also typically causes bilateral hilar nodes. CT scan may demonstrate nodal asymmetry, and anterior mediastinal involvement, more likely in lymphoma. Serological tests for sarcoid may help, and biopsy is needed to confirm lymphoma.

Other nodal groups
- E.g. para-aortic lymphadenopathy

Bone involvement
- Often sclerotic, but may be lytic

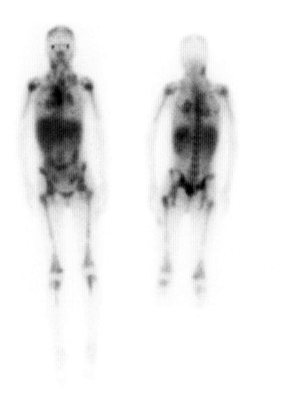

Fig. 12.3. Gallium scan, anterior (left) and posterior views, shows Stage IV HD, with cervical and hilar lymphadenopathy, marrow involvement and splenomegaly.

^{67}Gallium citrate scintigraphy
- ^{67}Gallium citrate is a non-specific marker of tumor and inflammation. It acts as an iron analog and is transported in the blood, bound to transferrin. Most lymphomas have transferrin receptors that avidly bind ^{67}gallium and facilitate incorporation into active tumor cells (Fig. 12.3).
- Normal distribution: salivary and lacrimal glands, liver, spleen, skeletal system, colon, nasal mucosa, breast, and genitalia.
- Indications:
  - Initial evaluation and staging of lymphoma – especially where lymph nodes are not enlarged.
  - To differentiate post-therapy residual fibrosis from active disease
  - To detect recurrent lymphoma
  - To predict disease prognosis – early response as judged by gallium is a predictor of longer term remission correlates

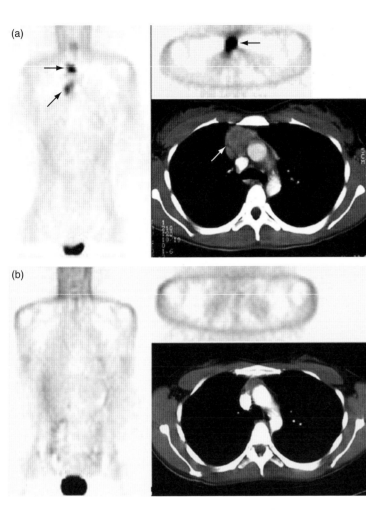

Fig. 12.4. CT and PET images in a patient with mediastinal HD. (a) Pre-treatment scans show an anterior mediastinal soft tissue mass on CT (arrow), and increased uptake on PET (arrows), corresponding to active tumor. (b) Post-treatment scans show a residual mass on CT that is smaller than the pre-treatment mass, but this could still represent active tumor. There is no uptake on the PET image, indicating that this represents inactive fibrosis.

- False positives:
  - Active inflammation, including post-therapy inflammation, thus follow-up study should be performed at least 1 month after therapy
  - Sarcoidosis
  - Other bony pathology, e.g. fracture, infection
  - No study should be interpreted without clinical history and examination
- False negatives:
  - Some low-grade lymphomas do not accumulate gallium, therefore a baseline pre-treatment study is important
  - Small volume disease

^{18}F-FDG PET scanning
- Availability has been more limited compared with gallium scans.
- Glucose analogue localized to active tumor, but not to fibrotic or necrotic tissues,

differentiating recurrence from treatment effect (Fig. 12.4).
- Higher resolution and less radiation to the patient compared to [67]gallium SPECT.

Complications of Hodgkin's disease
- Infections – especially lungs. Chemotherapy-related immunosuppression is common, and infection is the first consideration when lung abnormalities are present.
- Drug toxicity.
- Second malignancy, e.g. NHL, leukemia.

Non-Hodgkin's lymphoma (NHL)
Incidence and epidemiology
- NHL is more common than HD
- It affects all ages but peaks at 50 years
- Males > females

Table 12.1. Differences between HD and NHL

Hodgkin's	NHL
More often localized to single group of nodes	More often involves multiple peripheral nodes
Orderly contiguous spread	Non-contiguous spread
Mesenteric and Waldeyer's ring nodes rarely involved	Mesenteric and Waldeyer's ring nodes commonly involved
Extranodal involvement uncommon	Extranodal involvement common

Predisposing factors include
- HIV infection
- Celiac disease
- Organ transplantation
- Collagen vascular disease
- Congenital immunodeficiency

Presentation
- Similar to HD, but NHL does not follow an orderly anatomical progression, unlike HD.
- NHL is likely to be disseminated at the time of diagnosis.

Classification
- This is controversial and confusing, and several classifications have been used over the years. Details are beyond the scope of this text.

Staging
- The Ann Arbor classification is used for NHL (as in HD), but is less useful for prognosis.

Radiology of non-Hodgkin's lymphoma
Lymphadenopathy
- CT is routinely used for staging and follow-up. Lymphadenopathy is typical, but extra-nodal disease is also common, and the patient may present with symptoms referable to this.
- *Note:* CT cannot diagnose tumor in normal-sized nodes

Extra-nodal disease
- Soft tissue masses may be found in
  - Gastrointestinal tract – stomach, SI colon, pancreas, peritoneum
  - Chest – Lung nodules, pleura, heart and pericardium
  - Genitourinary tract – kidneys, testis, ovaries, uterus
- Bone
- CNS

- Liver, spleen
- Head and neck
- The imaging technique used to display lesions in different sites depends on the organ involved, e.g. for a bone lesion, work-up initially includes CXR, MRI, and possibly bone scan and CT. For a renal mass or cerebral symptoms CT is routine.

Once NIIL is diagnosed by biopsy, staging, and follow-up is usually with CT, with extra imaging depending on the primary site.

Complications
- As for Hodgkin's disease

Multiple myeloma
Clinical features
- This is the commonest primary malignant bony neoplasm in adults.
- It usually presents in the fifth to eighth decades, with 98% of cases seen over age 40.
- Two forms occur:
  - Disseminated form: usually >40 years, males > females
  - Solitary form: mean age 50 years
- Symptoms include: bone pain, anemia and other hematologic/serologic abnormalities, renal insufficiency, hypercalcemia, proteinuria.

Locations
- Disseminated form:
  - Scattered throughout axial skeleton (sites of red marrow): vertebrae, ribs, skull, pelvis, long bones in decreasing frequency.
- Solitary form:
  - Vertebrae, pelvis, skull, sternum, ribs in decreasing frequency.
  - Spinal plasmacytoma: vertebral bodies, not posterior elements (i.e. spares the pedicles, unlike metastases). Often causes paravertebral mass.

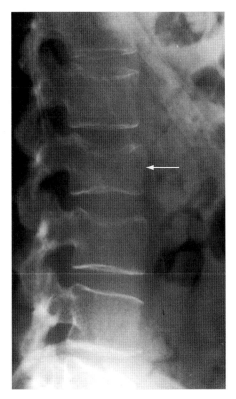

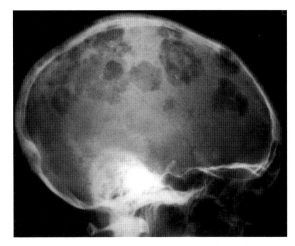

Fig. 12.6. Myeloma. Lateral skull view showing multiple destructive lucencies of varying sizes in the skull vault. The differential diagnosis includes metastases and myeloma.

Radiology in staging of malignant disease

Aims of staging

- Document extent (local and distant) of involvement before commencing therapy.
- Enable appropriate treatment choice (e.g. excision, radiotherapy, chemotherapy).
- Provide a baseline from which to measure treatment response or tumor recurrence.

Staging approach – overview

- The approaches used differ across the organ systems of the body.
- After the tissue diagnosis of neoplasm is made, staging examinations are usual. These are frequently plain radiographs, radioisotope scans, and CT scans of sites where metastases most often occur.
- Positron emission tomography (PET) is extremely useful in certain tumors and is often used to assess residual viable tumor when there is a residual mass on CT following therapy.
- The section below covers appropriate imaging strategies for various common specific malignancies, but individual hospitals and clinicians may prefer variations to that outlined. Availability of different techniques, e.g. PET, also affects the approach in different centers.

Fig. 12.5. Myeloma. Lateral view of lumbar spine shows diffuse osteopenia and collapse at L3 (arrow). These appearances could be due to generalized osteoporosis.

Radiological manifestations

- Generalized osteopenia, vertebral compression fractures (Fig. 12.5).

  Note: Multiple myeloma should be considered in the differential diagnosis of diffuse osteopenia, particularly in a male or relatively young patient with no identified risk factors for osteoporosis.

- Punched out lytic areas in axial skeleton. May be very widespread, and vary in size.

  Note: Should be remembered as a differential diagnosis for bony metastases.

- Large diffuse lytic areas.
- Soft tissue mass adjacent to bone destruction.
- Can involve the mandible.
- Staging and follow-up is usually with skeletal survey of the axial skeleton, i.e. radiographs of skull, whole spine, pelvis, chest, femora, and humeri (Fig. 12.6). Bone scans are less sensitive and are therefore not routinely used.
- Complications such as pneumonia and pathological fractures can be readily diagnosed by plain radiographs.

223

Lung cancer

- Tumors are often divided into small cell and non-small cell carcinomas, since they behave differently. Most small cell cancers will have spread by the time of presentation.
- Staging of lung cancer uses the TNM classification system.
- Many lung cancers are unresectable and the aim of the initial imaging is to determine whether this is the case. Reasons for unresectability include:
  - Extrathoracic metastases
  - Intrathoracic spread:
    - Malignant pleural effusion
    - Invasion of mediastinum
    - Contralateral mediastinal nodal disease.

Chest X-ray

- To assess size of tumor, location, lobar or segmental atelectasis, pleural effusion, and lymph node involvement.

CT

- Contrast-enhanced CT is usually performed from the lung apices down through the adrenal glands.
- Recognition of abnormal nodes is based on size, and is therefore not tissue specific. In the mediastinum, nodes >1 cm in size are usually regarded as abnormal. If mediastinal nodes are found, tissue confirmation is usually required before treatment. Similarly, an adrenal mass can be a coincidental benign adenoma and may need further imaging or biopsy.
- Limitations – not good for early chest wall invasion, and not tissue specific for nodal involvement.

Bone scans

- Only performed in selected cases, usually if skeletal symptoms or if PET suggests bony abnormalities.

^{18}F-FDG–PET

- More sensitive in staging the mediastinum than CT, and considered by most thoracic surgeons to be essential prior to surgery. Now usually combined with CT.

MRI

- Useful to assess the neurovascular bundle in Pancoast tumors.

Extrathoracic imaging

- Imaging of liver, skeleton and brain is performed for small cell carcinomas or patients with non-small cell carcinomas and symptoms such as weight loss.
- Adenocarcinoma and small cell carcinoma have a high rate of cerebral metastasis.

Follow-up of lung cancer

- CXR is routine.
- CT usually is reserved for investigation of specific symptoms or radiographic findings.
- Signs of radiotherapy (pneumonitis, fibrosis) affecting the lungs can complicate interpretation, but should be stable within 16–20 months following radiotherapy.

Gastrointestinal (GIT) malignancy
Esophageal carcinoma

- CT is routine. It can assess gross direct invasion of mediastinal structures and distant metastases.
- Lymph node metastases are also detected, but as with lung cancer, size is the criterion used. Therefore, one cannot distinguish between enlarged reactive nodes and tumor, or detect tumor in normal-sized nodes. This problem is substantially overcome with PET–CT which is now commonly performed if no distant metastases are found on initial CT.
- Endoscopic US can assess depth of tumor invasion, and adjacent lymph nodes, and can guide biopsy.

Gastric carcinoma

- CT used to assess lymph node and liver metastases, prior to surgical staging, but has limited accuracy for local invasion through stomach wall and lymph node involvement.
- PET–CT used in some centers.

Colorectal, liver, and pancreatic cancers (See Chapter 8)
Urinary tract

- Renal carcinoma (RCC)
  - Many are "incidental" findings on US or CT performed for vague signs and symptoms such as loss of weight, malaise, or anemia. Small tumors (<3 cm) are usually not advanced at the time of diagnosis, but overall approximately 30% of patients with RCC have metastases at time of diagnosis, often in lung or bone.

- Staging is usually by dynamic contrast enhanced CT ± MR.
- Venography is only occasionally required in equivocal cases of IVC or renal vein involvement. Angiography is performed only if embolization is required prior to surgery.
- Bone scan is the best test for skeletal metastases, with radiographs of abnormal areas.
- Bladder tumors
  - IVU or CT–IVU is performed to assess the remainder of the urothelium (i.e., pelvicalyceal system and ureters) because of a tendency for multiple tumors.
  - CT is routine, but MRI may be better for local tumor assessment. Local tumor assessment can also be performed by transurethral US.
  - In invasive disease, chest X-ray or chest CT is usually performed together with bone scan.
- Prostate carcinoma
  - Imaging modalities include CT, transrectal ultrasound (TRUS) and MRI. CT is relatively inaccurate for local extent and early invasion. MRI is probably best for local extent of disease, and is used increasingly.
  - Bone scans are frequently used, especially prior to radical prostatectomy, when there is rising PSA or for follow-up. Suspicious areas of increased uptake can be confirmed as metastases on plain X-rays.
- Testicular tumors
  - Most spread by regional lymphatics to retroperitoneal nodes, supra-diaphragmatic nodes and then extranodal disease (e.g. lungs). For staging, CT of chest and abdomen is usual.

Musculoskeletal and soft tissue tumors
- Tumor site affects the prognosis and choice of surgical resection. The intactness of anatomic and compartmental boundaries (e.g. fascia, periosteum) also affects prognosis.
- If a lesion appears aggressive on plain radiographs, then other imaging investigations are usually obtained before biopsy.
- Bone scan is used to identify multiple bony lesions or metastases.
- MRI is routine, as it readily defines tumor site and extent, the relationship of tumor to neurovascular bundles, and can sometimes aid diagnosis of tumor type.

- CT is sometimes useful for demonstration of tumor matrix and for detection of lung metastases.
- Angiography is occasionally performed for embolization prior to surgery.

ENT malignancies
- Both CT and MRI are routinely used. CT is standard for assessment of nodal disease and chest metastases. MR has superior soft tissue contrast and multiplanar capability, and is often better for assessing tumor extent and perineural spread.

Imaging for investigation of an unknown primary carcinoma

Patients may present with symptomatic metastases before the primary carcinoma has clinical manifestations. Some will have widespread metastases, and multiple organ involvement (e.g. liver, lungs and bones). Despite this, some disseminated tumors can respond to chemotherapy. Therefore, depending on the likely tumor and the general condition of the patient it can be important to perform clinical and pathological evaluation to identify the primary tumor.

Clinical presentation
Examples of metastases that may present early, before the primary tumor causes symptoms:
- Bone – pain or pathological fracture
- Lymph nodes – presents as a lump
- Cerebral – neurological symptoms and signs
- Liver – abdominal mass, loss of weight, jaundice, abnormal liver function tests
- Lung – cough, hemoptysis, dyspnoea

First, the diagnosis of carcinoma should be established, followed by a search for the primary site.

All patients should have a careful history and physical examination, and routine laboratory evaluation. A CT of the chest and abdomen is often performed at this stage.

Establishing pathological diagnosis
- The most accessible lesion should be biopsied. Open or core biopsies are sometimes preferable to fine needle aspiration for cytology, since a larger specimen allows better pathological evaluation.
- About 60% patients have adenocarcinomas. About 5% have squamous cell carcinoma (SCC).

- Some tumors have specific histological features (e.g. melanoma and some sarcomas).
- Many patients have poorly differentiated tumors, and specialized pathological techniques may be needed to identify treatable subgroups.
- The distribution and appearance of the metastases may also help, e.g. sclerotic bone metastases in a male should direct testing for prostate carcinoma.

Imaging and other diagnostic investigations

- Once the diagnosis is established, evaluation should be directed towards the likely sites of the primary tumor and other metastases.
- Specific symptoms, signs, and laboratory abnormalities should be investigated with appropriate imaging or endoscopy. Imaging of asymptomatic organs is usually unproductive, can be misleading, and is not cost effective.
- Further evaluation is necessary if there may be a treatable adenocarcinoma (e.g. breast, ovary, or prostate), even though these do not usually present with disseminated metastases.
  - Women with axillary lymph node metastases should have mammography.
  - Patients with SCC may present with cervical or supraclavicular lymph node metastases, and evaluation should include direct visualization of larynx/pharynx/upper esophagus.
  - Involvement of lower cervical or supraclavicular lymph nodes suggests a primary lung tumor, and chest CT and bronchoscopy are indicated.
- Poorly differentiated carcinomas more often involve the mediastinum, retroperitoneum, or peripheral lymph nodes. Work-up should include CT of chest and abdomen.

Interventional radiology in oncology

- In this section, some common interventional procedures are described, with their major complications.

Central venous catheters

- Different catheters can be used for central venous access, depending on the clinical indication.
- "Central" means that the internal end of the catheter lies in a large central vein rather than an arm vein. Some commonly used catheters are:
  - PICC line (peripherally inserted central catheter) – arm vein puncture; small

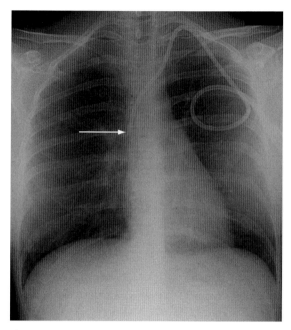

Fig. 12.7. Hickman's catheter has been inserted via left internal jugular vein (more often it is via the right) and the tip (arrow) is ideally located within the superior vena cava at the level of the right main bronchus.

caliber catheter for chemotherapy or antibiotics
  - Hickman line – jugular or subclavian vein puncture; high flow
  - Infusaport – jugular or subclavian vein puncture; implanted subcutaneously; long-lasting; lower risk of infection
- In general, if higher flow rates or more irritating drugs are required, the catheter tip should be more centrally positioned.
- Venous puncture for catheter insertion is frequently performed under ultrasound guidance, to lower the risks of arterial puncture, hematoma, and pneumothorax. Fluoroscopy is then used to ensure correct positioning of the catheter tip.
- A chest X-ray is usually performed (always performed if a line is inserted on the ward) following catheter insertion to ensure correct positioning, and check for complications (Fig. 12.7).

Complications of catheter insertion

- Hemorrhage – mostly at puncture site, but also mediastinum, or pleural cavity
- Inadvertent arterial puncture – uncommon with ultrasound guidance

- Infection – mainly in longstanding catheters, especially in immunocompromised
- Pneumothorax – uncommon with ultrasound guidance

Percutaneous biopsies

- Performed to obtain a tissue sample for diagnosis.
- Almost any body compartment can be biopsied under image guidance in radiology. The main exceptions are central nervous system (require surgical biopsy in theater), and intraluminal neoplasms (e.g. colon cancer) that usually require endoscopy.
- Imaging guidance allows precise lesion localization, thus minimizing trauma to surrounding tissues. Imaging is also important for some surgical biopsies, e.g. hook-wire localization of breast tumors.
- Biopsies include:
  - Fine needle aspiration (FNA) – uses 21–23-gauge needle and yields cells for cytology. For some tumors, e.g. lymphoma, FNA may not provide enough material, but for carcinomas, FNA is often enough.
  - Core biopsy – provides a larger tissue specimen for histology, using 14–20-gauge needles. Often an 18-gauge core biopsy yields enough tissue.
- The imaging modality chosen for biopsy is the one that best delineates the lesion and is considered the easiest and safest way to guide the needle to the lesion. For instance, CT is often used for lung, paraspinal, and retroperitoneal biopsies, whilst US is commonly used for breast, thyroid, and liver.
- Complications
  - The risk of complications is in general low but not negligible and it is important to balance the risk against the impact on management decisions.
  - In general, the smaller the needle, the lower the risk of complications. On the other hand, pathologists tend to prefer larger specimens. The type of needle therefore depends on site (likelihood of serious complications) versus pathologist requirements.
  - Hemorrhage is the commonest major risk. A coagulation screen should be performed before any biopsy and steps taken to correct any clotting defect.

- Other complications depend on the organ involved, and the anatomical structures traversed by the needle, e.g. pneumothorax with lung biopsy. Less common complications include air embolism, infection, and bile leaks.
- Seeding of tumors along the needle tract can occur with some neoplasms, and so percutaneous biopsy is sometimes avoided for this reason. The incidence of this is low.

Percutaneous tumor treatments

- Some inoperable tumors can be treated percutaneously under imaging guidance by radiologists. These are often liver tumors, e.g. hepatocellular carcinoma (HCC) or metastases.
- Two common techniques are:
  - Alcohol injections for HCC
  - Radiofrequency (RF) ablation for HCC, metastases, and some other tumors (e.g. renal cell carcinoma, lung cancers, osteoid osteoma).
- Both techniques aim to eradicate tumor from a well-localized region. Under imaging guidance (ultrasound or CT), a needle is advanced into the lesion, and then, either alcohol is injected slowly, or RF current is applied, to ablate the lesion. It is ideal for small lesions, if only one or a few are present.
- As for biopsies, individual cases must be discussed with the treating radiologist. A coagulation screen must be performed. The procedure requires sedation and analgesia as it is painful.

Tumor embolization

- Embolization works on the principle that malignant lesions require (and indeed stimulate) a good blood supply for ongoing growth. When a tumor is deprived of its blood supply, it may stop growing and undergo infarction/necrosis.
- Embolization aims to occlude some or all of the tumor arterial supply, and induce infarction and/or reduce tumor growth, or to reduce tumor vascularity prior to surgery to reduce the risk of hemorrhage or dissemination. Embolization is rarely curative as tumors are often angiogenic and rapidly recruit new vessels from adjacent vascular beds.
- Embolization is performed percutaneously as for angiography. It requires selective catheterization of the artery (arteries) that

supply the tumor and this may be technically difficult. Once the supplying vessel(s) has been catheterized, a variety of materials (metallic coils, particulate matter, glue) can be injected to thrombose the specific vessels. Ideally, the artery to be occluded should supply only neoplastic tissue, but it is usual that some normal tissue also infarcts. It is important, therefore, to perform selective catheterization to minimize loss of normal tissue.

- Chemoembolization is an extension of this technique used, for example, in the treatment of liver tumors, where arterial delivery of a cytotoxic agent is followed by occlusion of supplying arterial branches.
- Large or vascular tumors can be embolize prior to surgical excision, to decrease the risk of bleeding or dissemination. This is occasionally performed for large renal carcinomas, and some head and neck tumors. Occasionally, a whole organ (e.g. kidney) may be embolized prior to resection.

Complications of embolization
- Complications of angiography include: hematoma, false aneurysm, dissection, thrombosis, or embolism.
- Malposition of the deployed occluding agent resulting in undesirable infarction of normal tissue.
- Complications of the infarcted tissue:
  - Pain – can be severe but usually self-limiting; most severe in the immediate hours following procedure.
  - Pyrexia and general malaise are common, especially with a large volume of infarcted tissue.
  - Infection and abscess formation in the necrotic tissue uncommonly occur. This may require percutaneous drainage.

Dilatations and stent placement
- Tumors often encase tubular structures (ducts or vessels), resulting in luminal stenosis or occlusion, and clinical symptoms and signs including:
  - Jaundice from bile duct obstruction
  - Superior vena cava obstruction from mediastinal nodes
  - Dysphagia from esophageal obstruction

- Intractable vomiting from gastric outlet obstruction
- Symptomatic leg swelling from compressed iliac veins
- Strictures may also arise as result of treatment such as radiotherapy.
- Problematic strictures can sometimes be treated percutaneously by dilatation and/or stenting.
- For dilatation or stent insertion, the duct or vessel is cannulated percutaneously under imaging guidance. A fine wire is passed through the stricture or stenosis, followed by a balloon or dilating catheters to dilate the stenosis. Once a satisfactory lumen has been obtained, a stent may be inserted to maintain the lumen. Some stents can be changed while others are permanent.

Inferior vena cava (IVC) filter placement
- Patients with carcinomas have a tendency to develop deep venous thrombosis and may develop pulmonary emboli. Pulmonary embolism is usually treated by anticoagulation but if emboli persist or anticoagulation is contraindicated, an effective means of preventing further emboli from the leg veins or lower IVC is to place a filter in the IVC below the level of the renal veins.
- These filters may be permanent or temporary, and have various configurations. Access to the IVC is usually obtained via the non-occluded femoral vein or from above, via the jugular vein if the thrombus already extends into the IVC. The filter is placed below the renal vein, otherwise the renal veins may occlude with thrombus with resultant renal impairment.

Drainages and tube insertions
- Drainages are usually straightforward unless the collection is in an inaccessible location, or close to important structures, e.g. major arteries. The imaging technique (US or CT) chosen is the one that best shows the target collection or organ.
- Some common indications for imaging guided drainage/aspiration or tube insertion are:
  - For symptomatic relief of ascites or pleural fluid, when attempts at these procedures in the ward fail, for example, due to fluid loculation
  - Abscess drainage, e.g. intra-abdominal

- Percutaneous gastrostomy – percutaneous insertion into the stomach of a feeding tube.

Pain relief
- Occasionally, for intractable pain, sclerosing agents may be injected into, e.g. the celiac plexus. This may require imaging guidance.

Breast imaging
Commonly used tests:
- Mammography
- Ultrasound (US)
- Ultrasound guided fine needle aspiration (FNA)
- Hook wire localization of lesion using US or mammographic guidance
- MRI is not commonly used but is being used increasingly in patients at very high risk of carcinoma

Mammography
- Mammography requires dedicated equipment with special film that provides high soft tissue contrast and spatial resolution. Some systems now use digital mammography in place of film mammography.
- Standard views of both breasts are
  - Superoinferior (SI) – also called craniocaudal (CC)
  - Lateral oblique views – also called mediolateral oblique (MLO).
- These views are obtained using compression to reduce and even out the breast thickness. The mammogram must include all breast tissue back to the chest wall, and the axillary tail.
- Other common views include lateral views and "coned" magnified views. These help show a suspicious area in more detail.

Diagnostic versus screening mammography
- Diagnostic studies are performed for a particular clinical indication. The investigation is tailored to the clinical problem. They evaluate the area of clinical interest, as well as the remainder of the breasts.
- Screening mammography is performed in asymptomatic women, to detect early malignancy, and the investigation is performed according to set protocols (see below).

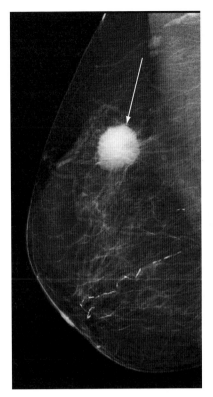

Fig. 12.8. Mammogram (MLO view) of a carcinoma – a large irregular mass (arrow), much denser than the surrounding parenchyma.

Mammographic signs of carcinoma
- Mass lesion – typically spiculated margins, but may be poorly defined or well defined (Fig. 12.8)
- Malignant microcalcifications
- Asymmetric density – parenchyma tends to be symmetrical between the two sides
- Architecture disturbance

Calcifications – malignant and benign
- Malignant microcalcifications are typically irregular, rod-shaped or branching (Fig. 12.9).
- Benign microcalcifications are common and often rounded.
- The distinction between benign and malignant can be very difficult.
- Fibroadenomas often show large clumps of calcification (Fig. 12.10).

How sensitive is mammography for detection of breast cancer?
- The sensitivity of mammography is not 100%, and referring doctors must expect that some lesions will be missed (i.e. some lesions are impossible to identify)

229

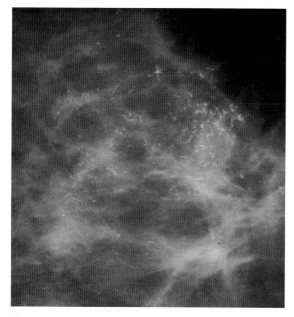

Fig. 12.9. Magnified view of typical irregular branching malignant microcalcifications.

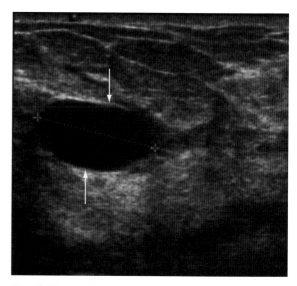

Fig. 12.11. An ultrasound of a patient with a smooth mobile lump shows a well-defined mass with thin smooth walls, anechoic contents and posterior enhancement, typical of a cyst (arrows).

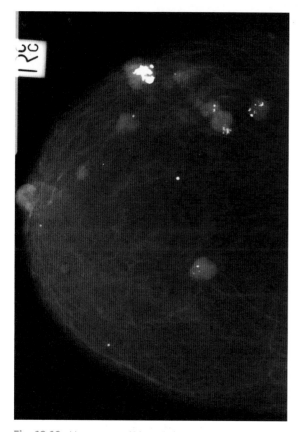

Fig. 12.10. Mammogram (CC view) shows multiple fibroadenomas some of which contain characteristic large calcifications.

- Approximately 10%–20% of carcinomas may be missed. On the other hand, mammography is the best available imaging modality that examines the entire breast.
- Missed diagnosis occurs for various reasons including very subtle or invisible lesions, technical difficulty and interpreter error.

Ultrasound
- Distinguishes between cysts (Fig. 12.11) and solid lesions.
- Helps characterize solid masses, and can diagnose some benign masses without biopsy (e.g. cysts and some fibroadenomas).
- Especially helpful if breast parenchyma is dense on mammogram. It may detect an invisible carcinoma in this situation.
- Used to investigate breast symptoms in younger patients, as mammographically dense parenchyma is common in this group.
- It is frequently combined with mammography to evaluate mammographically detected masses
- US is very operator dependent and should not be relied on to screen the entire breast.
- *Note:* Ultrasound cannot always differentiate benign from malignant lesions.

Fine needle aspiration (FNA)

- FNA is performed to obtain samples for cytological examination.
- It may be performed without imaging guidance in the case of clinically obvious masses, but frequently must be performed with ultrasound, or less often mammography, to guide the FNA.
- Both cysts and solid masses can be aspirated using this method.

Hook-wire localization

- This is usually performed immediately before surgery to allow excision of an impalpable lesion. Ultrasound or mammography is used for guidance, mammography being needed if microcalcification is the target for excision as these are generally not seen well with ultrasound.
- Prior to surgical excision, a wire with a hooked tip is passed into the lesion, and left in situ in order to guide the surgeon. The excised specimen is usually X-rayed to check that the suspicious region has been excised.

Carbon localization

- An alternative to hook-wire localization.
- A track of carbon emulsion injected under imaging guidance. It has the advantage that it can be done days or weeks before surgery.

How should you investigate a woman with a breast lump or other breast symptoms?

- The approach depends on a number of factors but age of the patient is very important:
  - >35 years – perform mammography ± US
  - <35 years – perform US first
- Why is there is an age dependent difference?
  - At younger ages the breast parenchyma is mammographically dense (Fig. 12.12) and it is difficult or impossible to detect masses (i.e. mammograms have a lower sensitivity; the false-negative rate may be as high as 20%!).
  - Mammograms are more likely to be diagnostic when fatty replacement of breast parenchyma increases in older women (Fig. 12.13). With increasing age, the overall density of the breasts typically decreases and focal masses are easier to see.
  - The likely diagnosis also depends to a degree on age.

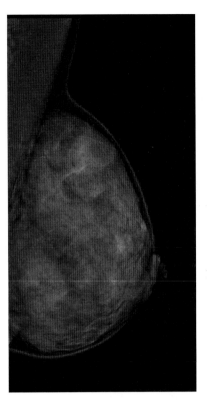

Fig. 12.12. Mammogram (mediolateral oblique view) of left breast showing mammographically dense parenchyma in a 32-year-old woman. It is difficult to detect small masses or calcifications in such dense breasts.

Common clinical problems
Palpable lump

- US is usually performed for this indication at any age. US-guided biopsy is also used.
- Mammographic findings depend on breast parenchymal density (patient's age) and nature of the lump.

Some typical scenarios of "palpable lump":

(1) 25-year-old with palpable lump
- Fibroadenoma is common and carcinoma unlikely. Perform US first and usually not mammography. If there is a characteristic appearance for fibroadenoma, the patient can be reassured.
- Do you perform a mammogram in a 25-year-old?
  - Generally not, because dense breast tissue gives poor visibility of lesions, and US is better for lumps at this age.
  - Sometimes mammography is appropriate, e.g. strong family history.

231

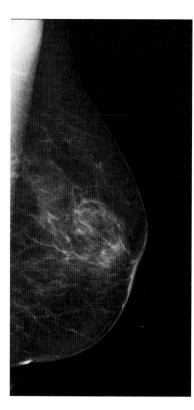

Fig. 12.13. Mammogram (mediolateral oblique view) of left breast in a 57-year-old woman showing little parenchyma with much of the breast being fatty and therefore of low mammographic density. Detection of masses or calcifications in this type of breast is easier.

- The radiation dose is higher for mammograms of dense breasts – important to consider in a young patient.

(2) 40-year-old with palpable lump

- Cysts are common. Differential diagnosis includes fibroadenoma and cancer.
- Use mammogram and US. Mammogram first to look for lump and any other pathology or calcifications.
- Then perform US. This can also guide biopsy or cyst aspiration.

(3) 60-year-old with palpable lump

- Carcinoma is more likely. Differential diagnosis includes fibroadenoma and cyst.
- Mammography first with US to further characterize the mass.
- US-guided FNA or core biopsy can be helpful in surgical planning even if the imaging diagnosis is carcinoma.

Pain

- If pain is generalized and related to menstrual cycle, usually no imaging is needed.
- If there are focal signs:

- < 40 years – ultrasound ± mammogram
- > 40 years – mammogram ± ultrasound
- Otherwise, imaging protocol is essentially the same as for breast screening guidelines.

Focal breast thickening

- Focal breast thickening may present at any age, and is quite common. The differential diagnosis includes normal breast, fibrocystic change and masses, including carcinoma.
- Imaging approach varies with age and breast texture, but is similar to the approach for breast pain (see above).

Breast screening
Why screen for breast cancer?

- Breast carcinoma has a high mortality and morbidity, and is the commonest cancer in women. Many cases occur in relatively young women.
- Several trials have shown a reduction in mortality as a result of early detection and treatment.
- Cancers detected by screening of asymptomatic patients are usually small with a good prognosis.
- Screening of a select population is cost-effective as it reduces the cost of morbidity and mortality of advanced carcinoma in that population.

Effectiveness of screening

- Screening may result in 30% reduction in mortality from breast cancer in women aged 50–69 years.
- Its impact is less in women aged 40–49 years because the incidence of breast carcinoma at this age is less. The cost-effectiveness is also less in women over 70 years, since other causes of death become more common.

Screening guidelines

- Screening guidelines vary between countries. A typical program is:
  - Women over 40 years can undergo free 2-yearly screening mammography.
  - Women aged 50–69 years are actively recruited and sent 2-yearly appointments.

Accuracy of breast screening

- Cancer detection rate on first screening the community as a whole is 5–8 per 1000.
- On screening the same population again after 2 years (and every subsequent two years), the detection rate is 3–5 per 1000.
- The rate of presentation of "interval" cancers that are diagnosed between the two-yearly screens is 10–15 per 10 000 patients. Some of these may represent "missed" diagnoses.
- The false-negative rate of screening mammography is about 10–20%.

Immunocompromised patients

Contents

The immunocompromised (non-HIV)
patient
Imaging in HIV infection

The immunocompromised (non-HIV) patient

Introduction

- Many secondary diseases (infections and tumors) occur in immune deficiency. The severity of these depends upon:
  - The degree of functional immune impairment
  - The therapy for the specific disease
  - The general state of the patient
- Deficiencies of neutrophil function, complement, immunoglobulins, and cell-mediated immunity occur, and result in differing patterns of disease. This discussion reviews only a few of these conditions.
- Overall, the commonest causes of immunosuppression are acquired causes in cancer patients, transplant patients and HIV-positive patients. These result in differing patterns of infection and tumors.

Thoracic disease

- Lung infections occur in 40% to 50%
- Infection can co-exist with other conditions, e.g. malignancy, drug reaction, radiotherapy.
- Often due to opportunistic organisms, e.g. gram-negatives bacteria, nocardia, fungi, viruses and *Pneumocystis carinii* (PCP).
- Sputum examination may be unhelpful.
- Clinical manifestations are often masked in the early stages due to the immunosuppression.

Common patterns

Three general patterns are seen on CXR (and chest CT):

Lobar (or segmental) consolidation
- Mostly bacterial pneumonia.
- Cavitation and abscesses are more readily seen by CT.
- If the CXR seems normal initially, despite clinical pneumonia, CT (HRCT), or gallium scans may detect early disease.

Rapidly growing nodules and/or cavities
- Often are due to fungi, e.g. aspergillosis, candida, mucormycosis, cryptococcosis; and nocardiosis. The commonest is aspergillosis, which often cavitates and there may be an air crescent sign (Fig. 13.1).
- The differential diagnosis includes metastases or lymphoma, but these do not usually develop as quickly.

Diffuse interstitial lung disease
- Often due to PCP or viruses, e.g. herpes, cytomegalovirus.
- PCP is the commonest, and typically has a central bilateral perihilar distribution that progresses to a homogeneous alveolar pattern. It can mimic cardiac failure, but the heart size is normal, pleural effusions are uncommon, and Kerley B lines are not features. If CXR is normal, HRCT may show "ground glass" opacification.
- The differential diagnosis for interstitial disease is long, e.g. non-specific interstitial pneumonitis, drug reactions, radiotherapy (XRT) and lymphangitis carcinomatosis (diffuse interstitial metastatic spread).
- Lymphangitis typically has basal septal lines (Kerley B lines), associated adenopathy, and frequent pleural effusions.

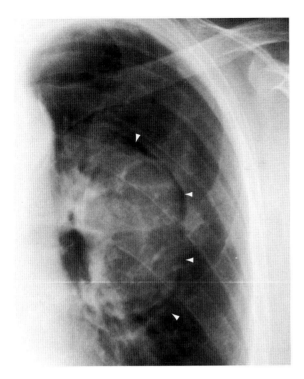

Fig. 13.1. Aspergillosis. A focal mass adjacent to the left hilum shows a typical fungus ball within a thin-walled cavity, outlined by a thin crescent of air (arrowheads).

- Radiotherapy usually causes focal (not diffuse) opacification, with sharply defined margins corresponding to the irradiated field.

Gastrointestinal (GIT) disease
- There is an increased incidence of GIT infection and cancer.
- Other post-transplant GIT complications include:
  - Peptic ulcers
  - Massive hemorrhage
  - Colon perforation, especially in diverticular disease
  - Fecal impaction
  - Obstruction or ileus
  - Pancreatitis – especially with steroid therapy.
- Plain films, contrast examination, and ultrasound and CT may be required to diagnose these acute conditions.

GIT inflammation following bone marrow transplantation
- May result from chemotherapy, graft versus host disease or infection.

Graft versus host disease (GVHD)
- Acute form affects skin, liver and GIT, especially small bowel
- Plain films and CT useful
- Chronic form affects skin and esophagus
- Barium swallow and small bowel follow-through for non-invasive detection

GIT infections following transplant
- Often bacterial or candidal, but viral and other fungal infections occur.

Neutropenic enterocolitis (typhlitis)
- Inflammation and/or necrosis of bowel, most common in cecum and ascending colon
- Features are abdominal pain, diarrhea (± PR blood), fever
- Occurs in leukemia, neutropenia, lymphoma, aplastic anaemia and post-renal transplantation
- Important to diagnose early, otherwise it may result in necrosis and perforation
- CT is most useful

Pseudomembranous colitis
- Increased incidence in immunocompromised.
- *Clostridium difficile* enterotoxin-induced colon inflammation.
- Colonic wall mucosal thickening better seen on CT than on plain abdominal X-ray ("thumb printing").
- CT better shows diffuse colon wall thickening.
- Endoscopy required for definitive diagnosis.

Abdominal lymphoma
- 20% of transplant patients.
- Usually B cell lymphomas, often with large masses at presentation.
- Clinical picture often ambiguous, and imaging is important for detection.
- Often aggressive and can occur soon after transplantation.
- Occurs anywhere within the abdomen, especially bowel, liver and lymph nodes. Increased incidence of spontaneous perforation, which may be the initial clinical manifestation.
- For detection and staging use CT.

General comments
- A multi-modality approach is often necessary for diagnosis of GIT disease in this setting.

235

- For mucosal abnormalities, endoscopy and culture are often used.
- Indications for CT and ultrasound include:
  - Diagnosis and staging of malignancies.
  - Evaluation of infection/abscesses.
- For evaluation of right upper quadrant pain or possible gynecological pain, ultrasound is often the most helpful first investigation. Otherwise, CT is usually more helpful.

CNS disease
- Use of steroids is associated with an increased incidence of unusual CNS infections.
- Diabetes is associated with increased risk of paranasal sinus fungal infections (e.g. mucormycosis and aspergillosis) that may extend into brain, especially following ketoacidosis. This has a poor prognosis.
- Transplant patients
  - Infections – increased risk of abscesses, meningitis, granulomas, PML (as in AIDS).
  - Neoplasms – often lymphoma (B-cell NHL). Often ring–enhancing masses with mass effect and edema. Since toxoplasmosis is not common (except in AIDS), a biopsy is usually performed.

Imaging in HIV infection
Introduction
- Complications of AIDS can be divided into four groups:
  - Diseases of the entire population, e.g. TB, HS, bacterial infections – presentation and course affected by degree of immune suppression.
  - Diseases resulting from re-activation of latent infection, e.g. toxoplasmosis, progressive multifocal leukoencephalopathy (PML), cytomegalovirus (CMV), *Pneumocystis carinii* pneumonia (PCP).
  - Diseases in immunocompromised patients caused by relatively non-pathogenic organisms, e.g. *Mycoplasma avium* complex (MAC), cryptococcosis.
  - Diseases unique to HIV infection, e.g. AIDS dementia complex.
- It is important to know the stage of infection (especially the CD4 cell count), as certain diseases

occur at different stages. Patient demographics, underlying risk factors (e.g. IV drug use) and previous therapy also affect the type and pattern of infection.
- In the imaging of AIDS it is important to remember that many infections and several tumors occur. This chapter concentrates on chest, central nervous system (CNS) and gastrointestinal (GIT) manifestations only.

Role of nuclear medicine in HIV
Gallium scan
- ^{67}Gallium citrate is a non-specific marker for tumor and inflammation.
- Useful for investigation of fever of unknown origin (immunocompromised and general population).
- Diagnosis and follow-up of pulmonary infections (e.g. *Pneumocystis carinii*).
- Evaluate abdominal infections.

Thallium scan
- ^{201}Thallium chloride has preferential uptake in certain neoplasms, and low avidity for infection.
- It is useful to differentiate cerebral toxoplasmosis from AIDS-related lymphoma.

Thallium–gallium scan
- A combination of the two tests.
- Can be used to differentiate PCP from Kaposi's sarcoma (KS) or lymphoma.

White cell scans
- Useful for detection of infective foci, provided the neutrophil count is $> 2000/\mu l$.

Pulmonary manifestations of HIV
- In AIDS, many infections cause pulmonary abnormalities. Atypical features are common. Multiple pathogens and diseases may co-exist.
- By correlating the radiographic appearance with the clinical presentation, CD4 cell count, underlying risk factors and previous therapy, diagnostic possibilities can be narrowed.
  - The CD4 count is the most important factor affecting the type and pattern of infection that occurs, and likelihood of complications.

- If the CD4 count is greater than 100 cells/mm^3, patients often develop PCP.
- If the CD4 count is less than 50 cells/mm^3, MAC and cytomegalovirus (CMV) are found.

Chest X-ray

Chest X-rays are usually the first investigation for pulmonary symptoms. Several radiographic patterns may be found:

- Normal CXR
  - If patient is symptomatic, consider PCP, disseminated mycobacterial or fungal infections, or interstitial pneumonitis.
- Diffuse interstitial disease
  - Consider PCP, KS, and interstitial pneumonitis.
- Focal consolidation
  - Consider mycobacterial, fungal, or bacterial pneumonias.
- Nodules
  - Consider lymphoma, and KS, *M. tuberculosis*, and fungi.
- Mediastinal and/or hilar adenopathy
  - Common
  - Infection or tumor, e.g. mycobacteria, fungi, KS, or lymphoma
  - Progressive generalized lymphadenopathy or lymphoid hyperplasia in the AIDS-related complex.
- Pleural effusions
  - Mycobacteria or complication of bacterial infection (empyema), KS or lymphoma.

CT – High resolution CT (HRCT)

HRCT is very useful:
- For early detection of PCP pneumonia, if CXR is normal
- To characterize pulmonary abnormalities, e.g. nodules, diffuse interstitial infiltrates
- To show complications, e.g. cavitation or cysts
- To monitor the disease and therapy
- To confirm adenopathy
- To plan biopsy sites
- To stage malignancies

Other tests

- Bronchoscopy is often necessary for definitive diagnosis.

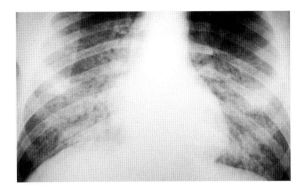

Fig. 13.2. CXR in a patient with *Pneumocystis carinii* pneumonia (PCP) showing bilateral finely granular fairly symmetrical opacity in the lung fields involving both mid and lower zones, including the perihilar regions.

- Percutaneous needle biopsies are sometimes appropriate for focal lung disease.
- Some patients require open lung biopsy.

Pneumocystis carinii pneumonia (PCP)

- The most common pulmonary infection in AIDS.
- A subacute, indolent presentation is typical.
- Typically produces bilateral perihilar and/or diffuse finely granular opacities (Fig. 13.2).
- Pleural effusions and adenopathy are not typical features of PCP.
- 10% have normal CXR at presentation – HRCT or gallium scans often useful here
- With successful treatment, chest X-ray changes clear in about 2 weeks.

Tuberculosis (TB)

- Usually re-activation infection
- Often occurs early, and may be the first manifestation of HIV.
- Contagious, so early diagnosis is important.
- Upper lobe pneumonia, cavities, ± bronchogenic spread.
- Usually confined to the lungs in early HIV.
- In advanced AIDS, TB appears more like the primary infection, with hilar and mediastinal lymphadenopathy, and diffuse opacification without cavitation or predilection for the upper lobes.
- Skin and sputum testing are often negative, and extra-pulmonary disease is common.

Other infections

Non-tuberculous Mycobacterium *infections*
- e.g. *Mycoplasma avium* complex (MAC)

Fungal infections
- Relatively uncommon.
- Cryptococcosis is the most frequent, and usually also involves the CNS.
- Candidiasis and aspergillosis can also involve the lungs.

Bacterial infections
- Common early in the course of AIDS
- Often *Staphylococcus, H. influenzae*
- Focal areas of consolidation (i.e. same as in pneumonia in general population)
- Usually readily differentiated from PCP.

CNS complications of AIDS
- CT and MRI are the most useful tests. Thallium scans can be useful.
- Most patients with CNS infections are symptomatic.

Toxoplasmosis
- The most common cause of a brain mass in AIDS.
- Typically ring-enhancing masses which may be multiple (Fig. 13.3).
- Differential diagnosis is cerebral lymphoma.

Cerebral lymphoma
- The second most common brain mass in AIDS is primary CNS lymphoma.
- Often is indistinguishable from cerebral toxoplasmosis.
- If a ring-enhancing mass is found, a trial of anti-toxoplasmosis therapy is commenced. Biopsy is reserved for unresponsive lesions after 1–2 weeks, or atypical or progressive lesions.
- Thallium scanning may help differentiate as it tends to be positive in lymphoma.

Other CNS infections
- Cryptococcosis and TB.
- Progressive multifocal leukoencephalopathy (PML) is an opportunistic infection due to the JC polyomavirus.

Gastrointestinal (GIT) complications of AIDS
- The GIT is a major site of symptomatic disease in AIDS patients.

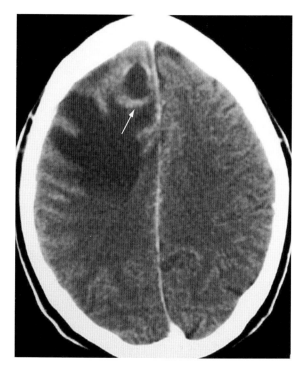

Fig. 13.3. Axial post-contrast CT scan in a patient with severe headache. There is a ring-enhancing lesion in the right anterior frontal lobe (arrow), surrounded by vasogenic (white matter) edema. This could represent either toxoplasmosis or lymphoma.

- Many opportunistic infections occur in bowel, e.g. *Candida, Herpes simplex*, TB, and *Cytomegalovirus* (CMV).
- Many are diagnosed by non-imaging methods, and the imaging is often non-specific.

Biliary disease
- Inflammation of the biliary tract can occur, thought to be due to *Cryptosporidium* or CMV.
- Patients with cholangitis typically have RUQ pain, and ultrasound is initially performed.

Intra-abdominal abscesses
- Due to a number of organisms, including PCP.
- Usually imaged by CT or US.
- Sometimes drained percutaneously under imaging control.

Abdominal neoplasms
- Lymphoma and KS.
- CT is the imaging modality of choice for staging.
- Percutaneous biopsy can be performed.

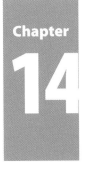

Endocrine disease

Contents

Thyroid masses

- Evaluation of a neck mass must address two questions:
  - What is the anatomic origin of the mass?
  - What is the pathology?
- Thyroid masses need to be differentiated from masses arsing from other structures in the neck including lymph node groups, salivary glands, congenital cysts, parathyroid glands, vascular masses and aneurysms, nerve masses, e.g. neurofibroma, muscular, or other soft tissues.

Normal thyroid variants

- The thyroid develops between pharyngeal pouches 1 and 2 and then migrates to its location in the neck.
- If this migration fails to occur, it remains in a lingual position near the foramen cecum in the posterior part of the tongue.
- More commonly, a small remnant of the descent persists as the pyramidal lobe.

Diffuse or multifocal thyroid enlargement

Causes:
- Physiological

- Multinodular goiter: iodine deficiency, enzyme deficiency, drugs
- Thyroiditis
- Graves disease
- Drugs, e.g. lithium
- Storage/infiltrative diseases, e.g. amyloidosis

Focal thyroid nodules

Causes:
- Multinodular goiter with a dominant nodule
- Thyroid adenoma
- Cyst
- Hemorrhage
- Focal thyroiditis
- Carcinoma
- Inflammatory

Cystic thyroid nodules

- Simple cysts – approx. 5%
- Degenerate benign adenoma or colloid nodules (Fig. 14.1) – approx. 80%
- Malignant – approx. 15%

Imaging approach to a neck mass

- Ultrasound is usually the first imaging test, and it can determine:
  - If the mass is in the thyroid.
  - If in the thyroid, whether it is a solitary nodule, multiple nodules or diffuse thyroid swelling.
- If a nodule is solitary, the approach is then influenced by the patient's thyroid function status as described below.

Focal thyroid nodule

Euthyroid patient

- The aim of investigation is to determine whether the nodule is benign or malignant.

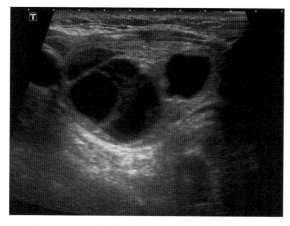

Fig. 14.1. Thyroid ultrasound shows several cystic colloid nodules.

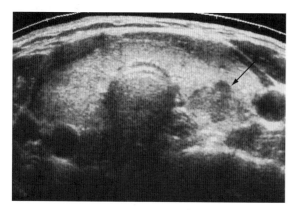

Fig. 14.2. Transverse ultrasound of thyroid shows a solitary hypoechoic nodule in the left lobe (arrow) which proved to be a papillary carcinoma on fine needle aspiration.

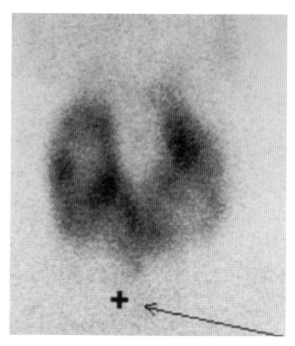

Fig. 14.3. Nuclear medicine thyroid scan (anterior view) of multinodular goiter with enlargement of right and left lobes and areas of reduced isotope uptake corresponding to the larger nodules. A marker is placed at the sternal notch (arrow) for anatomical marking of the thoracic inlet.

Thyrotoxic
- Nuclear medicine scan.

Hypothyroid
- Nuclear medicine scan.

Diffuse or multifocal thyroid enlargement
- Assessed by ultrasound in the euthyroid patient, and nuclear medicine scans in thyrotoxic patients.
- Generalized thyroid enlargement is frequently due to multinodular goiter (Fig. 14.3).

Retrosternal goiter
- Retrosternal extension of a goiter is more likely to produce compressive symptoms. The presence of retrosternal extension can be detected by ultrasound but assessment of the extent requires CT (Fig. 14.4).

Coincidental thyroid nodules
- Incidental nodules in the thyroid are common. At post-mortem, 37% of thyroids contain multiple nodules, and 12% contain solitary nodules. Nodules are therefore often incidental and usually

- If the nodule is a simple cyst on ultrasound, no further investigation is needed.
- However, if the nodule is solid or complex (mixed cystic/solid), further evaluation is required. 10% to 20% of these lesions greater than 1 cm will be malignant (Fig. 14.2).
- Fine needle aspiration cytology (FNA), often guided by ultrasound, is used for these.
- If there is diffuse thyroid enlargement without nodules, further evaluation is clinical and laboratory based rather than imaging.
- If ultrasound shows multinodular goiter, the nodules need to be assessed carefully. FNA is indicated where a lump(s) is dominant or increasing in size. Otherwise, imaging is mainly to assess possible retrosternal extension.

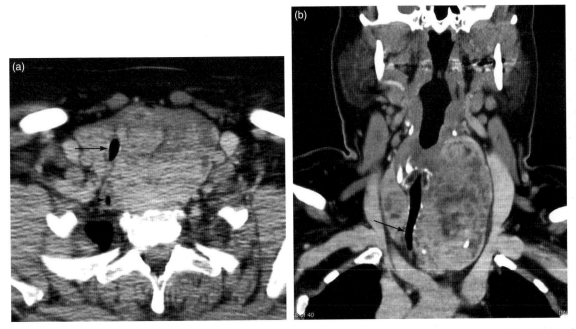

Fig. 14.4. Multinodular goiter with retrosternal extension. (a) Axial CT (without contrast) shows marked enlargement of the left lobe of the thyroid narrowing and displacing the trachea (arrow) and the esophagus (arrowhead). (b) Coronal CT shows extension of the left lobe in particular inferiorly through the thoracic inlet.

of no significance. They may be discovered, for example, during a carotid ultrasound examination.

Hyperthyroidism
- Suspected on clinical grounds: tachycardia, arrhythmia, irritability, and sweating.
- Diagnosis is confirmed by serum hormonal levels.
- The role of imaging is to provide a specific diagnosis as a guide to therapy.
- Nuclear medicine thyroid scanning helps discriminate between a hyper-functioning adenoma (Fig. 14.5) and Graves' disease, for example.

Hypothyroidism
- May be caused by an autoimmune disease, e.g. Hashimoto's thyroiditis. Ultrasound shows thyroid enlargement, and a diffuse hypo-echoic change.
- Radioactive ^{131}I treatment for thyrotoxicosis also causes hypothyroidism.

Hyperparathyroidism
- Parathyroid hormone is reliably measured in serum assay.

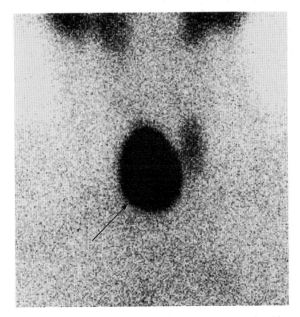

Fig. 14.5. Nuclear medicine thyroid scan. Autonomous thyroid nodule (arrow) with incomplete suppression of remaining thyroid tissue.

- Hyperparathyroidism may be primary, or secondary, often due to chronic renal failure.
- One cause of hypercalcemia. Other causes of hypercalcemia are:

- Malignancies involving bone, e.g. multiple myeloma
- Sarcoidosis

Primary hyperparathyroidism
- Causes are:
  - Parathyroid adenoma (single or multiple) – 82%
  - Diffuse hyperplasia – 15%
  - Parathyroid carcinoma – 3%
- The parathyroid glands are small (4 mm × 3 mm × 1.5 mm) paired structures, usually immediately posterior to the thyroid gland, but may be nearby or in the superior mediastinum.

Role of imaging
Normal parathyroid glands cannot be seen by current techniques, but are enlarged in hyper-function. The role of imaging is to attempt to identify the number and location of enlarged glands.
- Ultrasound – sensitivity up to 80%.
- Nuclear medicine scan with sestamibi, a protein labeled with ^{99m}technetium, that is injected intravenously. The hyperactive parathyroid glands accumulate the agent and retain it longer than the adjoining thyroid gland (Fig. 14.6).
- Sensitivity for localization of abnormally active parathyroid tissue is up to 90%.
- CT and MRI scanning of neck and mediastinum have lower sensitivities.
- The tests may be used in combination to improve localization rates.

Pituitary masses/dysfunction
- Pituitary abnormalities may present as intracerebral masses (generally non-hormone secreting) or smaller hormone secreting adenomas (macro- and microadenomas, the latter being <1 cm).
- MRI is the best imaging modality for the pituitary gland (see Chapter 10).

Adrenal mass/dysfunction
The adrenal glands comprise cortex (steroid hormone production) and medulla (chromaffin–catecholamine production). Endocrine abnormalities are determined by hormonal assays rather than imaging.

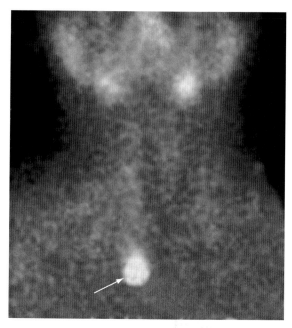

Fig. 14.6. Sestamibi scan showing adenoma (arrow) low in right side of neck.

The role of imaging is to identify and characterize mass lesions, and localize hormonally active components of the adrenals and related tissues.
- CT best defines adrenal anatomy but does not yield any information about hormonal function (Fig. 14.7).
- MRI has similar resolution to CT, and can help differentiate benign from malignant masses by the detecting fat content often associated with benign nodules.
- Nuclear medicine. Specific tracers can show specific endocrine abnormalities and provide functional imaging. MIBG (meta-iodo-benzyl-guanidine) demonstrates chromaffin tissue and catecholamine receptors and is useful for localizing pheochromocytoma. Occasionally labeled nor-cholesterol is used to target functioning cortical adenomas.

Osteoporosis
- Osteoporosis is the commonest generalized condition producing fragile bones. It is associated with an increased risk of fracture, most commonly, compression fractures of vertebral bodies (Fig. 14.8), femoral neck, and distal radius.

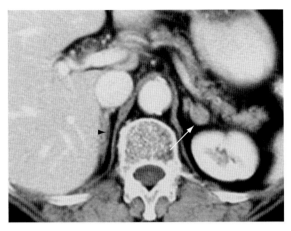

Fig. 14.7. CT showing a left adrenal adenoma (arrow). The patient had clinical and biochemical features of primary hyperaldosteronism. Normal right adrenal gland (arrowhead).

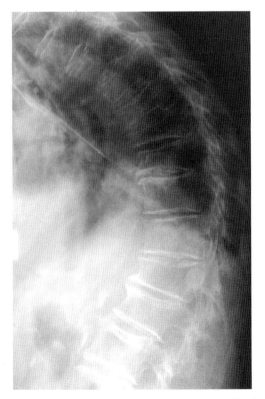

Fig. 14.8. Osteoporosis. Lateral view of thoracic and lumbar spine shows reduced bone density and wedge compression of several lower thoracic vertebrae as well as kyphosis.

Insufficiency fractures can also occur as a result of repeated minor trauma.

- Osteoporosis means reduced bone mass, both cortical and trabecular. It may be idiopathic or associated with nutritional disturbances, immobilization, endocrine disorders (e.g. hypogonadism), drugs, especially steroids, and generalized conditions such as rheumatoid arthritis.

Bone densitometry

- Assessment of bone density using low radiation X-ray absorption equipment, relies on the differential absorption of X-rays at different energies by bone and soft tissue.
- Osteoporosis is defined as 2.5 standard deviations below young adult control values.
- 50% of females at age 80 are osteoporotic.

Diabetes

There are many radiological manifestations of diabetes (some of these are discussed in other sections):

- Accelerated arterial disease, especially peripheral and coronary vascular disease
- Neuropathy including autonomic neuropathy leading to, e.g. neuropathic changes in the feet
- Fatty liver
- Renal parenchymal disease
- Large fetal size (macrosomia)

Pancreatic islet cell tumors

- Several tumor types can arise from pancreatic islet cells. These may secrete the hormone specific to that cell type with corresponding clinical features. The diagnosis is clinical and laboratory based. Imaging aims to localize the tumor for surgical resection, and to assess for malignancy and spread.
- They are typically less than 1–2 cm in diameter and frequently difficult to detect.
- CT is most commonly performed, but other modalities are often needed (see Chapter 8).

Carcinoid tumors

Carcinoid tumors may arise within the small bowel, bronchial tree, and other gut structures. Hormone secretions include serotonin, histamine, ACTH, and bradykinin. They may be benign or malignant. If metastases are present in the liver, the patient typically develops the carcinoid syndrome with flushing after certain stimuli.

Paraneoplastic endocrine states

- Paraneoplastic endocrine states can be associated with a variety of tumors. The appropriate imaging modality for locating the tumor is determined by the likely underlying tumor. Some of the recognized paraneoplastic states are listed below.
- Examples include:
  - ACTH secretion – lung carcinoma, malignant thymoma, pancreatic carcinoma
  - ADH secretion – lung carcinoma, intracranial neoplasms
  - Erythropoietin – renal cell carcinoma

Bone age

The patient's real age can be compared with their bone age, judged by the development of the secondary ossification centers, which follow a predictable time course. In certain hormone disturbances (e.g. growth hormone deficiency) bone age is delayed, and in other cases it is accelerated. Bone age is assessed using a wrist radiograph, which is then compared to a standard reference.

Contents

Chest
Interpreting the chest X-ray in children

- As with any radiograph a logical process should be followed so that abnormalities are not overlooked. The following should be checked:
- Check patient details (i.e. name, date of birth, date of examination)
  - Radiographic factors (i.e. side marker, penetration, centered, adequate field of view)
  - Mediastinal structures
  - Lung fields
  - Bones
  - Soft tissues
  - Easily missed areas – under the diaphragm, through the heart, lung apices, shoulders, neck soft tissues
- Some of the rules used when examining a child's CXR are different to those for an adult CXR

Heart size

- In neonates and infants the cardiothoracic ratio can be up to 60% (adult dimension is 50%).
- Measuring the heart size on an anteroposterior (AP) film is accurate in this age group as there is minimal magnification of the heart (unlike adult AP chest radiographs).
- Older children (and adults) require a posteroanterior (PA) film to measure the heart size.

Thymus

- The thymus is most commonly seen in the superior mediastinum in children under 2 years, but the thymus does not completely atrophy until adolescence (Fig. 15.1).
- The normal thymus can produce an unusual shape to the upper mediastinum and should not be mistaken for pathology. The classic appearance is called "the sail sign."
- In an unwell child the thymus can decrease in size and is often not seen.
- Lateral CXRs are infrequently performed. They often do not provide any additional information to the AP film.

The child with respiratory infection
Introduction

Acute respiratory infections are common in infants and children. Most involve the upper respiratory tract and rarely require imaging. Lower respiratory tract infections include:

- Croup
- Epiglottitis (rare)
- Acute bronchitis
- Whooping cough
- Acute bronchiolitis (e.g. respiratory syncytial virus)
- Pneumonia

  Not all lower respiratory tract infections require imaging. The need for imaging should be dictated by history and examination findings. For example, in a child with acute constitutional symptoms, fever and tachypnoea, with a presumed diagnosis of pneumonia, a CXR is warranted to confirm the diagnosis.

Acute bronchiolitis

- Most infants with the clinical diagnosis of acute bronchiolitis do not require a CXR. However, if the diagnosis of bronchiolitis is unclear

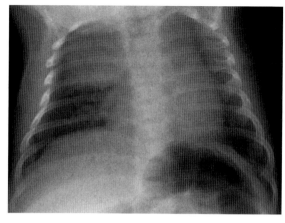

Fig. 15.1. Chest radiograph demonstrating a normal thymus in an infant. The apparent upper mediastinal widening is all due to normal thymus.

(e.g. congenital heart disease, pneumonia) a CXR could help clarify the diagnosis.

- In a severely unwell infant with bronchiolitis, who is receiving high inspired oxygen concentrations or who may need ventilation, a CXR is helpful to show secondary infection. Upper lobe collapse is common in bronchiolitis and does not generally indicate upper lobe pneumonia. However, lower lobe consolidation in bronchiolitis does suggest infection.

Whooping cough

- In a child with clinical evidence of whooping cough, a CXR can help show secondary pneumonia (often due to pertussis itself or adenovirus).

Chest X-ray findings in lower respiratory tract infections
Perihilar infiltrate

- There is loss of clarity of hilar vessels, and peribroncholar cuffing (ring-like thickening of perihilar bronchial walls) (Fig. 15.2).
- This pattern often occurs in viral infections, e.g. acute bronchiolitis.

Segmental/patchy consolidation

- There are ill-defined patchy peripheral lung opacities that irregularly involve several segments. It mostly occurs in secondary bacterial infection, viral infections and atypical pneumonias, e.g. mycoplasma.

Lobar consolidation and/or collapse

- This has typical appearances depending on the lobe affected (Figs. 15.3–15.5).

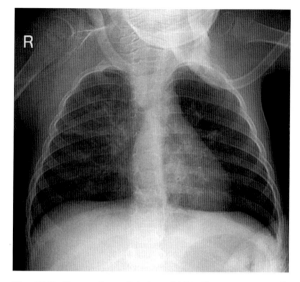

Fig. 15.2. Chest radiograph in bronchiolitis. There are interstitial perihilar changes and peribronchiolar cuffing (seen as white circles), and also some peripheral right upper zone consolidation.

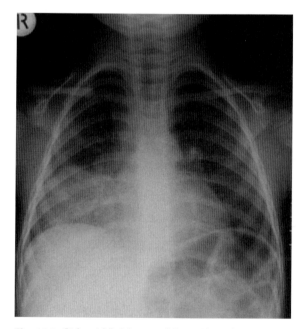

Fig. 15.3. Right middle lobe consolidation. The right hemidiaphragm is seen but the right heart border is obscured.

- In pneumonia, as well as consolidation, collapse can occur due to mucus/pus obstructing the lobar bronchus. Alternatively, an inhaled foreign body can cause obstruction, followed by secondary infection.

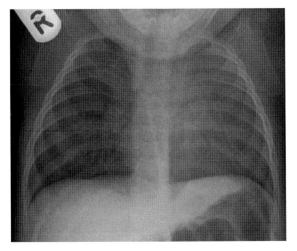

Fig. 15.4. Chest radiograph of left upper lobe collapse. As the left upper lobe collapses it forms a dense structure that runs roughly parallel to the anterior chest wall, which means that no sharp change in density is seen, but rather a diffuse hazy opacity is present over the hemithorax.

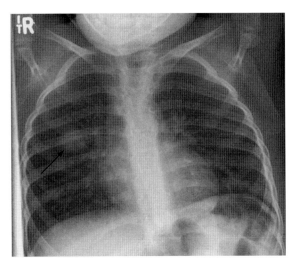

Fig. 15.6. Chest radiograph – Round pneumonia (arrow).

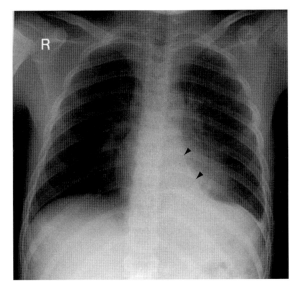

Fig. 15.5. Chest radiograph of left lower lobe collapse. As the left lower lobe collapses it forms a dense triangular shadow behind the heart (arrowheads). This is easy to overlook.

Round pneumonia
- Round pneumonia is only seen in children and represents acute consolidation secondary to infection, usually bacterial.
- It appears as a well-defined round lung opacity (Fig. 15.6). With treatment the initially sharply defined area becomes less well defined and then disappears.

Cavitation
- Several infections can cause lung cavities.
- Thin-walled cysts, or "pneumatocoeles", found after an episode of pneumonia are typically caused by *Staphylococcus*.
- A thick-walled cavity in a child is most likely due to tuberculosis.

Asthma
Introduction
- Asthma is common in children, and a common cause of hospital admission.
- Most children with asthma require no radiological investigation.
- Occasionally, in a child with atypical symptoms where the diagnosis is unclear, or when moderate to severe symptoms are present, a CXR may help to exclude other pathology.

Chest X-ray findings
- Most often, CXR is normal, apart from varying degrees of lung hyperinflation (Fig. 15.7).
- In acute attacks or severe asthma there may be lobar collapse, which is probably due to mucous plugging causing bronchial obstruction rather than bacterial infection.
- Pneumothorax is almost never seen in an acute attack unless there has been ventilatory intervention (e.g. mouth-to-mouth resuscitation or mechanical ventilation).
- Pneumomediastinum (Fig. 15.8).

247

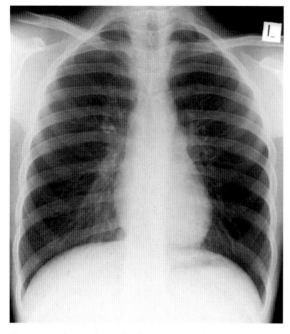

Fig. 15.7. Chest radiograph of an asthmatic showing hyperinflation (more than five anterior ribs are seen above diaphragm).

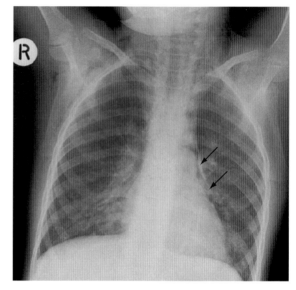

Fig. 15.8. Pneumomediastinum in an asthmatic. A thin line is seen running parallel to the mediastinum representing pleura lifted up by air in the mediastinum (arrows). The air has tracked up into the neck (surgical emphysema).

Pneumothorax
Causes
The commonest causes are:
- Trauma
- Idiopathic
- Congenital blebs
- Iatrogenic – mechanical ventilation or procedures.
- Neonates with:
  - Surfactant deficiency due to prematurity
  - Meconium aspiration
  - Mechanical ventilation
- Inhaled foreign bodies – either by a ball valve effect (most common) or by piercing the pulmonary parenchyma (very uncommon)

CXR findings
- Look for a collection of air between the lung and chest wall (Fig. 15.9).
- If the patient is erect, a small pneumothorax will be at the lung apex. With a larger pneumothorax, air is seen lateral to the lung.
- The air in the pneumothorax can be distinguished from lung parenchyma as it is slightly less dense (blacker) and contains no vessels.

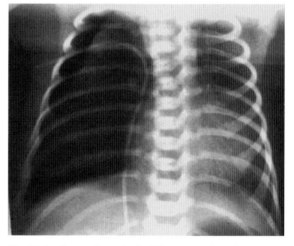

Fig. 15.9. Chest radiograph of a right pneumothorax in a neonate with surfactant deficit respiratory distress.

- A large pneumothorax causes the ipsilateral lung to collapse (become smaller and more dense).
- In neonates, who have supine CXRs, a pneumothorax lies anterior to the lung rather than laterally. This means that there is often only a subtle decrease in density over the lower lung.
- It is very important to diagnose and treat a tension pneumothorax.

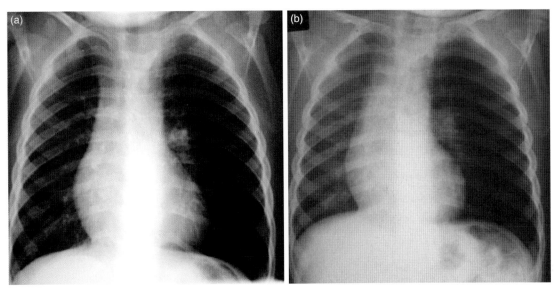

Fig. 15.10. (a) Inspiratory chest radiograph in a child with a foreign body in the left main bronchus. Note the decreased density of the left lung compared to the right due to air trapping. (b) Expiratory chest radiograph. Air trapping in the left lung prevents air being expelled during expiration, so the left lung remains more lucent (darker) and the mediastinum shifts to the right as the right lung decreases in volume.

Pleural effusion and empyema
Causes
- Exudates – pleural inflammation (e.g. infection or tumor)
- Transudates – secondary to oncotic pressure changes (e.g. cardiac failure, fluid overload and hypoalbuminemia).

In children, the most likely cause of an effusion is acute infection. This can either be a simple exudate or can be an empyema (pus and bacteria in the pleural space). The initial diagnosis of empyema always depends on clinical judgment.

Radiological appearances
- An erect CXR demonstrates a pleural effusion only when it becomes large enough to be seen above the diaphragm.
- On a supine CXR, pleural fluid lies posteriorly, causing increased density of the hemithorax, particularly towards the lung base.
- Fluid trapped in the oblique fissure or in loculated collections caused by adhesions produce localized densities and can be mistaken for masses.
- In children, ultrasound is useful for estimating the volume of pleural fluid. Importantly, ultrasound shows septations and fluid loculations, that can make percutaneous drainage difficult.

- CT can demonstrate the volume of pleural fluid, but septations are often not seen. CT can be used in complex cases where lung abscess or underlying tumor is suspected.

Foreign body and aspiration
Clinical features
- Most children who aspirate a foreign body are pre-schoolers (age 1 to 5 years).
- The most common foreign bodies are nuts, but any similar sized object can be inhaled (e.g. beads, plastic toys).
- Many children will not have a history of a choking episode, however acute choking, cough, breathlessness or wheeze may all indicate foreign body inhalation.

CXR findings
- A ball valve effect may occur when the foreign body partly obstructs a lobar bronchus so that air can be sucked into the lobe but is not expelled on expiration. This causes hyperinflation (air trapping) of the affected lobe that is more exaggerated on expiration. This can be demonstrated by taking inspiratory and expiratory films (Fig. 15.10).
- The most commonly affected lobes are the right lower lobe or right middle lobe due to the angle of the right main bronchus at the carina.

- *Note:* a child with an inhaled foreign body may have a normal CXR, hence if this suspected clinically, a bronchoscopy may be warranted even in the absence of clinical signs.
- Also, care must be taken to visualize all areas of the airway including the larynx and nasopharynx.
- Over time, if the inhaled foreign body is not removed, collapse of the lung distal to the obstructed bronchus develops. This can result in secondary infection and permanent damage, e.g. bronchiectasis.

Cystic fibrosis
Clinical features
- The most common suppurative lung disease in Caucasians.
- An autosomal recessive condition with variable clinical features.
- Recurrent or persistent cough may start in early infancy but often remains asymptomatic until late childhood or adolescence.

Radiological appearances
- A progressive disease.
- CXR changes include: hyperinflation, bronchiectasis and streaky fibrotic bands radiating from the hila.
- In acute infections, CXR can identify new changes or affected areas when compared to previous films.

Musculoskeletal
Fractures of childhood
Introduction
- Children have growing bones that contain a large cartilaginous component including a growth plate between the metaphysis and epiphysis. Their bones are more plastic and less brittle than adults and so pediatric fractures differ from adult fractures.
- The history and severity of trauma help determine if a fracture is likely, but young children may only present with disuse of the injured limb or in distress.
- Some fractures are more prevalent in different age groups. For example, infants previously able to walk may suddenly limp due to a subtle spiral fracture of the tibia (a Toddler's fracture)

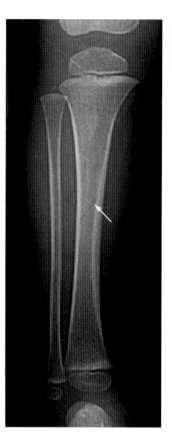

Fig. 15.11. Toddler's fracture of the tibia. The fracture is seen as a subtle oblique lucency in the tibial diaphysis (arrow).

Imaging principles
- Plain radiographs are standard for suspected fracture.
- In more complex injuries, particularly those involving a joint, a CT may be useful for assessing alignment and the exact course of a fracture line.
- In suspected or occult injury, a bone scan may reveal a site of injury, not seen on the radiograph e.g. in scaphoid injuries.
- If extensive soft tissue injury is suspected, e.g. in the cervical spine, an MRI can examine ligaments, tendons, muscle and the spinal cord.
- If the injury involves a joint then a joint effusion (particularly in the knee or elbow) is a useful sign indicating that a fracture may have occurred. At the elbow a joint effusion most likely indicates that a supracondylar fracture (younger child) or radial neck fracture (older child) has occurred.
- Fractures vary from the most subtle (Toddler's fracture, Fig. 15.11) to the most obvious with complete displacement of multiple fragments. In all cases careful examination of the cortex, which should normally be smooth, may reveal a small

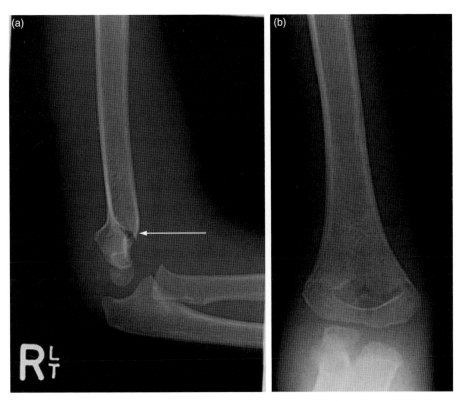

Fig. 15.12. (a) Lateral and (b) AP views of a supracondylar fracture (arrow) of the elbow.

deformity, i.e. a fracture. Toddler's fracture presents two problems, first because it can be difficult to see on initial films, but second because non-accidental injury may be wrongly suspected.

- Alignment – perpendicular films are needed to calculate the alignment of fracture fragments. A single view can underestimate the degree of angulation or displacement (Fig. 15.12).
- Stability depends as much on the soft tissues, e.g. ligaments, as the bone itself. Some fractures such as triplanar fractures of the ankle are unstable, requiring surgical intervention.
- Periosteal reaction around a fracture indicates healing, and means that the injury is certainly more than several days old.
- Repeat films – if there is suspicion that a fracture has occurred but none is definitely identified, repeat films in 7–10 days' time, or a bone scan may help.

Types of fractures in children
Mid-shaft or diaphyseal fracture
- As occur in adults

Torus or buckle fracture
- Often seen in the distal radial metaphysis. The cortex of the bone buckles producing a step in its normally smooth line. Torus fractures can be subtle.

Greenstick fractures
- Involve only one side of the cortex, whilst the other side bends so that a cortical injury can only be seen along one surface (Fig. 15.13).

Growth plate injuries (Salter–Harris fractures)
- Fractures involving the epiphysis and metaphysis are common in children. They are important because injury to the germinal layer of cells at the growth plate can result in abnormal bone growth and long-term disability.
- The Salter–Harris classification is often used to describe these injuries. There are five common types of Salter–Harris fracture (Fig. 15.14):
  - Type 1. A transverse fracture through the growth plate causes widening. The germinal layer is not generally damaged and growth disturbance is rare (Fig. 15.15).

251

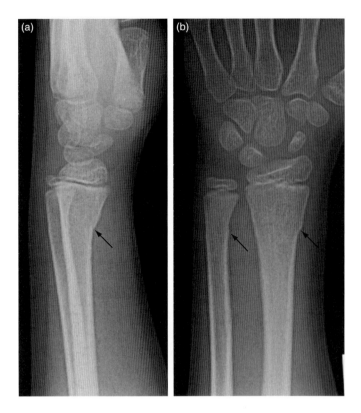

Fig. 15.13. (a) Lateral and (b) AP views of a greenstick fracture of the distal radius and ulnar. Note the buckled cortex (arrows).

- Type 2. A fracture through the metaphysis and along the growth plate. The germinal layer is usually not injured and growth is normal. (Fig. 15.16).
- Type 3. A fracture through the epiphysis and the distal growth plate. The germinal layer may be damaged with subsequent growth disturbance and deformity, although this is uncommon. As the epiphysis is fractured the joint surface is also involved. The epiphyseal fragment is often displaced.
- Type 4. A fracture through the metaphysis, growth plate and epiphysis. The growth plate is completely interrupted and so growth arrest may occur. The joint surface is also involved. Surgery is needed to restore alignment.
- Type 5. A crush injury to the growth plate is difficult to detect as the only initial findings can be soft tissue swelling. The injury is uncommon but results in abnormal bone growth.

Non-accidental injury

- In some situations non-accidental injury (NAI) is suspected on history and/or examination;

however, in other cases radiographs (see below) may first suggest NAI. When this happens, it is important to reassess the history and examination in the light of the radiographic findings.
- A number of fractures are considered pathognomonic indicators of NAI. A "bucket handle" or metaphyseal fracture occurs only in NAI (Fig. 15.17). It results from the forces exerted on bone when an infant is shaken and the limbs are left to flap.
- It is most important to compare the history of the injury with the clinical examination and radiological findings. If a fracture or injury is discovered it is a good basic principle to ask oneself "Could the child or infant have put themselves in a position to produce the force required?" For example, an immobile infant is not likely to be able to produce any force capable of causing a fracture.
- Fractures of different ages (i.e. at different stages of healing) without adequate explanation are highly suspicious for NAI.
- When NAI is suspected, referral to a senior member of staff is mandatory. Further radiological investigation of NAI will involve a

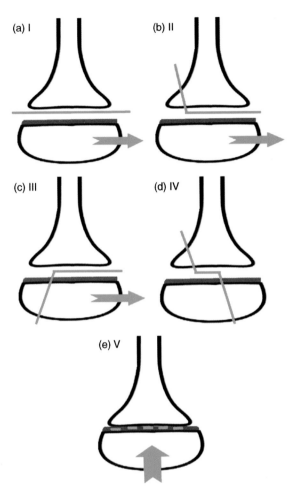

(a) I   (b) II

(c) III   (d) IV

(e) V

Fig. 15.14. (a)–(e) Salter–Harris fractures Types I–V. The germinal layer of the growth plate is shown in red, the fracture is shown in green, and the green arrow shows the direction of force required to produce the fracture.

full skeletal survey to look for other fractures and also a bone scan to identify any fractures too subtle to identify by radiography ("occult" fractures).

Osteomyelitis and septic arthritis
- The presentation, investigation, and management of acute osteomyelitis and acute septic arthritis overlap to a considerable degree in younger children.
- Infection can affect any joint or bone, but most commonly involve the lower limbs.
- Both are most commonly caused by *Staphylococcus aureus* but can be caused by group A β-hemolytic streptococci and *Haemophilus influenzae*.

- Osteomyelitis
  - This occurs in the metaphyseal ends of long bones.
  - It is usually due to hematogenous spread of the pathogen but may be due to direct spread from an infected wound.
- Septic arthritis
  - Acute septic arthritis generally occurs in a child who is systemically unwell with bacteremia.
  - Occasionally there is a history of a penetrating injury into or near a joint.
  - Clinical signs include fever, tenderness, warmth, and restricted range of joint movement.
  - Pain tends to be more rapidly progressive in septic arthritis and may occur on movement and on rest, whilst in osteomyelitis pain tends to progress more slowly and occurs on movement of the affected area. The range of movement tends to be more restricted in septic arthritis than in osteomyelitis.
  - The synovial joint environment responds to inflammation/suppuration by increased production of synovial fluid leading to an effusion.

Painful hip
Irritable hip (transient synovitis)
- The commonest reason for a limp in the pre-school age group is transient synovitis.
- It usually occurs in 3–8-year-olds, and may follow minor injury or viral illness.
- The child is usually afebrile and generally able to walk, but with pain.
- Symptoms of irritable hip overlap with those of septic arthritis and management is by exclusion of septic arthritis (and other conditions). Severe limitation of hip movement suggests septic arthritis. If there is any doubt, orthopedic consultation should be sought.

Perthe's disease
- Perthe's disease (avascular necrosis of the capital femoral epiphysis) occurs from 2–12 years (majority 4–8 yrs) (Fig. 15.18).
- 20% are bilateral.
- It presents with pain and limp. The child is afebrile.

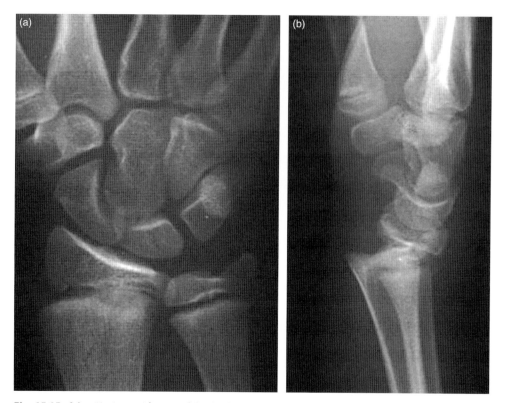

Fig. 15.15. Salter–Harris type I fracture of distal radius with epiphysis displaced posteriorly. (a) AP view, (b) lateral view.

Slipped capital femoral epiphysis

- This typically occurs in late childhood/early adolescence and affects boys more than girls (Fig. 15.19).
- Associated with obesity (weight often >90th centile).
- Presents with hip or knee pain and associated limp.
- Both hips may be involved.

Osteomyelitis and septic arthritis

Arthritis

- Juvenile chronic arthritis, arthritis associated with inflammatory bowel disease, psoriasis and ankylosing spondylitis may cause a painful hip. Other features of these conditions usually give clues to these diagnoses.

Investigation strategy for the painful hip

- Investigations usually include a full blood count and ESR.
- Plain X-ray of the hip may diagnose or exclude fractures, tumors, septic arthritis and

osteomyelitis. In osteomyelitis the changes may not be seen on plain X-ray for 7–10 days.

- Ultrasound of the hip shows an effusion. If an effusion is present, urgent drainage, gram stain, and culture of the fluid is arranged. Most often this is carried out in an operating theater under anesthetic so that arthroscopic washout or arthrotomy (treatment) can be carried out without delay. Systemic antibiotic therapy is required.
- Bone scan for early Perthe's disease in a child with persistent hip pain who has normal plain X-rays and ultrasound. It may also diagnose early osteomyelitis and synovitis due to irritable hip, as well as infective or rheumatological arthritis.

Clicky hip – developmental hip dysplasia

- The hips are routinely checked at birth for developmental dysplasia of the hip (DDH).
- DDH may produce anything from mild hip instability to dislocation.
- Early detection permits relatively simple treatment and excellent outcome.

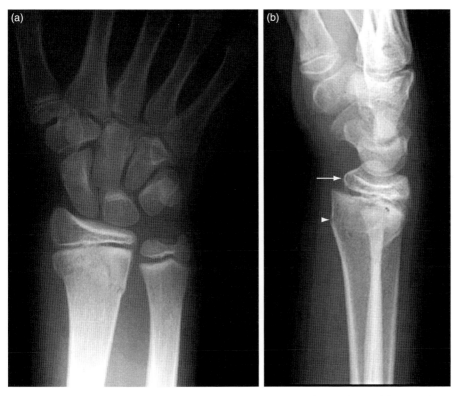

Fig. 15.16. Salter–Harris type II fracture of distal radius through the epiphyseal plate and the metaphysis (arrowhead). The epiphysis is displaced slightly posteriory (arrow). (a) AP view, (b) lateral view.

- Delayed diagnosis leads to secondary changes and dislocation, prolonged treatment and less than satisfactory results, with limp, pain and early osteoarthritis.

Diagnosis
Ultrasound
- DDH is usually suspected on the basis of clinical findings either at birth or soon after.
- The diagnosis is made by ultrasound. Infants with an abnormal clinical examination at birth and infants with risk factors for DDH undergo an early ultrasound. Routine hip ultrasound to check for DDH is performed on the following infants:
  - "Click" or instability on clinical examination
  - Other clinical suspicion of DDH (e.g. asymmetrical skin creases or leg lengths)
  - Family history of DDH
  - Breech presentation.
- Ultrasound is the best investigation because:
  - It demonstrates the unossified femoral head (the femoral head does not show up on X-rays until after 3 months)

- The position of the femoral head can be watched during stress maneuvers
- US does not use ionizing radiation.

Plain films
- Hip ultrasound does not yield useful information after the femoral heads are ossified, and only then is a pelvic X-ray performed (Figs. 15.20, 15.21).

Osteosarcoma
- Radiology can determine if a tumor has a benign or malignant appearance, and can define local and distant spread of disease.
- Osteosarcoma and Ewing sarcoma are the two commonest primary malignant bone tumors in childhood.
- Precise diagnosis can only be made by tumor biopsy, usually carried out by the orthopedic surgeon.
- Osteomyelitis can also produce an "aggressive" appearance and must be considered in the right clinical setting.

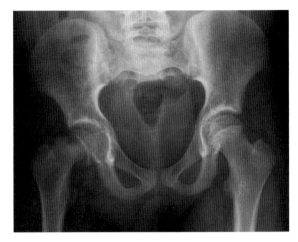

Fig. 15.19. Right slipped upper femoral epiphysis. Note the different position of the femoral head between the two sides.

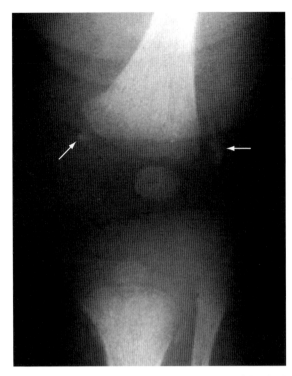

Fig. 15.17. Metaphyseal or corner fractures (arrows) of the distal femur in non-accidental injury.

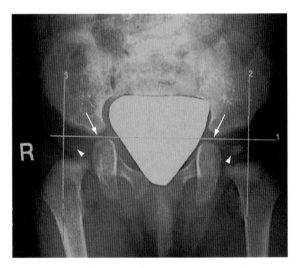

Fig. 15.20. AP pelvis of an infant demonstrating the lines used to determine the correct location of the femoral head. Line 1 is Hilgenreiner's line, drawn between the unossified triradiate cartilages (arrows). Lines 2 and 3 are Perkins' lines drawn perpendicular to line 1 at the edge of each acetabulum. The femoral head (arrowheads) should lie in the inferomedial quadrant.

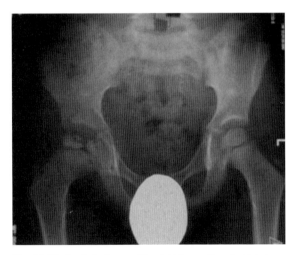

Fig. 15.18. Perthe's disease of the right femoral head which shows fragmentation.

- Osteosarcoma
  - Osteosarcoma usually presents with pain ± swelling in 5–20-year-olds.
  - It often arises in the metaphysis, most commonly around the knee.
  - Typically, it produces periosteal new bone formation and sclerosis.

- There are usually malignant features such as bone destruction and a florid spiculated periosteal reaction ("sunray appearance") (Fig. 15.22). The tumor may elevate the periosteum to form a "Codman's triangle."
- Following initial plain films, the following imaging techniques are routine for further evaluation:
  - Radionuclide bone scan for synchronous lesions or bone metastases
  - Chest CT for lung metastases

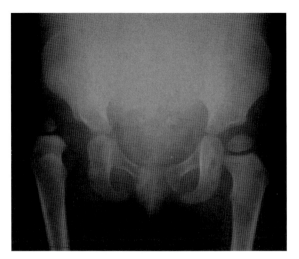

Fig. 15.21. AP pelvis in an infant showing dislocation of the right femur secondary to right acetabular dysplasia. Note the steeper angle and abnormal shape of the right acetabulum.

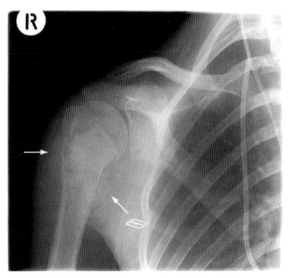

Fig. 15.22. Osteosarcoma of proximal humeral metaphysis. There is an irregular poorly defined lesion with a soft tissue mass and periosteal new bone formation (arrows).

- MRI for the marrow extent, soft tissue involvement, and extension across the physis or joint

Rickets

- Rickets is characterized by impaired mineralization of the growing ends of bones in childhood, with accumulation of cartilaginous matrix. It may cause marked bone deformities.
- Osteomalacia is the term used for the equivalent disorder in adults.

- The causes of rickets are vitamin D deficiency, abnormal metabolism of vitamin D, phosphate depletion and renal tubular acidosis.

Clinical features
- Physical signs may be subtle and easily overlooked.
- They include delayed closure of the anterior fontanelle, frontal and occipital skull bossing, rickety rosary, widening of long bone ends, and, in a mobile child, bowing of the legs.
- In young infants, vitamin D deficiency may cause convulsions.
- The diagnosis may be incidentally discovered when a chest X-ray performed for a chest infection shows thickening of costo-chondral junctions ("rickety rosary"). Blood tests show a high alkaline phosphatase, low serum phosphate and/or low serum calcium.

Radiological features
- Wrist and knee X-rays show metaphyseal cupping, fraying and splaying (Fig. 15.23), and CXR may show a "rickety rosary" (prominent costochondral junctions).

Urinary tract
Urinary tract infection
Clinical features
- Urinary tract infections are common in infants and children. Once diagnosed, further investigation and management are controversial. At present there is enormous variation in clinical practice due to lack of consensus about investigations and management.
- Symptoms of UTI are often non-specific and especially in younger children.
- Definite diagnosis can only be made by bacteriological culture of a properly collected urine specimen.
- Following treatment, further investigations are frequently performed to detect underlying urinary tract abnormality that could predispose to further UTIs and renal scarring, e.g. vesico-ureteric reflux (VUR), posterior urethral valves, ureterocoele, and other congenital abnormalities.

Imaging options
- Different opinions exist about when or whether prophylactic treatment is needed, and when and which investigations should be carried out.

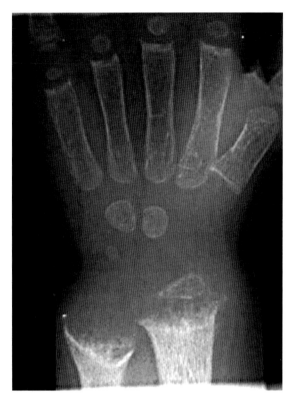

Fig. 15.23. Wrist in rickets. There is reduced bony density with coarse trabeculae, due to reduced mineralization, and loss of definition of the cortex due to secondary hyperparathyroidism. The metaphyses become "cupped" and "frayed" and the growth plates become apparently wider.

- The available investigations are:
  - Renal tract ultrasound
  - DMSA nuclear medicine scan
  - MAG₃ nuclear medicine scan
  - Nuclear medicine micturating cystogram
  - Fluoroscopic micturating cystourethrogram (MCU)

Ultrasound
- This is often the first line of investigation.
- It excludes major renal tract abnormalities such as scarring, renal duplication, renal size discrepancy, dilated collecting systems, bladder diverticula, and ureterocoeles.
- Bladder wall thickness and bladder emptying can also be assessed.
- A proper bladder examination requires a full bladder, to be emptied as required, so bladder ultrasound in children who are not toilet trained is variably successful.

DMSA scan
- This is performed to determine renal structure and relative function.
- An i.v. injection of technetium labeled dimercaptosuccinic acid (DMSA) is given and the child returns 2 hours later and must lie still on a bed over a gamma camera for around 20 minutes.
- It can be used to exclude focal scarring/inflammation or dysmorphic kidneys. Renal size and relative renal function is also determined.
- It should not be performed less than 6 weeks after an infection if scarring/dysmorphism is to be separated from focal inflammation.

MAG3 nuclear medicine scan
- This is used to obtain a physiological picture of renal function (uptake, clearance and drainage).
- An i.v. injection of technetium labelled mercaptoacetyltriglycerine (MAG₃) is given with the child on the gamma camera bed.
- The imaging starts immediately and the tracer (MAG₃) is followed for 45 minutes as it passes through the kidneys. After 15 minutes, an injection of frusemide is given to help differentiate obstructed from slow draining kidneys.
- At the end of the study, when the child has a full bladder, an indirect micturating cystogram (IMCU) can be performed if the child is toilet trained and can void when asked.

Nuclear medicine micturating cystogram (MCU)
- This detects vesico-ureteric reflux (VUR).
- It can be performed on neonates and infants, and requires bladder catheterization and the injection of radioisotope tracer into the bladder.
- Once the bladder is full, the child/infant micturates whilst on the table.
- In the investigation of infant boys with suspected posterior urethral valves a fluoroscopic MCU (see below) should be the initial investigation. Subsequent follow-up can then be with a nuclear medicine MCU. In girls a nuclear medicine MCU can be used as a first investigation if a lower dose of radiation is desired.
- A nuclear medicine MCU is approximately 2% of the dose of a fluoroscopic MCU.

Fluoroscopic MCU
- Allows accurate determination of bladder anatomy and severity of reflux (Fig. 15.24).

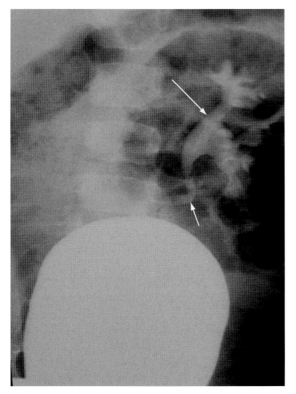

Fig. 15.24. Grade 2 vesico-ureteric reflux. An image from a micturating cystogram of a baby with vesico-ureteric reflux. Contrast is seen in the bladder and also in the normal caliber left ureter (short arrow) and non-dilated left renal pelvi-calyceal system (long arrow).

- The child is catheterized and iodinated contrast is injected into the bladder. The filling and micturating phases are observed.
- In general, this investigation should be performed only on children less than 1 year old since it is more traumatic for older children. In an older child, who is toilet trained, an indirect MCU following a MAG$_3$ is more appropriate.
- Fluoroscopic MCU is, however, the only imaging test that can reliably diagnose posterior urethral valves.

Wilm's tumor
- Wilm's tumor is highly malignant. It originates from embryonic renal tissue. Over 80% of cases present before 5 years of age.
- Children with Wilm's tumor often present with an abdominal mass.
- The differential diagnosis includes polycystic kidneys, neuroblastoma, hydronephrosis,

hepatoblastoma (if right-sided) and splenomegaly (if left sided).

Radiological diagnosis
- The lesion is initially confirmed by ultrasound.
- CT provides more detailed anatomical information for staging.
- Information required for staging includes the presence of metastases (frequently lung), the degree of local tumor spread and assessment of function of the contralateral kidney.

Gastrointestinal tract
Neonate
Esophageal atresia
- The mid-portion of the esophagus is missing, often with an abnormal communication between the lower esophagus and trachea: a distal tracheo-esophageal fistula.
- It should be suspected with polyhydramnios, or in any neonate who salivates excessively at birth. If suspected, the child must not be fed, to avoid milk aspiration.
- The diagnosis is confirmed by the inability to pass a firm catheter down the esophagus.
- Other congenital abnormalities are present in 50%, most of which form the VACTERL association (vertebral, ano-rectal, cardiac, tracheo-esophageal, renal, and limb abnormalities). Chromosomal abnormalities, e.g. trisomy 18 and 21 are seen in about 5%.
- Chest X-rays show a dilated proximal esophageal pouch, and may show cardiac and vertebral abnormalities. When a fistula is present, bowel gas will be seen, due to passage of air from the trachea to the distal esophagus.
- Barium studies are contraindicated due to the high risk of aspiration. If contrast is needed to outline the proximal pouch, air may be insufflated prior to the X-ray.

Small bowel obstruction
- May be recognized on antenatal ultrasound, or may present soon after birth with persistent vomiting, which is bile stained, unless the obstruction is above the ampulla of Vater. Bile stained vomiting can be due to malrotation with volvulus.
- Meconium passage is delayed or absent.

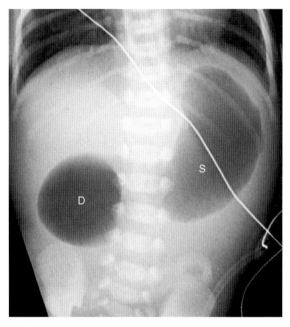

Fig. 15.25. Abdominal X-ray in a neonate with duodenal atresia, showing the classic "double bubble" of dilated stomach (S) and duodenum (D).

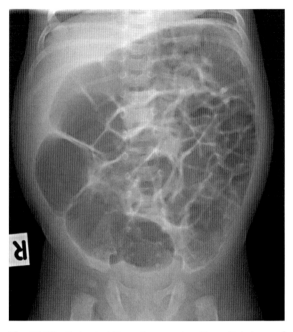

Fig. 15.26. Abdominal X-ray of a neonate with multiple loops of dilated gas-filled bowel secondary to obstruction from meconium ileus. There is no gas in the rectum.

- Abdominal distension is more prominent in distal obstructions.
- High lesions present soon after birth; distal lesions tend to present later.
- Bowel proximal to an obstruction becomes dilated and gas-filled. Therefore, the more distal an obstruction, the more loops of gas-filled bowel are present.
- Unlike adults, it is not possible to distinguish between dilated small and large bowel in neonates and infants.

Duodenal atresia/stenosis
- A third of these infants have Down's syndrome.
- Abdominal X-ray
  - The "double bubble" sign is characteristic, caused by gas in dilated stomach and duodenum (Fig. 15.25).

Jejunal atresia
- May be multiple atretic segments
- Abdominal X-ray shows multiple air–fluid levels. Distal jejunal atresia appears similar in appearance to obstruction from meconium ileus.

Meconium ileus
- Presents shortly after birth with vomiting and abdominal distention.
- Thick inspissated meconium obstructs the lower ileum.
- The colon is empty and no meconium is passed after birth.
- Most affected neonates have cystic fibrosis.
- Abdominal X-ray
  - Shows a small bowel obstruction with multiple gas-filled loops of bowel and an empty colon (Fig. 15.26).
- Contrast enemas (diagnostic and therapeutic)
  - Water-soluble contrast outlines the small-caliber colon ("micro-colon"), and the meconium plugs in the terminal ileum, and is often also therapeutic in dislodging the obstructing meconium.

Ano-rectal atresia
- Absence of the anus at the normal site.
- Classified as high or low relative to the levator ani muscle.
- In high lesions there is often a fistula to the bladder, urethra (boys) or vagina (girls). In low lesions there may be a fistulous opening to the skin.

- Forms part of the VACTERL association (see above).
- Abdominal X-ray
  - Shows a distal bowel obstruction. Vertebral abnormalities may be seen.
- Micturating cystourethrogram (MCU)
  - Shows any fistula between the bladder or urethra, and the rectum in high lesions.

Hirschprung's disease
- Absence of the rectal myenteric nerve plexus, which may extend proximally along the colon.
- Abnormal peristalsis in the affected segment, resulting in delayed passage of meconium (i.e. beyond 48 hours), or occasionally, an acute abdomen.
- Some children present later, with chronic constipation or acute enterocolitis.
- Full thickness rectal biopsy is required for definitive diagnosis.
- Barium enema may show the level of transition from abnormal to normal colon. The affected bowel starts from the rectum and extends proximally. The unaffected colon is dilated and a sudden transition to thin irregularly contracted bowel denotes the affected segment.

Necrotizing enterocolitis (NEC)
- This mostly occurs in premature neonates who undergo prenatal stress.
- Presenting features include vomiting, feed intolerance or abdominal distension, usually 2 days to 2 weeks after birth.
- Abdominal X-ray may be non-specific, with mildly dilated gas-filled bowel loops. Intramural bowel gas (Fig. 15.27), portal vein gas (branching pattern peripherally in the liver), and free intraperitoneal gas are all late findings in severe NEC.

Gastrointestinal tract in the infant and child
Hypertrophic pyloric stenosis
- Typically presents between 2 to 6 weeks of age with projectile vomiting.
- Males are affected five times more than females.

Clinical findings
- A thickened pylorus "tumor" in the epigastrium.
- Peristaltic waves may be visible.
- Dehydration.

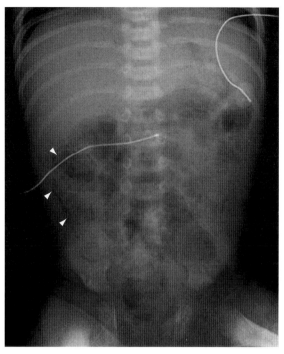

Fig. 15.27. Abdominal X-ray in necrotizing enterocolitis. Intramural gas produces "tram track" appearances in the bowel wall (arrowheads).

Ultrasound
- Should the diagnosis be in doubt, ultrasound will demonstrate the elongated thick-walled pylorus, and a full stomach with overactive peristalsis.

Barium meal
- Can be used, but ultrasound is easier, more accurate and does not involve ionizing radiation.

Small bowel obstruction
Midgut volvulus
- Volvulus in a neonate or child with malrotation causes a high bowel obstruction with bile stained vomiting.
- Any infant with bile stained vomiting should be presumed to have a volvulus until proved otherwise.
- Midgut volvulus can cause infarction of the entire small bowel, and is a medical emergency.
- A barium study must be performed urgently to confirm the diagnosis, unless there are signs of vascular compromise when an emergency laparotomy is needed.
- Abdominal X-ray findings are non-specific.

- Barium meal:
  - This confirms malrotation by demonstrating an abnormal position of the duodenal jejunal (DJ) flexure. The DJ flexure normally lies to the left of the spine at the level of the pylorus. In malrotation, the DJ flexure is not seen in its normal position.
  - In volvulus, a barium meal shows a corkscrew configuration of the distal duodenum and proximal jejunum as it twists (volves) around the root of the mesentery.
  - Often there is poor stomach emptying and dilatation of the proximal duodenum due to the obstruction at the site of the twist.

Intussusception

- Intussusception is commonest surgical cause of acute abdominal pain in the 3 to 18 month age group.
- In intussusception, the proximal bowel invaginates into the distal bowel, and is most commonly due to the distal ileum telescoping into adjoining cecum and colon. This causes intestinal obstruction.
- Clinical features
  - Paroxysms of severe colicky abdominal pain, pallor and vomiting.
  - Passage of "red-currant stool" (blood and mucus) is a late sign, along with abdominal distension and shock.
  - A palpable sausage shaped abdominal mass.
  - Resuscitation and reduction are urgent.
- Abdominal X-ray features include
  - Paucity of gas in the right lower quadrant
  - The impression of a soft tissue mass anywhere in the line of the colon (Fig. 15.28).
  - Note: The important role of the abdominal X-ray is to exclude bowel perforation prior to attempted non-operative reduction. Perforation is an absolute contraindication to the procedure.
- Ultrasound
  - Ultrasound can confirm the diagnosis by showing a target-shaped lesion in cross-section produced by the layers of trapped edematous bowel and mesentery within the colon.
- Air enema
  - If the child is adequately resuscitated and without evidence of bowel perforation,

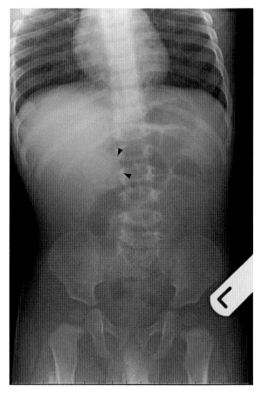

Fig. 15.28. Plain film in intussusception with some dilated gas-filled loops of bowel in the upper abdomen and a soft tissue mass of intussusception in the right upper quadrant (arrowheads).

non-operative reduction by air enema may be attempted.
- This is performed by a radiologist, with the attending surgeon, as there is a small risk of bowel perforation.
- The procedure is often successful, and no further treatment may be required.
- A long prodromal history, a very sick child, and ileo-ileal intussusceptions are all predictors of lower likelihood of success.

Hernias and adhesions

- As in adults, inguinal hernias can cause small bowel obstruction and should be detected clinically (Fig. 15.29).
- If there has been previous surgery, adhesions are the most likely cause of a new obstruction.

Appendicitis

- This occurs at any age but is rare before 5 years of age.

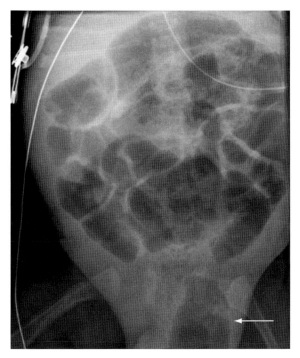

Fig. 15.29. An abdominal radiograph of an infant showing dilatation of bowel loops consistent with obstruction. Also note the bowel gas lying below the left inguinal ligament (arrow) in a left inguinal hernia. This is the cause of obstruction.

- The variability of symptoms and examination findings in children may hinder the diagnosis.
- Role of ultrasound and abdominal X-ray:
  - The diagnosis of appendicitis is largely clinical, but when the diagnosis is unclear, ultrasound can exclude mimicking conditions, e.g. a torted ovarian cyst in girls, and may demonstrate an enlarged inflamed appendix or complex peritoneal fluid collection.
  - The presence of an appendicolith and/or a soft tissue mass in the right iliac fossa on an abdominal X-ray can reinforce the clinical impression of appendicitis, but need not be present.

Paralytic ileus
- Post-operative
  - Following abdominal surgery, ongoing vomiting and abdominal pain (feed intolerance) may indicate a paralytic ileus.
  - Clinically, the abdomen will be silent, whereas in mechanical obstruction, bowel sounds are heard.
  - Abdominal X-ray

- In paralytic ileus, X-rays show dilated gas filled loops with multiple air–fluid levels.
- Gas will be seen right down to the rectum.
- The radiological differential diagnosis is a distal bowel obstruction.

Ingested foreign body
- Ingestion of foreign bodies is common in children.
- If the ingested foreign body is known to be radio-opaque, then radiographs are warranted to determine its site.
- Button batteries lodged in the esophagus need urgent removal.
- If the object has reached the stomach then no further imaging or review is necessary unless symptoms occur, as it will almost certainly pass spontaneously.
- If symptoms, e.g. drooling occur, surgical referral for endoscopic or surgical removal is needed.

Brain and head
Modalities
Ultrasound (US)
- US is used to image the infant brain. It is performed through the open anterior fontanelle, and cannot be performed after this has closed.
- As the fontanelle is a centrally placed, US shows central structures very well, e.g. ventricles and corpus callosum, but it is not good at examining posterior fossa contents, the brain surface, and surface subdural or extradural collections.
- US readily shows hydrocephalus, intraventricular hemorrhages in premature babies, and corpus callosum agenesis.

Computed tomography (CT)
- In pediatrics, CT is often used as a tool to quickly exclude large lesions, acute hemorrhages, abscess or fractures, but MRI is more sensitive. Many subtle lesions (e.g. encephalitis, acute disseminated encephalomyelitis, migrational anomalies) are difficult to identify on CT.
- Intravenous contrast is used to highlight blood vessels and tissue with increased vascularity, e.g. around an abscess or tumor.
- In unco-operative children, CT requires general anesthesia.
- A non-contrast head CT scan takes generally less than 30 seconds to perform.

263

Magnetic resonance imaging (MRI)

- MRI is the only accurate way of demonstrating cortical dysplasias, inflammatory lesions other than abscesses, and subtle changes of hypoxic ischemic encephalopathy. MRI is much better than CT when assessing the contents of the posterior fossa.
- Most children with complex neurological disease require an MRI.
- The drawbacks are:
  - Long examination time – usually requires general anesthesia for children under 6 years.
  - Poor visualization of cortical bone.

The fitting child

- Seizures are very common in childhood. About 7% of children have a verified seizure.
- Epileptic syndromes are often classified by the usual age of onset or presumed etiology.

Neonatal seizures

- These differ from seizures in older children, with different clinical manifestations and etiological factors.
- Causes include hypoxic-ischemic encephalopathy, intracerebral hemorrhage, metabolic disturbances, infections, developmental brain abnormalities, and benign familial neonatal convulsions.
- Thorough investigation should be undertaken, usually with US, and often with MRI.

Seizures in infancy and childhood

Febrile convulsions

- These occur in approximately 3% of infants.
- However, fever and convulsions may be present concurrently in CNS infections such as meningitis and encephalitis.
- It is important to exclude a CNS infection by careful history and examination, and where necessary by investigations, e.g. lumbar puncture and imaging.
- Children with fever and focal convulsions, an altered conscious state and/or abnormal neurological signs are at higher risk of cerebral infection.
- In children with febrile convulsions per se (i.e. CNS infection has been ruled out) imaging is generally not undertaken.

Infantile spasms

- Infantile spasms occur in the first year of life, may be difficult to control and frequently are accompanied by severe intellectual disability.
- About 5%–10% of these patients have tuberous sclerosis (TS).
- MRI is useful to show TS and other cerebral malformations.

Epilepsy

- Children with generalized epilepsy may warrant imaging to rule out treatable disease.
- Focal seizures warrant imaging to rule out a cerebral tumor or malformation.
- In temporal lobe epilepsy, mesial temporal sclerosis, developmental malformations or tumors may be detected.
- Imaging is not indicated after a single generalized seizure, unless there is evidence of a focal process on EEG.

Obstructive hydrocephalus

- Hydrocephalus is characterized by an increase in CSF volume associated with ventricular dilatation and elevation of intraventricular pressure.
- If the passage of CSF is obstructed within the ventricular system, the hydrocephalus is labeled "non-communicating" or obstructive.
- If the obstruction exists in the surface pathways (impaired absorption of CSF), the hydrocephalus is termed "communicating."

Clinical features

- Progressive increase in head circumference or a head circumference greater than the 97th percentile.
- Large bulging fontanelle
- Widening of the sutures.
- Upward retraction of the eyelids and a fixed downward gaze ("setting sun" sign) with fourth ventricle dilation.
- Neurological abnormalities vary.

Diagnosis

- Many lesions cause hydrocephalus, and cerebral imaging is required to ascertain the cause.
- *Note:* The radiologist must know whether the head circumference is normal or increased to interpret the presence of ventriculomegaly correctly. For example, a brain with ventriculomegaly could be

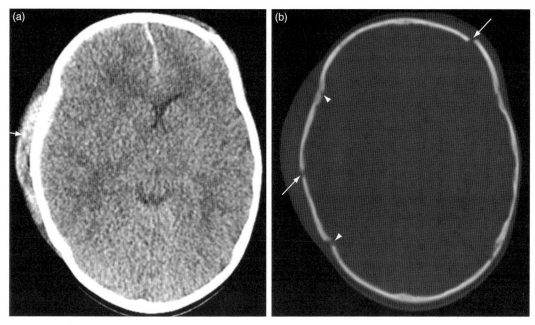

Fig. 15.30. Head CT in young child following injury. (a) Shows a large right frontoparietal scalp hematoma (arrow) and underlying subdural hematoma (arrowheads). (b) Bone windows reveal multiple fractures of the skull (arrows) and angulation of coronal and lambdoid sutures (arrowheads).

due to either CSF pathway obstruction, or a decrease in brain volume (i.e. clinically a large head in the first instance, and a normal or small head in the second).

Head injury
Introduction
- Head injuries are common at all ages. Causes include falls, sporting and road traffic accidents, and non-accidental injury.
- The primary examination should ensure that the child's airway, cervical spine, breathing, and circulation are secure.
- The child's mental state should be assessed.
- If the child is not responding to pain or responding non-purposefully then urgent intubation, head CT and intensive care/ neurosurgery consultation are required. Spine immobilization and lateral cervical spine X-rays are warranted.
- If the child is alert or responding purposefully to pain, but has focal neurological signs then urgent brain CT and neurosurgical opinion are warranted.
- Assessment should include other fractures and solid organ injuries. In non-accidental injury a skeletal survey and bone scan are warranted.

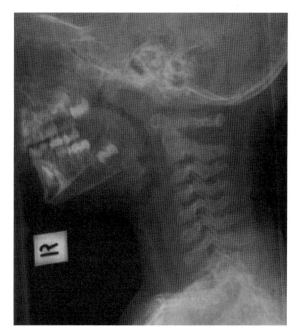

Fig. 15.31. Lateral cervical spine radiograph with pseudo-subluxation of C2 and C3. There is apparent non-alignment of the C2 and C3 posterior spinal line but this is just pseudo-subluxation. There is no soft tissue swelling.

CT head
- Injuries include cerebral contusions or lacerations, extradural or subdural hematomas, reduced cerebral perfusion from raised

intracranial pressure and cerebral edema (see Chapter 10).

- CT is best at identifying acute blood in the brain and extra-axial spaces. It can also show skull and skull base fractures (Fig. 15.30).

Cervical spine

- In trauma patients, a lateral cervical spine X-ray is often the only film that can be obtained.
- A normal appearance on a single lateral cervical spine film does not completely exclude a cervical spine fracture or ligamentous injury. Other films increase the chance of identifying a fracture but cannot absolutely exclude this, and the clinical assessment is very important in deciding whether further imaging is needed.

- In children, apparent non-alignment (pseudo-subluxation) of the posterior spinal line can occur normally. This most often occurs between the vertebral bodies of C2 and C3 (Fig. 15.31).
- For suspected cord damage, MRI is the investigation of choice, after neurosurgical consultation.

Skull X-ray

- If a CT scan is being carried out because of clinical head injury, then a skull X-ray is not indicated.
- In a clinically suspected skull fracture (e.g. boggy swelling) a skull X-ray can show a fracture, with a subsequent CT scan to assess brain injury. (Skull radiographs are still used in children in trauma, unlike adults, as they are often easier to perform than CT.)

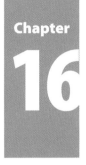

Obstetrics and gynecology

Contents

Introduction to ultrasound in obstetrics and gynecology

- In general, ultrasound is vastly superior to X-rays for imaging in obstetrics and gynecology because of the absence of ionizing radiation and better soft tissue definition.
- The place of magnetic resonance imaging in obstetrics and gynecology is still to be clearly defined. Its use is currently limited by availability and expense.

Indications for ultrasound in obstetrics and gynecology

The following are common indications for ultrasound in obstetrics and gynecology.

Obstetrics

First trimester

- Determine source of abnormal bleeding
- Confirm fetal viability and intrauterine location of gestation
- Screen for Down syndrome at approximately 12 weeks' gestation

Second trimester

- Fetal morphology – most women elect to have an 18–19-week ultrasound to exclude major fetal abnormalities. At the same time, the scan can also:
  - Confirm singleton or multiple pregnancy
  - Confirm gestational age
  - Identify initial placental site

  - Cervical length – may be of value as a prediction of potential prematurity

Third trimester

- Fetal well-being
  - Fetal biometry
  - Fetal activity (body movements, breathing movements and tone)
  - Amniotic fluid volume
  - Doppler assessment of umbilical blood flow
- Placental localization
  - Exclude placenta previa in the event of antepartum hemorrhage

Post partum

- Examination of the uterine cavity for retained products of conception

Guidance of procedures

- Guide procedures such as:
  - Amniocentesis
  - Chorionic villi sampling
  - Fetal blood sampling

Safety of obstetric ultrasound

- Although intense ultrasound exposure over long periods in experimental animals can have harmful effects, the levels of exposure employed in clinical diagnosis do not have any known adverse effects.
- Nevertheless, ultrasound exposure should be limited to the least required to achieve the desired clinical benefit.
- The most likely adverse clinical effect of obstetric ultrasound is thermal injury.
- In performing obstetric ultrasound, the following principles are advised:
  - Restrict to indications with defined clinical benefit
  - Limit duration intensity and frequency of exposure to US

- Particularly minimize pulsed Doppler ultrasound and focusing on a single focal area
- Recognize increased fetal susceptibility in the presence of:
  - A poor or absent blood supply – e.g. 6-week fetus
  - Highly absorptive tissue – bone, e.g. intracranial measurements
  - Maternal fever

Gynecology
- Ultrasound is invaluable in many clinical settings but particularly in the investigation of:
  - Pelvic pain
  - Abnormal bleeding
  - Pelvic mass

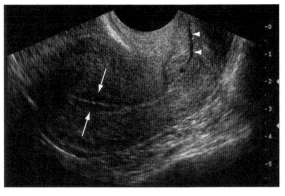

Fig. 16.1. Transvaginal longitudinal US of normal anteverted uterus in proliferative phase. Note the trilaminar appearance of the endometrium (arrows), and the small amount of fluid in the cervical canal (arrowheads).

Gynecology
Normal appearance of uterus
- The normal nulliparous uterus measures approximately $7.5 \times 5 \times 2.5$ cm. After the first pregnancy, all measurements increase by about 1.5 cm.

Endometrium
- The ultrasound (US) appearance of the endometrium changes with the phase of the menstrual cycle.
- In the menstrual phase, the endometrium thins and movement (i.e. bleeding) can be seen in the cavity.
- In the proliferative or follicular phase (first half of normal cycle) there is a trilaminar appearance and the endometrium thickens (Fig. 16.1).
- In the post-ovulatory or secretory phase the endometrium becomes thicker and partially loses its layered appearance (Fig. 16.2).
- After menopause the endometrium becomes thin with no discernible layers, and may be difficult to delineate from the surrounding myometrium (Fig. 16.3).

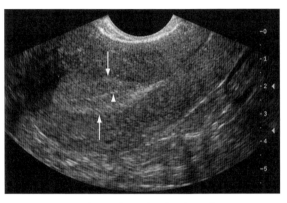

Fig. 16.2. Post-ovulatory phase of cycle. The endometrium (arrows) is more echogenic and the midline echo is still visible (arrowhead).

Normal appearance of ovaries
- The overall ovarian volume in women between menarche and menopause ranges between 3 and 8 cm^3.
- The ovaries also have features characteristic of the particular menstrual phase.

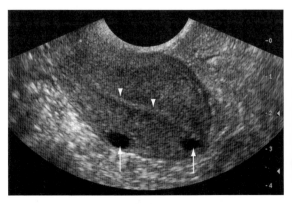

Fig. 16.3. Post-menopausal retroverted uterus with thin rather indistinct endometrium (arrowheads). The echo-free areas in the lower part of the image are blood vessels in cross-section (arrows).

- In the proliferative (follicular) phase, there will be several small follicles (<10 mm in diameter) in each ovary (Fig. 16.4). In an ovulatory cycle, a dominant follicle will become apparent. This reaches approximately 20–25 mm in diameter by the time of ovulation.
- Once ovulation has occurred, this follicle becomes the corpus luteum (CL).
- CL appearances vary from a collapsed cyst, a large hemorrhagic cyst, a simple cyst, or can mimic an ovarian malignancy.
- On color Doppler, there is low-resistance flow in the periphery of the CL, often referred to as the "ring of fire."
- The CL can be differentiated from neoplasms by repeating the US early in another menstrual cycle, when it will have disappeared.

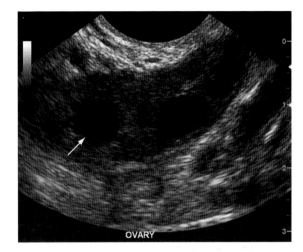

Fig. 16.4. Follicular phase ovary showing three follicles, maximum diameter 7 mm (arrow).

Abnormal uterine shape
- US can be used to determine uterine shape.
- Minor variations of normal (e.g. arcuate-shaped uterus) are more common than major abnormalities (e.g. uterus didelphys).
- 3D US can be useful in determining uterine shape.
- If an abnormal uterine shape is detected, then the presence and location of kidneys should be evaluated as 10% of these women have an associated renal anomaly.

Per vaginal bleeding disorders
Reduced bleeding – amenorrhea and oligomenorrhea
Primary amenorrhea
- US (transabdominal only in the young, sexually inactive female) helps to detect the presence of the uterus and ovaries, and if there is a blockage to menstrual flow (i.e. hematocolpos due to an intact hymen).
- It will also give information on ovarian activity.

Secondary amenorrhea/oligomenorrhea
- US can assess the endometrium and ovaries.
- A very thin endometrium suggests inadequate hormonal stimulation (consider hypothalamic causes).
- A very thin endometrium, with small areas of fluid "trapped" within the endometrial cavity in a woman whose amenorrhea followed a curettage after a pregnancy suggests Ashermann's syndrome (intrauterine synechiae)

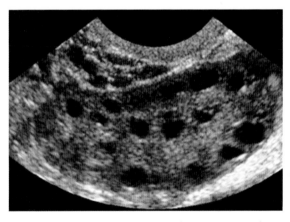

Fig. 16.5. Polycystic ovaries. Transvaginal US images. Note the small mainly peripherally arranged follicles, and the increased stroma. Ovarian volume is >12 cm^3.

- A very thick endometrium suggests anovulation in the presence of estrogen stimulation.
- Although serum and urine hCG levels are the most sensitive detectors of pregnancy, US may occasionally detect the pregnancy that has been the cause of the secondary (or primary) amenorrhea.

Imaging of the ovaries may also provide clues:
- Large ovaries (>12 cm^3 in volume) with more than 15 peripherally-placed follicles, and increased ovarian stroma fulfill the US criteria for polycystic ovaries (PCO) (Fig. 16.5).
- 20% women have ovaries that fulfill these criteria, although far fewer have the syndrome associated with PCO.

- Therefore, US diagnosis of PCO must be correlated with the clinical and hormonal features, before a true diagnosis of polycystic ovarian syndrome can be made.
- Very small ovaries, with no follicular activity, may suggest ovarian failure (i.e. menopause). This is not an US diagnosis, but US suspicion would prompt appropriate hormonal investigations.

Irregular bleeding – intermenstrual and post-coital bleeding
- This may be caused by anovulation (see above) in the presence of unopposed estrogen (e.g. PCO, obesity, estrogen-only hormonal therapy).
- Without regular progesterone (intrinsically or extrinsically supplied) the endometrium becomes very thick and sheds irregularly.

Endometrial polyps
- Endometrial polyps may also cause irregular bleeding, and can be detected by US.
- If there is doubt about the presence of a polyp, a saline-infusion sonohysterography can be undertaken. This involves insertion of a fine feeding tube through the cervix into the uterine cavity. Under US vision, a small amount of warmed normal saline is infused through the tube, separating the two endometrial layers. Any polyp is easily seen projecting into the fluid.
- US is not useful for the detection of ectocervical lesions. Speculum examination and visualization of the cervix is the investigation of choice

Excessive bleeding – menorrhagia
- US can confirm or exclude several possible causes or contributing factors for menorrhagia.

Leiomyomas (fibroids)
- Fibroids are circumscribed areas of fibrous and smooth muscle tissue within the uterus. Most commonly they are multiple, and vary in size.
- They are often described according to their position relative to the endometrium and serosal surface (submucosal, intramural, and subserosal).
- The symptoms they cause will usually depend on their position, size, and rate of growth.
- US does not reliably detect small intramural fibroids (<3 cm in diameter). Larger fibroids are usually readily seen, although the shadowing and the refraction they cause may interfere with visualization deep to the fibroid (Fig. 16.6).

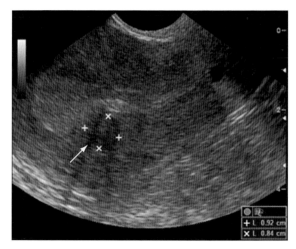

Fig. 16.6. A 9 mm intramural fibroid (arrow) impinges on the posterior layer of endometrium, displacing it anteriorly.

- Submucosal and sometimes intramural fibroids tend to cause or contribute to menorrhagia. Subserosal fibroids, if they are symptomatic, are more likely to cause pressure symptoms.
- US is useful in determining the feasibility of hysteroscopic resection of submucosal fibroids, by measuring the diameter and distance of the fibroid from the serosal surface.

Post-menopausal bleeding (PMB)
Menopause is, by definition, no bleeding for 12 months.
- A short-lived resurgence of ovarian activity is not uncommon in the first few years of menopause. These women often describe the return of premenstrual symptoms (breast tenderness, bloating, moodiness) prior to this type of bleed, which will still be labeled "post-menopausal bleeding." US is particularly useful in this scenario as it can often make this diagnosis (resumption of ovarian activity), and hence reduce anxiety for clinician and patient. US may detect a corpus luteum in one ovary, and other smaller follicles, plus a thin endometrium (if bleeding has just finished). This supports a non-pathological cause for the bleed.
- Most PMB occurs several years into the menopause.
- PMB can be a sign of an endometrial malignancy. This is present in 10% of women with PMB.

- However, many women present with PMB because of atrophy rather than hypertrophy/neoplasia of genital tract tissues.
- US can be very useful in distinguishing between these two opposing causes of PMB, e.g. if the endometrial thickness is ≤5 mm, the chance of an endometrial carcinoma is said to be about 1%.

Tamoxifen

- This drug is used as adjunctive treatment, or in prevention of, breast carcinoma, and increases the risk of endometrial carcinoma.
- US appearances of the endometrium and myometrium in women taking Tamoxifen are often difficult to interpret. Endometrial polyps and US changes in the sub-endometrial myometrium occur commonly.
- US is best for those with symptoms, rather than a screening tool for carcinoma.

Pelvic pain
Adenomyosis

- This usually develops late in a woman's menstrual life. Small islands of endometrial cells grow within the myometrium, and undergo normal menstrual changes (including bleeding). This typically causes uterine tenderness and dysmenorrhea.
- On US the uterus is bulky and the posterior wall often thicker than the anterior wall (because of the predilection of adenomyosis for the posterior uterine wall). Furthermore, the uterus is often quite tender to pressure from the US probe (transvaginal US).

Endometriosis

- The most common finding is that of pin-head sized black-brown spots in the Pouch of Douglas and on the utero-sacral ligaments at laparoscopy. US cannot visualize these lesions. The only US clue may be marked tenderness to pressure from the vaginal probe.
- Less commonly, endometriosis involves the ovary, in which case US may visualize lesions as areas of hemorrhage. This may be fresh hemorrhage in an ovarian cyst, but the classical finding in long-standing endometriosis is the so-called "ground-glass" appearance within a cyst (Fig. 16.7).

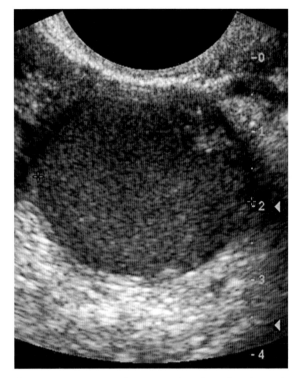

Fig. 16.7. An ovarian endometrioma. Note the uniform "ground glass" appearance.

Pelvic inflammatory disease (PID)
Acute PID

- Often no distinctive signs on US. The transvaginal probe may cause extreme discomfort. Other signs of inflammation such as fluid in the Pouch of Douglas may be seen.
- *Note:* Normal fallopian tubes are usually not seen on US. They become evident if diseased.
- Tubo-ovarian abscess
  - US appearances are of a complex mass with internal septations and fluid collections. Ovarian follicles may be identifiable within the mass.

Chronic PID

- US may show a tubular, fluid-filled structure(s) in the adnexal region.

Contraceptive devices and related issues
Intrauterine contraceptive devices (IUCDs)

- IUCDs are usually plastic and metal, so they reflect US waves, allowing visualisation.
- US is often used to locate an IUCD when the strings are no longer visible through the cervical

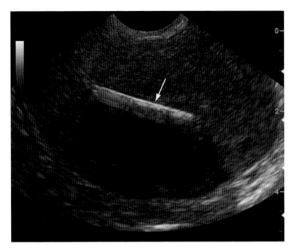

Fig. 16.8. IUCD in uterus appears as an echogenic line (arrow) with posterior acoustic shadowing.

os. Usually the IUCD is still present within the uterus.

- US can also determine if the IUCD is appropriately situated within the uterus. Occasionally it may dislodge, and sit low in the uterus or cervical canal. When this happens, its contraceptive effect will be less, and it may cause dysmenorrhea (Fig. 16.8).
- If the IUCD is not visible within the uterus, then there are two possibilities:
  - It has fallen out
  - It has "migrated" out of the uterus into the peritoneum. As US cannot see through the bowel, an abdominal X-ray is required to locate it.

Essure
- US can visualize the spirals in the cornual portion of the fallopian tubes used in this non-reversible form of sterilization.

Implanon
- This recently released, slow-release progestagen contraceptive is inserted within a tiny rod into the flexor aspect of the forearm.
- When the woman wishes it to be removed, US of the upper arm may help locate it if it is impalpable.

Tubal ligation
- US cannot locate the clips used in laparoscopic tubal sterilizations.

Infertility
- US can assess the size and shape of the uterus and endometrial cavity. It can assess the ovaries to exclude such things as PCO or endometriomas.
- If in the second half of the cycle, there is an appropriately thickened echogenic endometrium and a corpus luteum evident, this is very suggestive of normal ovulation.
- US may be used to "track" a menstrual cycle. This requires several US examinations in the one cycle, following the development of the endometrium, and the growth of the dominant follicle. An endometrial thickness of 8 mm and a dominant follicle of at least 20 mm in diameter suggests that ovulation is imminent.
- Tubal patency may be assessed radiologically (a hysterosalpingogram) or at laparoscopy by instilling dye through the cervix and checking that it flows through, and out, of the tubes.
- US can also assess tubal patency. Using US, an ultrasonic contrast agent is instilled through the cervix using a fine catheter. Its progress is then monitored as it passes through and out of the tubes. The advantage of this over the other methods is that it does not require pelvic radiation or an anesthetic.

Ovarian cysts
- A cyst is a localized collection of fluid. Ovarian cysts can be benign or malignant.
- As the previous discussion and images have highlighted, ovarian cysts are a normal, ongoing part of a woman's life in reproductive years. A dominant follicle may well reach 2.5–3 cm in diameter. Thereafter, the corpus luteum (CL) mimics all sorts of cysts: solid, cystic, hemorrhagic.

Benign epithelial tumors
Serous cystadenoma
- These comprise approximately 15%–20% of all ovarian tumors. They are usually 5–10 cm in diameter. Most commonly they contain one or two loculations. The cyst walls are usually smooth and the fluid within the cyst is echo-free.

Mucinous cystadenoma
- 15%–20% of ovarian tumors are of this type. They may become extremely large before they are detected. They are often multiloculated and the fluid within them is often echogenic.

Mature teratomas (dermoid cysts)

- Mature teratomas can often be visualized with US. 10% are bilateral.
- They are recognizable by localized areas of different echotexture within the one ovary that are caused by the different tissues that comprise a dermoid cyst (e.g. hair, sebum, teeth, neural tissue).
- They may occasionally be missed because of difficulty differentiating them from adjacent bowel.

Other adnexal cysts

- Various other cystic structures (non-ovarian) may be evident on US.

Ovarian/adnexal torsion

- This is a gynecological emergency. The ovary (with or without the fallopian tube) twists on its pedicle and in so doing cuts off the blood supply. If this is not rectified quickly, the ovary (and tube) will necrose. For an ovary to tort, there usually needs to be a cyst within it. It occurs more commonly in pregnancy.
- The symptoms of torsion are those of increasing severity of pain, associated with nausea and vomiting.
- US may just find a mass, or thickened cyst walls, and edematous stroma.
- Doppler studies may show absent flow; but the presence of flow does not exclude the diagnosis.

Malignant ovarian tumors

- A malignant ovarian tumor shows multiloculation, thickened septations and papillary excrescences projecting from the cyst wall into the fluid. On Doppler interrogation, there is usually low resistance flow. There is often free fluid within the peritoneal cavity.

Endometrial hyperplasia/carcinoma

- Endometrial hyperplasia is often caused by unopposed estrogen stimulation and US detects a thickened endometrium.
- US cannot distinguish between benign or atypical hyperplasia: it merely alerts the clinician to the need for a histological examination of the endometrium.
- The US appearance of endometrial carcinoma is usually that of an extremely thickened

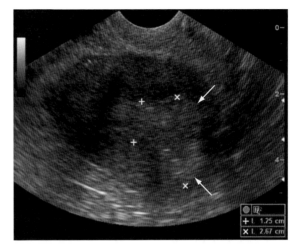

Fig. 16.9. Endometrial carcinoma. The endometrium is thickened and is extending locally into the myometrium (arrows), suggestive of endometrial carcinoma.

endometrium (often >18 mm bi-layer thickness). In more advanced carcinoma, the endometrial/myometrial interface may become ill-defined as the tumor extends outwards through the myometrium towards the serosal surface (Fig. 16.9).

Obstetrics
Ultrasound in the first trimester

- Ultrasound (US) may be used to assess early pregnancy. It is possible to determine:
  - Site of the pregnancy (i.e. intrauterine or ectopic)
  - Presence of a fetus and heart pulsations
  - Number of fetuses
  - Gestational age (this is most accurately estimated in the first trimester)
  - Presence of cysts or fibroids
- *Note:* the most sensitive test for pregnancy is serum β-human chorionic gonadotrophin (βhCG) (detectable approximately 10 days after conception).

Normal development in early pregnancy

- An intrauterine pregnancy is not ultrasonically visible until at least 4½ weeks of amenorrhea (i.e. 2½ weeks of embryonic age). At this very early stage the pregnancy is best seen using a transvaginal US probe.

273

- The first evidence of pregnancy is a gestational sac within the endometrium. At 4½ weeks gestation, the sac measures approximately 3 mm in diameter.
- By 6 weeks a fetal pole can be seen. The measurement used is the crown–rump length (CRL)
- By 7 weeks the fetus is much clearer (Fig. 16.10).
- Around this time, fetal heart activity is evident. M-mode (motion mode) can be used to record and measure this.
- Limb buds are evident by 7–8 weeks, as are fetal movements (Fig. 16.11).
- By 12 weeks, the fetus is fully formed. The fetal bladder and stomach can be identified.

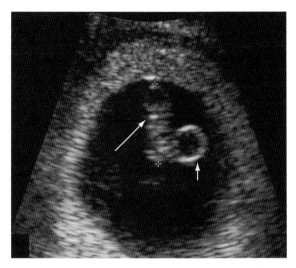

Fig. 16.10. Fetus (long arrow) and yolk sac (short arrow) within the gestational sac. The CRL is 13 mm.

Threatened miscarriage
- In this situation, there is vaginal bleeding but no pain. The cervical os is closed.
- US findings shows an apparently normally developing pregnancy, although there may be signs of blood collecting behind the membranes or developing placenta.

Miscarriage
- Occurs in 10%–20% of clinical pregnancies
- Is often heralded by vaginal bleeding.
- Vaginal bleeding occurs in about 20% pregnancies.

Missed miscarriage
- Also referred to as missed abortion, an embryonic pregnancy, and blighted ovum.
- The embryo or fetus has ceased to grow, and heart activity has ceased (or never commenced).
- May be asymptomatic or present with PV bleeding, or decrease in symptoms of pregnancy (e.g. nausea, breast tenderness).
- The diagnosis is made by US, which shows an empty sac ≥20 mm in diameter, or a CRL ≥6 mm without fetal heart activity.

Complete/incomplete miscarriage
- This presents with heavy bleeding and pain, often with a history of having passed a lump of tissue.
- US shows either an empty cavity (complete miscarriage), or irregular echoes within the endometrial cavity suggesting retained products of conception (incomplete miscarriage).

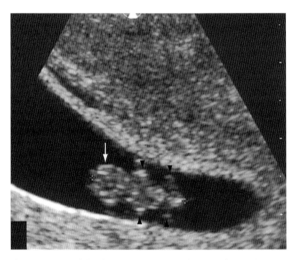

Fig. 16.11. Limb buds (arrowheads) and fetal head (arrow) are evident.

- The final decision regarding whether a miscarriage is complete or incomplete depends on the combination of symptoms and US findings, not on US alone.

Ectopic pregnancy
- Describes a pregnancy outside the endometrial cavity.
- Most commonly occurs in the fallopian tube, but also occurs in the ovary, the cornu of the uterus, the cervix, a cesarean section scar, or intra-abdominally.

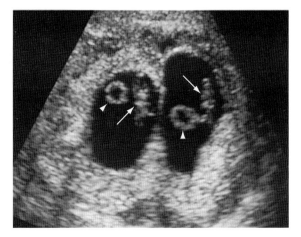

Fig. 16.12. Dichorionic diamniotic twins at 7 weeks. Two gestational sacs, two fetuses (arrows), two yolk sacs (arrowheads).

- US shows an empty uterus and sometimes, a mass between the uterus and ovary. There may be free fluid (blood) in the Pouch of Douglas.
- The presence of a positive pregnancy test, with a serum hCG level >1000 IU, an empty uterus, even without other signs, means an ectopic pregnancy until proven otherwise.

Molar pregnancy
Complete mole
- Only placental tissue is present (i.e. no fetus).
- All genetic material comes from the father.
- US shows mixed echogenicity within the endometrial cavity, consistent with many small cystic spaces (the grape-like vesicles seen macroscopically).

Partial mole
- Contains both a fetus and molar placental tissue.
- The karyotype is triploid.

Multiple pregnancy
- The first trimester is the best time to determine chorionicity; the number of chorions, amnions and fetuses should be determined (Fig. 16.12).
- This is important as monozygotic twins have a poorer prognosis (increased risk of abnormalities, twin–twin transfusion syndrome) and the increased surveillance required.
- If two sacs or fetuses are identified, a diligent search is made for a third!

Third trimester scanning and fetal welfare assessment
Ultrasound can provide valuable information about:
- Placental site
- Fetal lie and presentation
- Fetal size and growth
- Fetal well-being, including amniotic fluid volume, biophysical assessment of the fetus and Doppler studies of both the umbilical and fetal circulation.

Clinical indications for US in the third trimester include:
- Known low-lying placenta in the mid-trimester
- Antepartum hemorrhage
- To confirm fetal lie and presentation
- Assessment of liquor volume
- Concerns about fetal growth and well-being.

Known low-lying placenta in the mid-trimester
- 5% placentae lie within 2 cm of the internal os in the mid-trimester. By term, most of these will have "moved away" from the cervix as the lower uterine segment forms.
- At term, the prevalence of placenta previa is <1%.
- If the placenta is previa at 34 weeks, it is unlikely to move further, and a cesarean section is indicated.

Antepartum hemorrhage
Bleeding after 20 weeks of ≥15 ml is termed antepartum hemorrhage (APH). Causes include:

Placenta previa
- Bleeding is generally bright and painless.
- It is maternal bleeding and generally unassociated with fetal compromise, except where maternal shock occurs.
- Associated with a high head or a malpresentation, because the low-lying placenta stops the head entering the pelvis.
- Any patient with an APH should not have a vaginal examination until US has excluded placenta previa.
- To define exactly where the placenta is in relation to the cervix, both transabdominal and transvaginal scanning may be necessary.

275

Placental abruption

- Consider in any patient with an APH, particularly if associated with uterine contractions, and uterine tenderness between contractions.
- May be complicated by preterm labor.
- The bleeding is maternal, but results from premature separation of the placenta.
- May occur with trauma, e.g. motor vehicle accidents and, particularly, seat belt injuries.
- Risk factors include hypertension (including pre-eclampsia), smoking and vaso-active illicit drugs, e.g. cocaine.

The loss of functioning placental bed means this is more likely to result in fetal compromise.

The role of US is to:

- Exclude placenta previa.
- Examine the entire placenta for retroplacental clot (*Note:* Placental abruption is essentially a clinical diagnosis, and most patients with a clinically significant abruption will not have this US finding).
- Confirm fetal well-being, including fetal growth, biophysical assessment and Doppler studies.
- Ensure placental abruption has not caused preterm labor (confirm cervix is long and closed).

Vasa previa

- Bleeding from a vasa previa generally occurs late in labor when the membranes rupture and a fetal vessel crossing the membranes ahead of the presenting part tears.
- Fetal hemorrhage is generally catastrophic, and US has no role in this situation, which is suspected clinically and confirmed with cardiotocography.
- Nevertheless, antenatal US may suggest a vasa previa before labor and allow appropriate delivery.

Incidental hemorrhage

When the cause of an APH is not demonstrated (previa or abruption), the bleeding is termed "incidental."

At times, the bleeding arises from a local cause, e.g. cervical erosion or polyp. If no local cause is found, it is often assumed there has been bleeding from the placental edge (a so-called "marginal hemorrhage").

Although considered low risk, these pregnancies nevertheless require continued follow-up for adequate fetal growth and well-being.

Confirm fetal lie and presentation

- As term approaches, knowing the lie and presentation of the fetus is critical.
- A lie other than longitudinal suggests placenta previa, or other pelvic mass preventing the presenting part from engaging.
- If the lie is longitudinal, it can sometimes be difficult to differentiate clinically between a cephalic or breech presentation.
- Given the hazards of vaginal breech delivery, the presentation needs to be confirmed by 36 weeks, so appropriate management can be discussed. 5% fetuses are in breech presentation at term.

Assessment of liquor volume

- This may be indicated when clinical examination suggests too little or too much liquor.
- Too little liquor is called oligohydramnios, and too much liquor, polyhydramnios.

Causes of oligohydramnios

- Prelabor rupture of the membranes, either at term or preterm. This is usually a clinical diagnosis, but US confirmation of oligohydramnios may be useful.
- Insufficient liquor production
  - In the third trimester, this most commonly results from reduced fetal urine output due to reduced renal perfusion, in the setting of uteroplacental insufficiency. Other evidence of uteroplacental insufficiency, e.g. impaired fetal growth, abnormal Doppler examinations, and abnormal biophysical assessment should be sought.
  - May result from fetal kidney disease, although renal abnormalities are usually suspected in the mid trimester survey.

Causes of polyhydramnios

- Increased production, particularly among diabetics.
- Reduced swallowing, due to atresia (e.g. duodenal or esophageal atresia), neurological disorders (e.g. anencephaly) or neuromuscular disorders.

Different standardized methods are used to estimate the liquor volume on US. Indices such as the amniotic fluid index (AFI) and maximal vertical pocket (MVP) are measured.

Concerns about fetal growth and well-being

US may be indicated to assess fetal growth and well-being in patients known to have risk factors for intrauterine growth restriction, including:

- Hypertension
- Diabetes
- Renal disease
- Multiple pregnancy
- Antepartum hemorrhage
- Clinically small fetus
- Diminished fetal movements
- Abnormal cardiotocograph

Growth tracking of small babies is important because they have a worse perinatal outcome.

In a suspected "small for gestational age" fetus, US can:

- Confirm the presence of intrauterine growth restriction, by performing biometry.
- Help confirm the underlying cause (e.g. raised vascular resistance in the placental bed)
- Detect fetal compensation in the face of uteroplacental insufficiency: oligohydramnios, impaired growth, cerebral blood flow redistribution
- Detect fetal decompensation: abnormal biophysical profile or cardiac function.

Slowing of fetal growth/growth restriction

- Fetal biometry: important measurements include:
  - Biparietal diameter (BPD)
  - Head circumference
  - Femur length
  - Abdominal circumference (AC).
- These measurements are then used in a multiparameter regression equation to generate an "estimated fetal weight." This weight can then be compared to birthweight centiles for that gestational age.
- A fetus below the tenth centile for live births, a fetus who is "crossing centiles," or a fetus with an abdominal circumference below the fifth centile for gestational age is considered at high risk for "uteroplacental insufficiency" and increased fetal surveillance should be instituted.

Umbilical artery blood flow

- In normal pregnancy, the feto-placental circulation is a "high flow, low resistance" circuit,

with continuous flow in both the systolic and diastolic components of the cardiac cycle.

- Doppler US of the umbilical artery provides information about this circulation
- In placental pathology, such as vascular sclerosis and poor development (or obliteration) of terminal villi, increased placental bed resistance develops, resulting in:
  - Initially reduced flow during diastole (raised systolic-diastolic ratio)
  - As pathology becomes more severe, absence of diastolic flow occurs and
  - Finally, reversal of flow occurs (almost always associated with severe fetal compromise).

This progression is associated with progressive deterioration in placental gas exchange and a stepwise increase in perinatal mortality.

Evidence of fetal compensation for intrauterine hypoxia

In the presence of hypoxia, little or no change in cardiac output occurs, but there is redistribution of blood flow favouring the essential organs

US features:

- Cerebral vasodilatation
- "Carcass" vasoconstriction results in reduced renal blood flow with oligohydramnios, and further growth impairment.

Fetal decompensation for acidosis and asphyxia

- When the fetal compensatory mechanisms reach their limit, "hypoxic heart failure" occurs
- US features:
  - Precordial veins (IVC, DV, hepatic veins) reflect the increased ventricular after-load and end diastolic pressure.
- Once the disease reaches this decompensatory phase, the fetus is at high risk of dying and of developing multi-system organ failure.

Biophysical profile (BPP)

- As originally described, the BPP was used to "score" fetal behavior (0, 1 or 2) in each of the following areas:
  - Fetal tone
  - Fetal movement
  - Fetal breathing movement
  - Amniotic fluid volume assessment – amniotic fluid index (AFI)
  - Cardiotocography (CTG).
- A perfect score was 10/10.

277

- Reduced liquor, a non-reactive CTG, and a reduction in "non-essential fetal activity" are suggestive of fetal hypoxia and acidosis.
- Although the AFI and CTG remain mainstays of fetal growth and well-being assessment, the formal BPP is used less commonly, partly because it is time-consuming. The fetus must be observed for over 40 minutes since absence of fetal movements occurs commonly at times of fetal sleep.
- A biophysical assessment may still be useful, however, in the fetus with a persistently non-reactive CTG when preterm or under the influence of maternal drugs. A well-grown and active baby on US in these circumstances excludes hypoxia as a possible cause.

Ultrasound screening for Down syndrome

- Down syndrome (Trisomy 21) is the single most common aneuploidy among live births.
- Risk factors for aneuploidy
  - Maternal age
  - Past history of chromosomal abnormalities – consider if recurrent miscarriages or stillbirth with abnormalities
    - Family history of chromosomal abnormalities
- Most pregnancies affected with Down syndrome have no identifiable risk factors, because most occur as a result of a random non-dysjunction, an unpredictable and unavoidable event.
- 70% of Down syndrome fetuses are born to women under the age of 37 years, because these women form the majority of the child-bearing population.

Rationale for screening

Screening aims at secondary prevention, i.e. the antenatal detection of affected fetuses. In order to detect most fetuses with Down syndrome, genetic screening needs to be applied on a population basis, and offered to all couples in early pregnancy.

The aim of antenatal detection is to identify affected fetuses before 20 weeks' gestation. This enables parents to make an informed choice about continuing or terminating the pregnancy. Even for parents who have no interest in termination of pregnancy, genetic screening should still be discussed, as there may be value in identifying affected fetuses antenatally, in order to:

- Perform a targeted ultrasound (US) for associated structural abnormalities e.g. congenital heart defects

- Discuss neonatal and childhood issues with a pediatric team before delivery
- Identify with support groups etc.

Pregnancies with a "high risk" result on screening should then be offered a diagnostic test (e.g. amniocentesis or chorionic villus sampling) to establish with certainty whether the fetus is affected.

Screening tests – maternal age

The options for genetic screening for Trisomy 21 include:

- Maternal age alone
- The 18-week ultrasound
- Nuchal translucency screening.

Maternal age alone

- As discussed above, offering diagnostic testing based on maternal age alone, has a 30% sensitivity for detecting Down syndrome. This sensitivity is very low.

Screening tests – the 18 week US

The mid-trimester US is performed for a number of reasons. It:

- Confirms the expected due date
- Localizes the placenta
- Excludes a hitherto undiagnosed multiple pregnancy
- Allows detailed examination of the fetal anatomy. This review searches for both structural anomalies (e.g. spina bifida, diaphragmatic hernia, exomphalos, structural cardiac disease) and so-called "soft markers" of chromosomal abnormalities. These soft markers are not structural anomalies that threaten the babies' health or life per se, but are US features of phenotypic abnormalities noted in newborns with Down syndrome. These include:
  - Short long bones, particularly humerus and femur
  - Thickened nuchal fold
  - Echogenic bowel
  - Renal pelviectasis.

The relative risks for aneuploidy when these "soft markers" are seen varies, but given that the age-related risks for Down syndrome are known, it can be multiplied by the relative risks for the given soft marker to approximate an individual's level of risk.

The sensitivity of the 18-week US for the detection of Down syndrome is approximately 50%. A completely normal US (no structural abnormalities or soft markers) reduces the risk of Down syndrome by 50%.

Nuchal translucency screening

- An increased thickness of the fluid filled space at the back of the fetal neck (the so-called "nuchal translucency") can be observed in fetuses with Down syndrome.
- The nuchal translucency (NT) measurement, the maternal age and the crown–rump length can be used to calculate the risk of Down syndrome affecting a pregnancy. This can then guide the use of diagnostic testing.
- The NT measurement can be performed on 98%–100% of pregnancies between 10 and 13 weeks' gestation.
- How well does the test perform?
    - Where the risk of 1:300 or greater is used for invasive testing, the sensitivity (i.e. Down syndrome detection rate) is 77% if the false-positive rate is set at 5%.
- What if the NT is abnormal, but the karyotype returns as normal?
    - A number of other causes of increased NT exist.
    - Fetuses with an increased NT but normal karyotype have a 20%–30% risk of unfavourable outcome. Approximately 10% have structural anomalies (most commonly cardiac), 10% have single gene defects, and there is an increased association with spontaneous abortion and perinatal death.
    - Patients with an increased NT should at least be offered a referral for a specialized follow-up mid-trimester scan to exclude a structural anomaly not associated with aneuploidy.

Combined first-trimester screening

- This test combines biochemical and US features to generate a Down syndrome risk. The biochemistry is the Pregnancy Associated Plasma Protein A (PAPP A) and human Chorionic Gonadotrophin (hCG).
- These tests are performed at approximately 10 weeks' gestation, the results withheld until combined with the NT measurement, performed at approximately 12 weeks' gestation. A combined risk is generated that can be used to guide diagnostic testing.

How does the test perform?

- The combined first trimester screening test has improved sensitivity (90%) when compared with either second trimester biochemistry or NT measurement alone.
- This is achieved with the same level of false positives (5%) with a "high-risk" result (recommending invasive testing) of 1:300 or more.

Second trimester biochemistry

- This is performed between 14 and 20 weeks, and generates an estimate of risk of Down syndrome and neural tube defects.
- It is not applicable for multiple pregnancies, where a NT scan should be offered instead.
- The sensitivity of this screening for Down syndrome is 65%, with a false-positive rate of 5% and a high-risk result (recommending invasive testing) at 1:250 or greater.

Diagnostic tests

- Diagnostic testing is reserved for those found to be high risk on any of the above screening tests. This is because any invasive testing carries a risk of miscarriage.
- Chorionic villus sampling (CVS)
    - This can be performed from 10 weeks' gestation.
- Amniocentesis
    - This can be performed after 15 weeks' gestation. It is performed with US guidance.

Preterm labor and cervical incompetence

- Preterm labor (PTL) is defined as labor prior to 37 completed weeks gestation.
- 7% of babies are born before 37 weeks and 2% before 32 weeks.
- Before 23 weeks' gestation, neonatal survival is very uncommon. Survival ranges from approximately 40% at 24 weeks, to over 90% at 28 weeks. Over the same gestational period, the expected rate of some disability is close to half of all children born.

Background physiology

- Maintaining the fetus in the uterus depends on the cervical integrity and the absence of uterine contractions.
- Although individual cases of premature delivery may be due primarily to failure of the cervix or to

uterine activity, it is increasingly apparent that a similar molecular environment promotes both uterine activity and cervical failure.

- When delivery occurs in the relative absence of uterine contractions and weakness of the cervix appears paramount, the condition is termed "cervical incompetence." This may be idiopathic (presumably congenital) in origin or arise from previous cervical injury e.g. cone biopsy or cervical tear.

Factors predisposing to preterm delivery

- Previous preterm birth
- Uterine structural anomalies
- Preterm premature rupture of the membranes (preterm PROM)
- Over distension (multiple pregnancy, polyhydramnios)
- Infection (systemic, adjacent, intrauterine)

- Antepartum hemorrhage
- Foreign body (suture, IUCD)
- Fetal compromise or abnormality
- Systemic disease, e.g. renal disease
- Cervical incompetence

Early diagnosis of cervical changes preceding preterm birth

- Cervical shortening may precede preterm delivery by days or weeks, and ultrasound assessment of cervical length sometimes help predict premature labor. This is not always the case as some women deliver very soon after a normal ultrasound, but in many others, the detection of cervical shortening allows interventions (e.g. a cervical suture) to be made.
- Screening of cervical length is commonly performed fortnightly from approximately 14 weeks' gestation in women at increased risk of cervical incompetence.

Index